AF685456

Janet & Barry,

Thank you for your continued support of the Frances McClelland Institute.

I hope you enjoy reading about my research on improving lives of young people.

In partnership,

Andrea

Youth-Community Partnerships for Adolescent Alcohol Prevention

Andrea J. Romero
Editor

Youth-Community Partnerships for Adolescent Alcohol Prevention

Springer

Editor
Andrea J. Romero
Family Studies & Human Development
The University of Arizona
Tucson, Arizona, USA

ISBN 978-3-319-26028-0 ISBN 978-3-319-26030-3 (eBook)
DOI 10.1007/978-3-319-26030-3

Library of Congress Control Number: 2015957588

Springer Cham Heidelberg New York Dordrecht London

Printed on acid-free paper

Springer International Publishing AG Switzerland is part of Springer Science+Business Media (www.springer.com)

Contents

Contributors

Josefina Ahumada, M.S.W. School of Social Work, Arizona State University, Mesa, AZ, USA

Payal Anand, M.P.H. Family Studies and Human Development, The University of Arizona, Tucson, AZ, USA

Jaime Arrieta, M.P.H., C.H.E.S. Carondelet Health Network, Tucson, AZ, USA

Sofia Blue Pima County Public Library Sam Lena Branch, South Tucson, AZ, USA

Juvenal Caporale, M.A. Mexican American Studies, University of Arizona, Tucson, AZ, USA

Oscar Ceseña Pima Community College, Tucson, AZ, USA

Ana Fonseca, M.A. Family Studies and Human Development, The University of Arizona, Tucson, AZ, USA

Alejandro Gallego John Valenzuela Youth Center, Tucson, AZ, USA

Gloria Hamelitz-Lopez John Valenzuela Youth Center, Tucson, AZ, USA

Robby Harris, M.S. University of New York, New York, NY, USA

Elisa Meza, M.S.W. San Francisco Unified School District, San Francisco, CA, USA

Joel A. Muraco, Ph.D. Human Development and Women's and Gender Studies, University of Wisconsin-Green Bay, Green Bay, WI, USA

Michele Orduña, M.Ed. House of Neighborly Service, Tucson, AZ, USA

Luis Perales, M.S. Mexican American Studies, University of Arizona, Tucson, AZ, USA

Jesi Post, M.S. Mel and Enid Zuckerman College of Public Health, University of Arizona, Tucson, AZ, USA

Juan "Johnny" Quevedo Pima Community College, Tucson, AZ, USA

Andrea Romero, Ph.D. Family Studies and Human Development, The University of Arizona, Tucson, AZ, USA

Maricruz Romero-Ruiz, M.S. United Way of Tucson and Southern Arizona, Tucson, AZ, USA

Kimberly Sierra-Cajas Office of Undergraduate Research, The University of Arizona College of Science, Tucson, AZ, USA

Michal Urrea John Valenzuela Youth Center, Tucson, AZ, USA

Patty Valera, L.M.S.W. Department of Veteran's Affairs, Tucson, AZ, USA

Chapter 1
Youth-Community Partnerships for Adolescent Alcohol Prevention: "We Can't Do It Alone"

Andrea Romero

Abstract Adolescent alcohol use proves to be a continued challenge for public health, given that approximately 35 % of the USA's high school age youth used alcohol in the past 30 days. This book describes an innovative collective approach to create community transformational resilience, which we define here as the ability of a community collective group to work together to transform ecological factors in order to limit risk factors and to promote protective factors. A low-income ethnic enclave community transformed themselves from a low level of community readiness rooted in denial and tolerance of adolescent alcohol use to institutionalization of community-level prevention activities. Over an 8-year period, the South Tucson Prevention Coalition evolved from Phase 1, building youth leadership and critical consciousness through after-school programs to Phase 2, building a youth-community coalition to change alcohol norms and alcohol availability. South Tucson Prevention Coalition was successful in developing a functioning coalition whose participatory action research led to critical consciousness of the environmental context surrounding adolescent alcohol use which spurred collective action for change.

Keywords Community • Transformation • Resilience • Alcohol prevention • Critical consciousness

This is a story about how one community went from denial and tolerance of adolescent alcohol use to organizing and mobilizing community members to transform their city in order to prevent underage drinking. The goal of sharing this inspiring story of creating sustainable adolescent alcohol prevention through coalition building is to reach other similar communities who are struggling with adolescent alcohol use and the associated consequences. Through collaboration and participatory

A. Romero, Ph.D. (✉)
Family Studies and Human Development, University of Arizona, 650 North Park Avenue, Tucson, AZ 85719, USA
e-mail: romeroa@u.arizona.edu

A.J. Romero (ed.), *Youth-Community Partnerships for Adolescent Alcohol Prevention*, DOI 10.1007/978-3-319-26030-3_1

action research, the community was able to create sustainable changes for adolescent alcohol prevention through changing community alcohol norms and limiting alcohol availability. During Phase 1, the youth became empowered to become community leaders, and during Phase 2 partnerships were forged that brought together researchers, law enforcement, nonprofit leaders, and youth. In this way, the community was able to raise awareness about adolescent alcohol use that led to changes in their physical environment through city policy to prevent new liquor licenses. Yet, most importantly, our results demonstrate how youth and community perceptions of minority adolescents changed from "the problem" to "the solution." ***Truly, it was the fact that not only youth, but also adult allies among community leaders and researchers, learned to work together which led to enhanced alignment and system-level changes in order to achieve a healthier community with less alcohol availability.***

Fundamental to this work is that youth and adults both developed a critical consciousness about how adolescent alcohol use is influenced by the reality of societal inequalities associated with economic and cultural factors. Yet, building on community cultural assets and collective strength, they worked together to create more positive development opportunities for youth and also to limit the risk factors they identified within their community. Once this critical consciousness was developed, it became clear to the community that prevention of adolescent alcohol use cannot be achieved alone by youth or by single agencies. In fact, the thing that brought them together to work on changing the status quo of their community in terms of adolescent alcohol use was the conclusion that "***We can't do it alone,***" which lead to coalition efforts to transform their environment in a manner that created greater resilience within their community.

Alcohol is the substance most often used by adolescents of all ethnic backgrounds (Centers for Disease Control, 2014), and it is linked with illegal substance use and risky sexual behavior (Centers for Disease Control, 2014). Alcohol use among adolescents starts early and increases with age. A higher percentage of youth aged 12–20 years use alcohol (29 %) than tobacco (24 %) or illicit drugs (14 %), making underage drinking the leading public health problem among adolescents in the United States. Adolescent alcohol use has been found to impair brain development during adolescence, particularly among youth who engage in binge drinking and heavy consumption (Squeglia, Jacobus, & Tapert, 2009). Although the general trend for adolescent alcohol use has decreased over the past 10 years, it still remains over 35 % for use in the past 30 days (see Fig. 1.1, Centers for Disease Control, 2014). Additionally, over the past 10 years Latino youth across the USA tend to consistently report higher rates of alcohol consumption than White youth (Centers for Disease Control, 2014).

The majority of adolescent prevention programs are focused on individual adolescents, and they are most often delivered through after-school programs during a few brief sessions. It is rare that prevention programs situate the adolescent within their community contexts, despite the fact that low-income neighborhoods are often fraught with multiple hazards such as adult alcoholics, pervasive alcohol advertising,

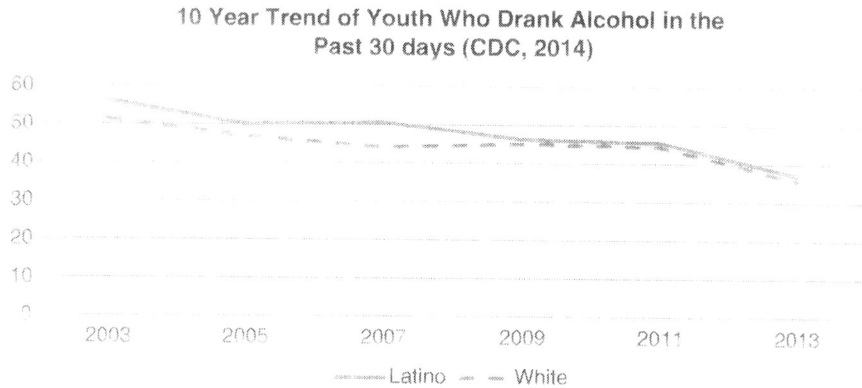

Fig. 1.1 The 10-year trend of youth 30-day alcohol use

and easily accessible alcohol. Moreover, few studies place the adolescent in an active role in negotiating their neighborhood community or as agents of change within their community (Chaskin, 2008). In the current book, we discuss how one city changed from a low level of community readiness for adolescent alcohol prevention to a level of institutionalization and expansion of prevention activities (Oetting et al., 1995). This was achieved through a 8-year project for the prevention of adolescent alcohol use in an urban low-income US/Mexico border city. We will specifically discuss the interconnected influence of after-school programs, community coalition development, and participatory action research that led to city-level policy changes to ban outdoor alcohol advertising and to limit new alcohol licenses.

Some of the key findings we will discuss are:

1. **Coalition building** is critical to the success of preventing underage drinking because it provides a supportive resilience-promoting environment that links youth with access to health resources and limits exposure to risk factors.
2. The utility of **participatory action research** to guide coalition building through principles of inclusion of diverse community members (youth, community-based organizations, police, schools, and faith communities), equality of participation of all members, dialogue before decision making, critical consciousness about the societal context of adolescent alcohol use within low-income communities, and collective action prevention strategies.
3. The relevance of the Community Readiness Model for Change not only to develop youth-focused programs but also to **identify when a community is ready to join collective action efforts to create community transformation resilience** that promotes community resources for positive youth development changes and also limits risk factors, such as alcohol availability and community norms of tolerance.

Prevention programs targeted at individuals in isolation are not enough—community-level change is required through group efforts that represent a cross-section of the community in order to reframe community-level norms, align resources, and reduce risk factors. In order to change the status quo, there is a need for community members themselves to be aware of and to be leaders in changing the existing ecological systems. ***Specifically, in order for community-level change to be effective it MUST include those who are most affected, in particular adolescent alcohol prevention must include youth and community as equal partners.***

1.1 Place-Based Community Approach

By taking a place-based approach, we specifically identify the current and historical economic, political, and social contexts of youth as a way to understand and prevent adolescent alcohol use. Community context matters for adolescent alcohol prevention (Oetting et al., 1995). In particular, Latino youth on the US/Mexico border report that they begin drinking alcohol at earlier ages (Almodovar, Tomaka, Thompson, Mckinnon, & O'Rourke, 2006; Breslau & Peterson, 1996; Chassin, Curran, Hussong, & Colder, 1996; McKinnon, O'rourke, Thompson, & Berumen, 2004; SAMSHA, 2004). Early alcohol and drug use are predictors of future alcohol and drug addiction (Breslau & Peterson, 1996; Hingson, Heeren, & Winter, 2006; Chassin et al., 1996; SAMSHA, 2004). Moreover, ethnic minority girls who live in US/Mexico border areas have reported greater severity of substance use at entry into substance use treatment programs (Stevens, Estrada, Murphy, McKnight, & Tims, 2004; Stevens et al., 2003). The US/Mexico border has higher rates of immigrant youth who were born in Mexico; however, existing data suggests that immigrant youth have lower rates of substance use, particularly girls, which indicates the diversity even within regions that must be considered in prevention programs (Bacio, Mays, & Lau, 2013; Bettes, Dusenbury, Kerner, James-Ortiz, & Botvin, 2008; Carvajal, Photiades, Evans, & Nash, 1997; Otero-Sabogal, Sabogal, Perez-Stable, & Hiatt, 1995).

It is for these reasons that we took a place-based approach to focus on context and community-level factors over a 8-year period (2003–2010) of adolescent alcohol prevention activities. ***South Tucson is a community with many preexisting strengths, such as youth Safe Havens, belief in their own children, strong community affiliation, a positive view of ethnic heritage, and many passionate and committed service providers.*** While there was a history of civic engagement to reduce liquor licenses, there was little to no history of substance use or alcohol use prevention among adolescents. Despite the concentration of needs in this city, there is a distinct sense of pride and identity that connects people within the tight-knit community. It is for these reasons that this city was identified in order to build on strengths that will have impactful long-term consequences.

1.1.1 City of South Tucson Description

The City of South Tucson (CoST) is a 1.2 square mile incorporated city surrounded by the City of Tucson, giving it an inner city ethnic enclave character. When research collaborations began in 2000, CoST had a population of 5490, comprised of 81.2 % people of Latino descent and 9.1 % people of Native American descent (U.S. Census Bureau, 2000a). The demographic profile changed little during this period; in 2010 the total population of 5,652 included 78.5 % Latino descent individuals and 10.7 % Native American descent individuals (U.S. Census Bureau, 2010a). Poverty is a consideration given that, in 2000, 54 % of families with children lived below the poverty line in South Tucson, compared to 15.2 % of families with children under 18 years old in the state of Arizona (U.S. Census Bureau, 2000b, 2000c). In 2010, 54.4 % of families with children under 18 years old in South Tucson were living below the poverty level compared to 17.2 % of families in the state of Arizona (U.S. Census Bureau, 2010b). Associated poverty factors include crime in the local neighborhood; according to the South Tucson Police Department, 12 gangs existed in this area, and the number of juvenile arrests related to underage alcohol possession more than doubled from 2003 to 2004. In a Door-to-Door survey conducted in 2008 by Primavera Foundation, crime and other safety issues were listed as the worst things about the neighborhood. 93 % reported having experienced (seen/heard) violent acts between adults, and violent acts were experienced by 1/3 of residents in past 12 months, the majority which were drug related, auto theft, or home vandalism. However, 70 % of residents felt that police were responsive to calls.

Education rates in South Tucson were lower than state averages with 41.1 % of adults in the community who report having a high school diploma or higher compared to 81 % in Arizona in 2000 (U.S. Census Bureau, 2000a). Furthermore, 3.7 % of South Tucson adults had a bachelor's degree or higher compared to 23.5 % of adults in the state of Arizona in 2000. These trends did improve by 2010 when 58 % of the South Tucson adult community had a high school degree or higher compared to 86 % of Arizona's population (U.S. Census Bureau, 2010c). Yet, the rates of bachelor's degrees went down slightly; 2.5 % of South Tucson's adult population had a bachelor's degree or higher compared to 26.9 % of Arizona in 2010. Not surprisingly, there was also a general mistrust of university researchers, perhaps in part because of the lack of experience and exposure to higher education.

In the City of South Tucson, there were three Safe Havens for youth: House of Neighborly Service (HNS), Project YES, and the John Valenzeula Youth Center (JVYC). Each one provided a variety of different youth programs, and each made a unique contribution to the community; however, none of these agencies offered substance use prevention programing. All of the agencies did offer after-school tutoring; most of the youth in the tutoring program functioned far below their grade level. Project YES and HNS provided a tutoring program for youth from their feeder school, Mission View Elementary. JVYC provided tutoring for students from Ochoa Elementary school; the tutoring programs had wait lists because the need for academic assistance was so high. This means many children did not have access to the resources that they needed to improve their academic performance. HNS offered a tattoo removal program to ex-gang members in order to help them move on to a better life with better employment opportunities. HNS also offered basketball, dance classes for young women, services for the elderly, and the only Native American youth program in the city. JVYC offered a variety of physical activities, such as basketball, volleyball, and a drop-in after-school program, for teens. Project YES also offered a program for adjudicated youth with a community service component.

1.2 Context of Historical Trauma and Need for Community-Led Strategies

We acknowledge that the income, health, and educational challenges in the CoST are interrelated and rooted in issues of generational poverty and historical trauma of both the Native American and Mexican American families that are represented in this community. Thus, there is a need to consider the historical context in order to provide insight into the ways in which societal infrastructure influences contemporary health disparities and also to identify existing strengths and sources of resilience (De la Torre & Estrada, 2001; Ungar et al., 2007). The tragedies over the past 500 years for Native Americans and Mexican Americans have resulted in a lack of access to education, health care, and economic opportunity; however, it has also resulted in community-embedded sense of resilience and maintenance of culture (Rodriguez, 2014; Walters & Simoni, 2002). Both groups have survived hundreds of years of discrimination and oppression while maintaining their identity and their cultural rootedness throughout the southwest regions of the United States (Rodriguez, 2014).

South Tucson is located on the northern edge of the US/Mexico border and has historically been considered an immigration corridor, and approximately 27 % of South Tucson residents are foreign born. Since 9/11, there has been a dramatic change in immigration policy and their associated debates (Esses, Dovidio, & Hodson, 2002; Hines, 2002; Puar, 2007); in the 5 years between 2005 and 2010, over 6000 immigration policies were proposed in the United States and 976 became law (Kohout, 2012) with the majority of them being focused on the US/Mexico border and Latinos of Mexican descent (Johnson, 1997). During this time, Arizona was at the national forefront, with many new laws that limited access to resources and emphasized the need to demonstrate citizenship. This is one specific and recent way in which the environment in South Tucson was being shaped by larger forces that increased power inequity among immigrants, their families, and their allies (Tseng & Yoshikawa, 2008). Unfair treatment across Arizona institutions only further engrained stigma of individuals of Mexican descent, and such stigma is known to be associated with one's social position and has been linked to pervasive stress and poor health (Allport, 1954; Diaz, Ayala, Bein, Henne, & Marin, 2001; Gee, Ryan, Laflamme, & Holt, 2006; Noh & Kaspar, 2003; Romero, Carvajal, Valle, & Orduna, 2007; Romero, Martinez, & Carvajal, 2007). While bilingualism and cultural pride are considered some of the greatest assets by the South Tucson community, the K-12 public school system has consistently invalidated the interests of Mexican-American and Native American families by imposing its Euro-centric curriculum that many consider alienating to their lives and values. The history of the people has been consistently excluded from the curriculum in the public schools, along with the literary and artistic expressions of their rich and enduring culture.

It is the context of prejudice and negative expectations of youth of color that further reinforces the importance of the work done by the South Tucson Prevention Coalition to fully engage youth and adults in their community in a manner that led to positive community changes. Moreover, there is a significant amount of research on the self-fulfilling prophecy, which states that "we become what people expect us to be"; in other words, it is too easy for adolescents to begin behaving in ways that fulfill the negative stereotypes that the world has of them (Niemann, 2004). Specifically, this has a negative impact on Native American and Latino youth because of the stereotypes that are specific to their overuse of substances, selling of substances, and risky behaviors that include violence and risky sexual behavior (Niemann, 2004).

In many ways, the historical denial of access to resources and the continued silencing of ethnic minority voices highlights the radicalness and the necessity of programs to develop youth voice and community partnerships that can lead to changes in the system that will promote health and provide access to supportive resources for positive ethnic minority youth development (Fine & Torre, 2004). Participatory action research is a meaningful way to conduct research that helps researchers reject deficit models based on traditional methodologies and allows space to listen and reflect on the sources of resilience and the development of resiliency among marginalized groups and within their environments (Brown & Rodríguez, 2009; Ungar et al., 2007). These approaches are also described as facilitating the re-membering of an oppressed and silenced history through a process of unveiling privilege and power (Cahill, Rios-Moore, & Threatts, 2008; Fine & Torre, 2004). Far too often, research has focused on the negative aspects of low income neighborhoods and the associated risk factors. This deficit-based perspective limits our understanding of the reality of the experiences of adolescents who are developing in these types of environments; it also limits the discussion of the sense of agency among adolescents living in poverty (Wandersman & Nation, 1998). In this book, we will discuss how individual and collective resilience factors interact to reinforce each other and how this approach to working with low-income and minority community is essential because it acknowledges existing adversity while also indicating individual and collective agency to overcome challenges and create a better future for adolescents.

City of South Tucson has a strong history of civic engagement, and there is a distinct sense of pride and identity that connects people to this tight-knit community, despite the magnitude of the concentration of needs. Moreover, and most importantly, despite multiple factors of distress, the South Tucson community sees the promise in their children and families. The community has a unique sense of pride, identity, and connectedness rooted in the City of South Tucson. ***Based on these community strengths of a history of civic engagement, community connection, and the desire of parents to offer their children a better future***, we approach community change from a strength-based approach rather than a deficit model. Building on the strengths through a community-led perspective was central to the successful transformation of the ecological context of adolescent alcohol use.

1.3 South Tucson Prevention Coalition: Phase 1 and Phase 2

We will discuss in this book the creation of The South Tucson Prevention Coalition (STPC) that began working together in 2003 and continued until 2010. STPC had a Phase 1 and a Phase 2. Phase 1 was an after-school youth substance use prevention program to develop critically conscious youth leaders; yet there was minimal community integration in this program. However, Phase 2 was marked by coalition broadening and development, youth leadership, participatory action research, civic engagement, and sustainable policy changes. The STPC and the work of the coalition are at the heart of the community change. STPC represented several sectors of the South Tucson community, including schools, churches, service agencies, universities, local government, police, fire, youth, and parents. STPC organized annual community events in order to change community alcohol norms; these events will be described in terms of planning, organization, implementation, and integration of community-led research. We will also describe youth advocacy to raise community awareness of alcohol norms and to prevent new liquor licenses from being approved. One particularly powerful story that will be described is how this community stopped a new liquor license from a major corporation. Despite a challenging journey of collective action that included over 200 signatures on petitions, two city council meetings to reach decisions with overflow attendance, and a trip of youth and community advocates to the state liquor license board, the final result was that their community was only one of two licenses denied to this corporation, out of over 100 granted in the state. This event demonstrates the ability of a community to overcome adversity in order to create community transformational resilience.

1.4 Community Transformational Resilience

Far too often research has focused on the negative aspects of low income neighborhoods and the associated risk factors. This deficit-based perspective limits our understanding of the reality of the experiences of adolescents who are developing in these types of environments; it also limits the discussion of the sense of agency among adolescents living in poverty (Wandersman & Nation, 1998). Resilience theory is one way to understand how individuals living with adversity are able to overcome challenges (Luthar, Cicchetti, & Becker, 2000). Early definitions of resilience focused only on internal individual-level characteristics (Luthar et al., 2000). However, many researchers have contested original views of resilience that focus solely on individual-level factors and overlook the important shaping context of political and structural systems and infrastructures that often contribute to poverty (Pearson, Pearce, & Kingham, 2013).

More recent definitions of resilience based on qualitative and quantitative research with international samples of adolescents indicate that resilience is an interaction between the individual and their environment (Ungar & Liebenberg, 2011). Efforts to define and understand collective resilience have often group efforts to survive crises such as 9/11 (Freedman, 2004), bombings (Drury, Cocking, & Reicher, 2009), political violence (Fielding & Anderson, 2008; Sousa, Haj-Yahia, Feldman, & Lee, 2013), or war (Hernández, 2002; Vindevogel, Ager, Schiltz, Broekaert, & Derluyn, 2015). However, most of this work on collective resilience has primarily focused on how individuals access resources that already exist in the physical environment (Pearson et al., 2013), such as positive mentors, safe settings, passive contagion effects, or social support (Wandersman & Nation, 1998). A few discuss how individuals come to create solidarity and then rely on social support for resilience (Chaskin, 2008; Drury et al., 2009; Ebersöhn, 2014; Hernández, 2002). Previous research has primarily focused on existing community infrastructure, but not on community member's ability to change it.

In this book, we develop a new concept of **Community Transformational Resilience**, *which is defined here as a community's ability to overcome adversity through changing their community infrastructure in ways that can promote positive youth development by increasing resources and access to resources while also limiting accessibility to risky behaviors*. Key components of this concept that will be highlighted are (1) development of community through personalismo-based relationships, (2) development of transformational capacity through participatory action research that links critical consciousness to collective action, and (3) development of community-level factors of resilience for adolescent alcohol use that promote positive factors and limit risk factors. In this book, we will discuss how STPC created community transformational resilience utilizing participatory action research and community readiness model of change focused on their own specific community.

1.5 Community Readiness Model for Change

Often a pivotal component for sustainable change is community support for prevention programs. Yet, no matter the quality of the planning and implementation of the program, it may fail merely because the community was not ready to receive the program. Community is defined as people and groups who are involved in local production/distribution/consumption of goods and services, socialization, social control, social participation, and mutual support (Oetting et al., 1995). ***Community readiness is defined as the shared norms, values, group decision making, and leadership that contribute to the identification of the need for change based on discrepancies between expectations and reality*** (Thurman, Plested, Edwards, Foley, & Burnside, 2003). Actions in response to identified need are marked by group decision making. The explicated multiple levels of readiness in this theory guide not only our description of implementation but also the extent of community-level change over several years. We used strategic processes of participatory action research embedded within Community Readiness Theory to identify the appropriate strategy for the community level of receptivity.

1.6 Participatory Action Research Principles

The South Tucson Prevention Coalition utilized a participatory action research approach (Cousins & Earl, 1992) as a means of primary prevention for adolescent alcohol use because delaying onset of use is an effective way to reduce other risky behaviors and to reduce later issues with addiction. At beginning stages, the level of integration of participation action research (PAR) was low; however, over time the level of PAR increased steadily, to the point of community-led research and action. This method is particularly useful when researchers desire a balance between technical rigor and responsiveness to stakeholder needs, through the following methods (1) the researchers, the program staff and community stakeholders, and the recipients and key informants of services jointly share the control of the research, (2) number of stakeholders is limited to those with program responsibility or a vital interest in the program, and (3) members of the collaborative effort are involved at all stages of the research including designing and preparing the project proposal, defining the design, selecting/developing instrumentation, collecting data, processing and analyzing data, and reporting and disseminating results. Over time, the STPC members moved from being more of an advisory council to being directly involved in joint analysis and dissemination of findings. This book will discuss the process of change over 10 years and the key steps that helped facilitate this progression.

Participatory action research strategies to work with youth and communities was utilized to guide the development of a youth–adult coalition, youth-led research, and community-led research. These participatory strategies helped to guide basic assumption of equality of all members and also to guide the problem-posing dialogue. The use of PAR strategies was essential to working effectively with adolescents who were viewed as equals in the discussion and decision-making processes and with historically oppressed groups, such as Mexican American and Native Americans. Eventually, these strategies led to youth leaders who helped created community change. Often adults had preconceptions about youth of color based on negative stereotypes, but the development of their own critical consciousness and humanization of adolescents was fundamental to the effective coalition work.

We use a Freirian (1968) approach to our work with youth to understand how they create knowledge and that by facilitating opportunities for problem posing within multiple contexts, they will understand how their environment shapes their experiences (Freire, 1968; Ginwright & Cammarota, 2006; Watts & Guessous, 2006). Freire's (1968) work, based on the concept of praxis, represents not only critical awareness of societal inequities but also an element of action (Cammarota & Fine, 2008). The critical awareness and analysis that considers privilege and power is essential to engaging minority youth in creating critical change. In one study, Watts and Guessous (2006) found that youth who engaged in more critical analysis to understand societal inequities, and those who were committed to a collective action approach were more likely to report commitment to civic involvement. It is this focus on social justice through analysis that contributes to the development of critical consciousness among youth (Freire, 1968; Ginwright & Cammarota, 2002).

In the following chapters, there are several comments about how the adults and youth had moments when they gained a critical awareness of youth and alcohol use and also moments when they became conscious that working together as a community could be transformative for collective resilience. This process of awakening to consciousness is what Freire (1968) termed *conscientización*, where individuals come to view themselves as active participants in society and with the capacity to change existing structures. What is challenging also about this process is the conscious acknowledgement of the previous denial of problems or acceptance and tolerance of stereotypes and negative portrayals of youth and their connection to hopelessness within the community. The critical consciousness moves individuals away from the cultural-deficit model, blaming their culture as the problem, and it always resituates their perspective, so they are no longer blaming themselves for the problems they experience and witness within their communities (Romero et al., 2008).

As such, youth involvement must be based on a critical form of consciousness that acknowledges the existing problems and systemic racism that continues to marginalize minority youth (Watts & Guessous, 2006). Thus, we also worked together to identify environmental strategies to create youth-led community transformation to prevent alcohol use. In this way, rather than perceiving youth as victims of the existing economic and political forces surrounding their development, they are perceived as able to improve their own community through leveraging the access and capacity that they already have at hand within their families, schools, peers, community centers, and city.

We will demonstrate through the course of several chapters and research over several years that participatory action research principles were central to nurturing hope and collective action in order to change city infrastructure in a manner that could promote and nurture adolescent health and limit access to alcohol (Cammarota & Fine, 2008). The tenets of PAR are essential to our work on adolescent health promotion because it situates youth within a broader context, and rather than putting the entire burden on them to continually negotiate a risky environment, it reminds them of the power already within **their own capacity to connect with others to create change in their environments. This is the heart of the message of our book "*We can't do it alone.*"**

1.7 Basic Structure of the Book

The basic structure of this book will be to tell the story of *the transformation of this community over an 8-year period that came about as a result of concerted collaborative efforts to prevent adolescent alcohol use*. We provide a mixed method analysis over the 8-year period to document city-level changes that occurred and the factors that contributed to these sustainable changes. Specifically, we present longitudinal in-depth survey data with youth, city-level data for youth attitudes, qualitative youth semi-structured interviews, community interviews, participatory action research youth-led alcohol mapping city-level analysis, and city-level policy analysis. Through using mixed methods, we shed light on the developmental process of critical civic praxis that occurred among youth, community leaders, and researchers (Ginwright & Cammarota, 2002) that ultimately led to changes in daily practices and city-level policy. There is no singular hero here, but the collective voice and effort of the community shine forward with stories of successes and feelings of progress and unity.

Chapter 2 provides an overview of the 8 years of community-level change through the use of the Community Readiness Model to explain community receptiveness to adolescent alcohol prevention. Identification of community readiness helped determine the most appropriate and tailored interventions in order to ensure community support, effectiveness of strategies, and assist in advancing to the next level of community readiness. This chapter describes some of the tensions that arose as the coalition members grew in scope to additionally include police officers, school representatives, new nonprofit agencies, and government officials. Specifically, this chapter addresses the changes over time in trust, or lack of, between community partners and researchers.

Chapter 3 describes participatory action research principles that guide the majority of the work in this book. We make the argument for the importance of using participatory action research principles with marginalized communities and with youth of color. The key principles of equal participation, open dialogue, research, reflection, and action are described in detail. Additionally, this chapter includes the positionality statements of university researchers who collected interview survey data with STPC key stakeholders who are quoted in this book.

Chapter 4 presents South Tucson Prevention Center (STPC): Phase 1 of adolescent alcohol prevention activities. This was an after-school adolescent-focused program (entitled Omeyocan YES) that *developed youth critical consciousness of health and economic inequities* in their community utilizing a Frierian pedagogy model. It also taught them community-organizing skills as a means to combat these challenges. Triangulated evaluation data is presented that represents youth program leaders, youth quantitative longitudinal survey data, and youth qualitative responses.

Chapter 5 discusses the transitions and breaking down of silos that were necessary to build the coalition. We will present the in-depth interviews with directors of local nonprofit agencies who discuss how they overcame agency competition and existing silos of services that were not accessible to all adolescents throughout the community.

The directors also discuss the role of research and researchers at this stage as well as the development and submission of a federal grant as a collaborative project.

Chapter 6 will present adult perspectives on the role of youth prevention programs and the evolution of thinking and programing that led to youth-led strategies for alcohol prevention. Based on in-depth interviews and ethnographic observations of youth-led events, we discuss the challenges in fulfilling the youth-led participatory research principles as adults began this transition. The continued infrastructure opportunities for youth to participate and lead after-school programs was foundational to building generations of youth who were prepared to take a stand as community leaders and create policy change. We also discuss specific strategies that eased this transition from the intensive after-school prevention program, Omeyocan YES to the youth-led program, Youth 2 Youth (Y2Y). Community leaders discuss the transformative moments of accepting youth as equal partners and positive leaders.

Chapter 7 presents the youth perspectives on the development of the Y2Y program from in-depth interviews with youth leaders from two different generations of Y2Y youth. Comments are analyzed to find themes of targeting community alcohol norms, youth leadership, critical community pedagogy, and sustainable youth development. Furthermore, there are specific examples provided about the implementation of Freirian (1968) dialogue-based youth-community partnerships for problem solving and collective action for community change.

Chapter 8 describes how the youth-community partnership began to tackle larger community interventions to raise awareness about alcohol norms and community perspectives of adolescent alcohol use. Historical documents of the STPC are analyzed to describe and critically discuss the community readiness strategies of alcohol prevention. We describe how community partners, both youth and adults, came together to develop activities to raise awareness about adolescent alcohol prevention. This period is marked by a shift from not only preventing risky behaviors but also promoting positive youth health opportunities.

Chapter 9 describes the development of community-led research, and historical documents of community surveys and reports of research are presented. Evaluation of changes in community alcohol norms are presented based on the community-led longitudinal survey research. This period is marked by coalition members embracing *the use of local data survey collection as a means to create unity around collective action for change.* We also discuss the presentation of findings to the local city council to contribute to discussions of city policy on the availability of alcohol and access to local parks.

Chapter 10 describes a pivotal youth-led participatory action research project to map the city for local liquor licenses and youth attractions. The use of external funding and partnership with the city planners is discussed. We provide the final map and analysis of the findings provided by students. This section also goes into detail about how youth took several steps to share their findings at city council meetings, and local town hall meetings, as well as presenting their findings at a national conference. Interviews with youth and STPC leaders are analyzed to understand their use of research and relationship to the city government.

Chapter 11 presents in-depth interviews with multiple adult community leaders who participated in the coalition and describes and analyzes their retrospective understanding of the coalition and youth involvement. This chapter discusses the foundational influence of critical consciousness of coalition members that led them to believe in collective approaches to adolescent alcohol prevention. The overlap in the mission and the passion of the coalition members is described in terms of keeping the core group committed to the larger cause of providing a better future for young people in South Tucson. Specifically, this chapter describes the personalismo-relationship-based approach to building coalitions that was the foundation of the success of this coalition.

Chapter 12 summarizes the results of the 8 years of work in the City of South Tucson. Recommendations are offered for other communities across the world about how to create community transformational resilience as a means to create and sustain a functional and productive coalition of youth-community partnerships for adolescent alcohol prevention. Some of the key findings will be further discussed such as building community, transformational capacity, and key resiliency factors. The utility of participatory action research and community readiness will be discussed as a means to reduce health disparities of Latino adolescents and their communities. It is our aim to share both the challenges and success so that other researchers and communities may learn ways to reduce and eliminate adolescent alcohol disparities.

References

Allport, G. W. (1954). *The nature of prejudice*. Reading, MA: Addison-Wesley.

Almodovar, A., Tomaka, J., Thompson, S., Mckinnon, S., & O'Rourke, K. (2006). Risk and protective factors among high school students on the US/Mexico border. *American Journal of Health Behavior, 30*(6), 745–752.

Bacio, G. A., Mays, V. M., & Lau, A. S. (2013). Drinking initiation and problematic drinking among Latino adolescents: Explanations of the immigrant paradox. *Psychology of Addictive Behaviors, 27*(1), 14–22. doi:10.1037/a0029996.

Bettes, B. A., Dusenbury, L., Kerner, J., James-Ortiz, S., & Botvin, G. J. (2008). Ethnicity and psychosocial factors in alcohol and tobacco use in adolescence. *Child Development, 61*(2), 557–565.

Breslau, N., & Peterson, E. L. (1996). Smoking cessation in young adults: Age at initiation of cigarette smoking and other suspected influences. *American Journal of Public Health, 86*(2), 214–220.

Brown, T. M., & Rodríguez, L. F. (2009). *New directions for youth development: Youth in participatory action research*. San Francisco, CA: Jossey-Bass.

Cahill, C., Rios-Moore, I., & Threatts, T. (2008). Different eyes/open eyes: Community-based participatory action research. In J. Cammarota & M. Fine (Eds.), *Revolutionizing education: Youth participatory action research in motion* (pp. 89–124). New York, NY: Routledge Press.

Cammarota, J., & Fine, M. (2008). *Revolutionizing education: Youth participatory action research in motion*. New York, NY: Routledge Press.

Carvajal, S. C., Photiades, J. R., Evans, R. I., & Nash, S. G. (1997). Relating a social influence model to the role of acculturation in substance use among Latino adolescents. *Journal of Applied Social Psychology, 27*(18), 1617–1628.

Centers for Disease Control. (2014). Fact sheets – Underage drinking. Centers for Disease Control. http://www.cdc.gov/alcohol/fact-sheets/underage-drinking.htm

Chaskin, R. J. (2008). Resilience, community, and resilient communities: Conditioning contexts and collective action. *Child Care in Practice, 14*(1), 65–74. doi:10.1080/13575270701733724.

Chassin, L., Curran, P. J., Hussong, A. M., & Colder, C. R. (1996). The relation of parent alcoholism to adolescent substance use: A longitudinal follow-up study. *Journal of Abnormal Psychology, 105*(1), 70.

Cousins, J. B., & Earl, L. M. (1992). The case for participatory evaluation. *Educational Evaluation and Policy Analysis, 14*(4), 397–418.

De la Torre, A., & Estrada, A. L. (2001). *Mexican Americans and health: Sana! Sana!* Tucson, AZ: University of Arizona Press.

Diaz, R. M., Ayala, G., Bein, E., Henne, J., & Marin, B. V. (2001). The impact of homophobia, poverty, and racism on the mental health of gay and bisexual Latino men: Findings from 3 US cities. *American Journal of Public Health, 91*(6), 927–932.

Drury, J., Cocking, C., & Reicher, S. (2009). The nature of collective resilience: Survivor reactions to the 2005 London bombings. *International Journal of Mass Emergencies and Disasters, 27*(1), 66–95.

Ebersöhn, L. (2014). Adding 'flock' to 'fight and flight': A honeycomb of resilience where supply of relationships meets demand for support. *Journal of Psychology in Africa, 22*(1), 29–42.

Esses, V. M., Dovidio, J. F., & Hodson, G. (2002). Public attitudes toward immigration in the United States and Canada in response to the September 11, 2001: "Attack on America". *Analyses of Social Issues and Public Policy, 2*, 69–85.

Fielding, A., & Anderson, J. (2008). *Working with refugee communities to build collective resilience*. Perth: Association for Services to Torture and Trauma Survivors.

Fine, M., & Torre, M. E. (2004). Re-membering exclusions: Participatory action research in public institutions. *Qualitative Research in Psychology, 1*, 15–37.

Freedman, T. G. (2004). Voices of 9/11 first responders: Patterns of collective resilience. *Clinical Social Work Journal, 32*(4), 377–393. doi:10.1007/s10615-004-0538-z.

Freire, P. (1968). *Pedagogy of the oppressed*. New York, NY: Seabury.

Gee, G. C., Ryan, A., Laflamme, D. J., & Holt, J. (2006). The relationship between perceived discrimination and mental health among African descendants, Mexican Americans and other Latinos in the New Hampshire REACH study: The added dimension of immigration status. *American Journal of Public Health, 96*(10), 1821–1828.

Ginwright, S., & Cammarota, J. (2002). New terrain in youth development: The promise of a social justice approach. *Social Justice, 29*(4), 82–95.

Ginwright, S., & Cammarota, J. (2006). Introduction. In S. Ginwright, P. Noguera, & J. Cammarota (Eds.), *Beyond resistance!: Youth activism and community change: New democratic possibilities for practice and policy for America's youth* (pp. xiii–xxii). New York, NY: Routledge Press.

Hernández, P. (2002). Resilience in families and communities: Latin American contributions from the psychology of liberation. *The Family Journal, 10*(3), 334–343. doi:10.1177/1068070201000301l.

Hines, B. (2002). So near yet so far away: The effect of September 11th on Mexican immigrants in the United States. *Texas Hispanic Journal of Law and Policy, 8*(37), 37–46.

Hingson, R. W., Heeren, T., & Winter, M. R. (2006). Age at drinking onset and alcohol dependence: Age at onset, duration, and severity. *Pediatrics, 160*, 739–746.

Johnson, K. (1997). The new nativism: Something old, something new, something borrowed, something blue. In J. F. Perea (Ed.), *Immigrants out!: The new nativism and the anti-immigrant impulse in the United States*. New York, NY: New York University Press.

Kohout, M. (2012). Local anti-immigration politics in California's inland empire. In M. Verea (Ed.), *Anti-immigrant sentiments, actions and policies in North America and the European Union* (pp. 137–156). Mexico, DF: Centro de Investigación sobre América del Norte (CISAN) de la Universidad Autónoma de Mexico (UNAM).

Luthar, S. S., Cicchetti, D., & Becker, B. (2000). The construct of resilience: A critical evaluation and guidelines for future work. *Child Development, 71*(3), 543–562. doi:10.1111/1467-8624.00164.

McKinnon, S. A., O'rourke, K. M., Thompson, S. E., & Berumen, J. H. (2004). Alcohol use and abuse by adolescents: the impact of living in a border community. *Journal of Adolescent Health, 34*(1), 88–93.

Niemann, Y. F. (2004). Stereotypes of Chicanas and Chicanos: Impact on family functioning, individual expectations, goals, and behaviors. In R. J. Velasquez, L. M. Arellano, & B. W. McNeill (Eds.), *The handbook of Chicana/o psychology and mental health* (pp. 61–82). Mahwah, NJ: Lawrence Erlbaum.

Noh, S., & Kaspar, V. (2003). Perceived discrimination and depression: Moderating effects of coping, acculturation and ethnic support. *American Journal of Public Health, 93*, 232–238.

Oetting, E. R., Donnermeyer, J. F., Plested, B. A., Edwards, R. W., Kelly, K., & Beauvais, F. (1995). Assessing community readiness for prevention. *International Journal of the Addictions, 30*, 659–683.

Otero-Sabogal, R., Sabogal, F., Perez-Stable, E. J., & Hiatt, R. A. (1995). Dietary practices, alcohol consumption, and smoking behavior: ethnic, sex, and acculturation differences. *Journal of the National Cancer Institute. Monographs, 18*, 73–82.

Pearson, A. L., Pearce, J., & Kingham, S. (2013). Deprived yet health: Neighborhood-level resilience in New Zealand. *Social Science and Medicine, 91*, 238–245.

Puar, J. (2007). *Terrorist assemblages: Homonationalism in queer times*. Durham, NC: Duke University Press.

Rodriguez, R. C. (2014). *Our sacred maiz is our mother: Indigeneity and belonging in the Americas*. Tucson, AZ: The University of Arizona Press.

Romero, A., Cammarota, J., Dominguez, K., Valdez, L., Ramirez, G. & Hernandez, L. (2008). "The opportunity if not the Right to See": Social justice education project (pp. 131–151). In Cammarota, J. & Fine, M. (Eds.), *Revolutionizing education: Youth participatory action research in motion*. New York, NY: Routledge Press.

Romero, A. J., Carvajal, S. C., Valle, F., & Orduna, M. (2007). Adolescent bicultural stress and its impact on mental well-being among Latinos, Asian Americans and European Americans. *Journal of Community Psychology, 35*(4), 519–534.

Romero, A. J., Martinez, D., & Carvajal, S. C. (2007). Bicultural stress and adolescent risk behaviors in a community sample of Latinos and Non-Latino European Americans. *Ethnicity and Health, 12*(5), 443–463.

SAMSHA Administration. (2004). *National survey on drug use and health: National findings*.

Sousa, C. A., Haj-Yahia, M. M., Feldman, G., & Lee, J. (2013). Individual and collective dimensions of resilience within political violence. *Trauma, Violence, and Abuse, 14*(3), 235–254. doi:10.1177/1524838013493520.

Squeglia, L. M., Jacobus, J., & Tapert, S. F. (2009). The influence of substance use on adolescent brain development. *Clinical EEG and Neuroscience, 40*(1), 31–38.

Stevens, S. J., Estrada, B., Murphy, B. S., McKnight, K. M., & Tims, F. (2004). Gender difference in substance use, mental health, and criminal justice involvement of adolescents at treatment entry and at three, six, 12 and 30 month follow-up. *Journal of Psychoactive Drugs, 36*(1), 13–25.

Stevens, S. J., Hasler, J., Murphy, B. S., Taylor, R., Senior, M., Barron, M. … & Powis, Z. (2003). La Cañada adolescent treatment program: Addressing issues of drug use, gender and trauma. In S. J. Stevens & A. R. Morral (Eds.), *Adolescent substance abuse treatment in the United States: Exemplary models from a national evaluation study* (pp. 183–209). Binghampton, NY: The Haworth Press.

Thurman, P. J., Plested, B. A., Edwards, R. W., Foley, R., & Burnside, M. (2003). Community readiness: The journey to community healing. *Journal of Psychoactive Drugs, 35*(1), 27–31.

Tseng, V., & Yoshikawa, H. (2008). Reconceptualizing acculturation: Ecological processes, historical contexts, and power inequities. *American Journal of Community Psychology, 42*(3–4), 355–358.

U.S. Census Bureau. (2000a). Profile of general demographic characteristics: 2000 census 2000 summary file. http://factfinder.census.gov/faces/tableservices/jsf/pages/productview.xhtml?src=bkmk

U.S. Census Bureau. (2000b). Profile of selected economic characteristics: 2000 census 2000 summary file. http://factfinder.census.gov/faces/tableservices/jsf/pages/productview.xhtml?src=bkmk

U.S. Census Bureau. (2000c). Profile of selected economic characteristics: 2000 census summary file – Arizona. http://factfinder.census.gov/faces/tableservices/jsf/pages/productview.xhtml?src=CF

U.S. Census Bureau. (2010a). Profile of general population and housing characteristics: 2010 demographic profile data. http://factfinder.census.gov/faces/tableservices/jsf/pages/productview.xhtml?src=bkmk

U.S. Census Bureau. (2010b). Selected economic characteristics: 2006-2010 American Community Survey 5 year estimates. http://factfinder.census.gov/faces/tableservices/jsf/pages/productview.xhtml?src=bkmk

U.S. Census Bureau. (2010c). State and county quick facts: South Tucson, Arizona. http://quickfacts.census.gov/qfd/states/04/0468850.html

Ungar, M., Brown, M., Liebenberg, L., Othman, R., Kwong, W. M., Armstrong, M., & Gilgun, J. (2007). Unique pathways to resilience across cultures. *Adolescence, 42*(166), 287–310.

Ungar, M., & Liebenberg, L. (2011). Resilience across cultures using mixed methods: Child and youth resilience measure. *Journal of Mixed Methods Research, 5*(2), 126–149. doi:10.1177/1558689811400607.

Vindevogel, S., Ager, A., Schiltz, J., Broekaert, E., & Derluyn, I. (2015). Toward a culturally sensitive conceptualization of resilience: Participatory research with war-affected communities in northern Uganda. *Transcultural Psychiatry, 52*(3), 396–416. doi:10.1177/1363461514565852.

Walters, K. L., & Simoni, J. M. (2002). Reconceptualizing Native women's health: An "indigenist" stress-coping model. *American Journal of Public Health, 92*(4), 520–524.

Wandersman, A., & Nation, M. (1998). Urban neighborhoods and mental health: Psychological contributions to understanding toxicity, resilience and interventions. *American Psychologist, 53*(6), 647–656.

Chapter 2
Community Readiness Stages of Change to Achieve Community Transformational Resilience

Andrea Romero, Payal Anand, Josefina Ahumada, Sofia Blue, Gloria Hamelitz-Lopez, Michele Orduña, Maricruz Romero-Ruiz, Juan "Johnny" Quevedo, and Kimberly Sierra-Cajas

"Local people are likely to have the greatest and most sustainable impact in solving local problems and in setting local norms" (Oetting, Jumper-Thurman, Plested, & Edwards, 2001).

A. Romero, Ph.D. (✉) • P. Anand, M.P.H.
Family Studies and Human Development, University of Arizona, 650 N. Park Avenue, Tucson, AZ 85719, USA
e-mail: romeroa@u.arizona.edu; payala1@email.arizona.edu

J. Ahumada, M.S.W.
FSC, School of Social Work, Arizona State University, Tempe, AZ, USA
e-mail: josefina.ahumada@asu.edu

S. Blue
Pima County Public Library Sam Lena Branch, South Tucson, AZ, USA
e-mail: quetzazul@gmail.com

G. Hamelitz-Lopez
John Valenzuela Youth Center, Tucson, AZ, USA
e-mail: gloriahamelitz@hotmail.com

M. Orduña, M.Ed.
House of Neighborly Service, Loveland, CO, USA
e-mail: miorduna@gmail.com

M. Romero-Ruiz, M.S.
United Way of Tucson and Southern Arizona, Tucson, AZ, USA
e-mail: mrruiz1@gmail.com

J.J. Quevedo
Pima Community College, Tucson, AZ, USA
e-mail: Tucsonhigh12@yahoo.com

K. Sierra-Cajas
College of Science, University of Arizona, Tucson, AZ, 85719, USA
e-mail: kjsc@email.arizona.edu

A.J. Romero (ed.), *Youth-Community Partnerships for Adolescent Alcohol Prevention*, DOI 10.1007/978-3-319-26030-3_2

Abstract The Community Readiness Model for Change describes nine stages of incremental changes for community prevention. In this chapter, we utilize this model to describe 8 years of change led by South Tucson Prevention Coalition (STPC) that transformed one community from a level of tolerance of adolescent alcohol use to a level of professionalization of prevention strategies. This model helps to identify the incremental changes over time in community alcohol norms that indicate how ready the community is to receive different prevention strategies. The Community Readiness Model for Change requires community involvement to develop prevention strategies that are rooted in community strengths. This model also requires that the community assesses their own level of readiness for change in order to develop their capacity to determine the type and level of intervention that would be most appropriate. In this chapter, we describe the model and then apply it to 8 years of work by STPC to highlight changes in community alcohol norms, changes in prevention strategies, and integration of research techniques. Utilizing community readiness interviews and retrospective interviews with coalition members, we describe the community transformations that occurred.

Keywords Community readiness • Coalition • Adolescent alcohol prevention • Community transformation

Community prevention of underage drinking is an important and necessary work, as identified by researchers (Burrow-Sanchez, 2006; Plested, Edwards, & Jumper-Thurman, 2006). Communities are not all "ready" to engage in prevention activities; the readiness of the community refers to the degree to which they are equipped and have the capacity to take action on issues of health promotion and disease prevention (Plested et al., 2006). When prevention strategies are a mismatch with the readiness of the community, they are more likely to be rejected, to fail, or to not be sustainable (Oetting et al., 1995). Community Readiness is a research-based model that describes how interventions can and should be tailored to be appropriate to make incremental changes in the current community norms for adolescent alcohol use (Thurman, Plested, Edwards, Foley, & Burnside, 2003). When prevention efforts are appropriately matched to the community level of readiness, adolescent alcohol and substance use prevention is more likely to be effective and sustainable (Kelly et al., 2003). In this chapter, we describe 8 years of work by the South Tucson Prevention Coalition (STPC) to transform their community in order to enhance community transformational resilience to prevent adolescent underage drinking.

A central component of the Community Readiness Model for Change is to help communities mobilize for change through the cyclical use of assessment as a tool to guide intervention strategies (Edwards, Jumper-Thurman, Plested, Oetting, & Swanson, 2000). One of the strengths of this model, and one of the reasons it was chosen by the STPC, was so that the community themselves could assess their own readiness for change as a source of empowerment to improve adolescent health. This model also highlights the importance of community involvement at every level of prevention, which is particularly key with minority communities. Walters, Canady, and Stein (1994) identify several common errors in prevention with minority youth which include: (1) lack of community participation, (2) inappropriate reading levels and jargon, (3) disregard of differences between and within cultures, (4) no consideration of specific behaviors associated with risky behavior within cultures, and (5) inappropriate use of language, symbols, and visual images of culture to portray values. STPC highlights the role of community involvement and adolescent involvement in the creation and implementation of prevention programs for their own community.

This chapter will first describe The Community Readiness Model for Change and then apply it to examine adolescent alcohol prevention strategies over a period of 8 years in one city with a high rate of poverty and predominantly Mexican and Native American families (see Chap. 1 for city description). We describe how STPC Phase 1 began with adolescent after-school prevention programming and minimal community involvement and evolved into STPC Phase 2 which was driven by coalition activities that raised awareness, integrated research to focus strategies, and ultimately resulted in transformation of community infrastructure to promote positive factors and reduce risk factors. Specifically, STPC was successful in professionalizing positive youth-led after-school programs, blocking new liquor licenses, and working with the local city government to develop neighborhood preservation strategies such as limiting alcohol availability and alcohol advertising.

2.1 Why Community-Level Change Is Necessary for Adolescent Health

The focus on community-level change is critical because it shifts the prevention focus from the individual instead to their ecodevelopmental contexts (family, school, neighborhood, policy, society), which have repeatedly found to be highly influential on health, development, and overall well-being (Bronfenbrenner, 1986; Minkler & Wallerstein, 2011). Adolescent alcohol use is shaped by multiple facets of the community, including community alcohol norms of disapproval/permissiveness, alcohol availability, alcohol regulation, alcohol advertising, knowledge of risks of alcohol use, and adult role models of alcohol use. Adolescents in low-income communities (see Chap. 1 for description of community economic context) have even less infrastructure to support the continuance of adolescent positive youth development or involvement in prevention activities. Adolescents living in low-income neighborhoods are typically exposed to more than the average amount of ecological stressors, such as noise, traffic, trash, and other hazards. Additionally, lower income neighborhoods are also more likely to have higher access to alcohol, higher rates of public drunkenness, and more availability of alcohol (Pearson, Pearce, & Kingham, 2013; Wandersman & Nation, 1998). Additional research (Castro, Boyer, & Balcazar, 2000) also cites the central role of the normative influence of parents, older family members, and community members as an important consideration of health behaviors for Mexican adolescents. Youth living in impoverished neighborhoods are more likely to report less familial monitoring of adolescent's out of school time and alcohol norms that contribute to more adolescent alcohol use (Trucco, Colder, Wieczorek, Lengua, & Hawk, 2014). Thus, youth in low-income neighborhoods are more likely to face more risks more often and find that they have less support for continued positive health behaviors (Milam, Furr-Holden, Cooley-Strickland, Bradshaw, & Leaf, 2014). It is this combination of higher access/availability and community alcohol norms that can be destructive for adolescent health.

However, most prevention programs do not include community members or environmental change prevention strategies. In fact, most prevention programs are run by a single community-based organization (CBO), and many agencies act in isolation from each other, and it is this silo-ed effect we attempted to change with STPC (Kania & Kramer, 2011; Merves, Rodgers, Silver, Sclafane, & Bauman, 2015). Too often prevention is fragmented because time and resources are devoted to the same issue by different agencies who have the same goals, but who do not collaborate. Based on STPC's coalition work, we will demonstrate that collaboration can increase agency's potential to reach more people and use their resources more effectively and with greater impact. Furthermore, silo-ed approaches to adolescent alcohol use prevention ultimately contribute to the lack of sustainability of public health change because without a coordinated approach there is not going to be continued support for adolescent involvement in alcohol use prevention.

Thus, for these reasons we argue that community-level change is important and that by bringing multiple sectors of the community to work together on prevention strategies it is much more likely to be effective as compared to one segment of the community. On a very concrete level, bringing together diverse groups to discuss the issue provides broader societal insight into the health issue, each individual or agency has expertise within the perspective of their own group, yet they often have less experience or exposure to alternative viewpoints. Understanding resources outside of one's own agency can help bring a community together to coordinate prevention efforts. STPC created community transformational resilience, by transforming their community to create new protective factors, aligning existing resources, and reducing risk factors, such as alcohol availability and alcohol advertising. Thus, we demonstrate how we applied the Community Readiness Model for Change to understand how community infrastructure changes were achieved through coalition building strategies that linked readiness levels to prevention strategies.

2.2 Community Readiness Model for Change Stages

The Community Readiness Model for Change (Oetting et al., 2001) was originally based on theories of individual behavior change, such as, social action process (Beal, 1964) and innovation decision-making process (Rogers, 1983). Both previous theories are based on five stage process models that begin with awareness of behavior and then describe a process of change that moves through decisions to act and finally to reflections on behavior change (Beal, 1964; Prochaska, DiClemente, & Norcross,

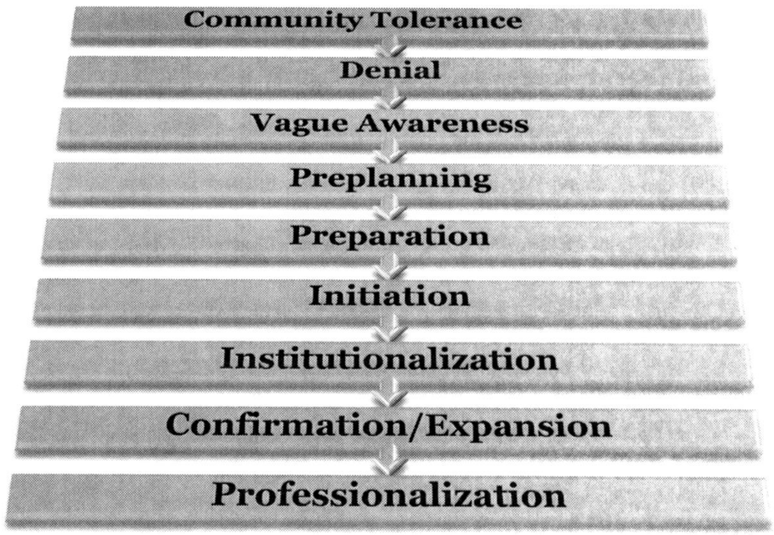

Fig. 2.1 Community readiness model

1992; Rogers, 1983). The stage model for Community Readiness expanded the original five-stage process models for individual change to a nine-stage model for community change (Oetting et al., 2001). The stages describe progressively more receptive levels of (1) current community norms and, (2) appropriate prevention strategies given the current norms. The flow of this public health change process is recognition of the health issue as a problem and the resulting motivation to change the issue. The following are the primary stages that describe representative community norms at each level (see Fig. 2.1)

1. Community Tolerance or No Awareness: "health issue is normal and acceptable"
2. Denial: "belief the health issue does not exist or that change is impossible"
3. Vague Awareness: "recognition of health issue, but no motivation to change"
4. Preplanning: "recognition of health issue and agreement that something needs to be done"
5. Preparation: "active planning to change the health issue"
6. Initiation: "implementation of a program to change the health issue"
7. Institutionalization: "1–2 prevention programs are operating and stable"
8. Confirmation and Expansion: "recognition of limitations and attempts to improve the prevention program"
9. Professionalization: "sophistication, training, and effective valuation of the prevention programs"

Previous research has found that the psychological readiness to change is fundamental to success, because if an individual is pushed to change their behavior before they are ready or aware of need/desire to change their behavior the efforts to create change are most likely to fail (Oetting et al., 2001; Prochaska et al., 1992). This may be due to resistance to change, denial about the need to change, or lack of sufficient skills to sustain the behavior change. Thus, the Community Readiness model applied models of individual level behavior change to a community-level public health change approach. As such, the model is based on first understanding community norms around the health issue and then working to move the needle on those norms incrementally by targeting interventions to the existing normative state (Oetting et al., 2001). This model advocates for intervention strategies to be rooted in collaborations with community decision-makers in order to assess readiness, develop strategies to act, and community-led evaluation of prevention efforts. Continuous community-led evaluation is also essential to this process of change as a tool for reflection on results, which can lead to informed modification of prevention strategies.

2.3 Prevention Strategies Linked to Readiness Stage

This model also describes the most appropriate prevention or intervention strategies at each level of community readiness in order to create effective incremental change that will naturally lead to the next stage of community readiness. The intervention strategies that are linked with the first four stages are aimed primarily at raising awareness about adolescent alcohol use as a problem. At *Stages 1 & 2 of tolerance and denial*, the intervention approaches focus more on descriptive community-based examples and rely less on statistics, or do not include statistics at all. Effective strategies include small one-to-one settings, small group discussions/focus groups, home visits, or talking circles (Oetting et al., 2001; Plested et al., 2006). Local anecdotes have been found to be much more effective at communicating with community members, who are often in a state of denial that the issue exists in their own community, this is one reason why statistics, particularly national or large-scale statistics or research are often not as effective in these stages and may even be counter-productive.

During *Stage 3, vague awareness with some recognition of the problem but no motivation to change,* strategies can grow to larger settings that include small group events, newspaper articles, or local survey data (Plested et al., 2006). Targeted one-to-one outreach to community leaders, such as government officials, school officials and parents, may be effective to raise awareness, particularly with those who may be hesitant to admit the existence of adolescent alcohol use in their community. In the early stages, the primary focus is still on increasing awareness about the issue at a local level and introducing the idea that these issues are changeable. At these early stages (1–3) the broader community may not be prepared to receive interventions to create change, because they may deny the problem exists or feel that there is no need to change. Some community members may even feel that change may not be possible because the issue is too big, too long-standing, or because they have accepted that something such as adolescent alcohol use is a normative aspect of development. Once awareness about the local problem of adolescent alcohol use is raised then the community can move to the next *Stage 4, preplanning and taking stock of existing prevention programs*. It is important to acknowledge that not all community members are likely to be at the same stage at the same time; moreover, it is not necessary that the majority of community members reach Stage 4 in order to begin preplanning. As long as a strong cohort of community leaders and influential community members is ready then preplanning can begin (Plested et al., 2006).

At *Stage 5 and 6, preparation & initiation*, the community is ready to begin gathering and sharing community-specific information, such as local data. The focus during this stage is to develop community-specific strategies that incorporate a broader representation of the community. During the initiation stage some of the appropriate activities include prevention training for professionals and further needs assessment about existing services, effectiveness, and gaps in service (Plested et al., 2006).

Stage 7 and 8, institutionalization, confirmation and expansion, are continuation of these activities at stages 5 and 6, but at a higher level of sophistication and quality. For example, this may be represented by the collaboration with an external evaluation service to develop a comprehensive community database. It may also include formalizing relationships with local business sponsorship in order to diversify funding. These stages can then more easily lead to the institutionalization stage where one or two programs are being implemented on a regular basis. During the final stages comprehensive evaluation plays a more central role in that it should be integrated and used as a key decision-making tool (Oetting et al., 2001). While data at these stages are regularly shared publicly, it is expected that the community climate is open, but always critically questioning the meaning of data trends. The *9th final stage of professionalization* where the results of the prevention efforts have been confirmed, formalized and professionally maintained throughout larger segments of the community.

2.4 Community Readiness and Assessment

A firm understanding of the community's readiness through continual and community-led assessment can aid in building on existing cultural strengths and neighborhood resources. Oetting et al. (2001) propose *six dimensions for assessment, which include existing community efforts, community knowledge of efforts, leadership, community climate, community knowledge about issue, and resources for prevention issue*. A principal way to assess the six dimensions is through key informant interviews (Kelly et al., 2003; Plested et al., 2006). The key informant interviews are best conducted, analyzed, and interpreted by community members, themselves. If the community members are trained in using these protocols and are able to allow the interviewees to share information with minimal bias and validity. This can be a highly challenging task for community members to interview each other. The interview serves as a tool to understand the community level of readiness, and the results can be utilized for community discussion and reflection on existing strengths and resources as building blocks to advance to the next stage of community change.

The ultimate goal of assessment within a Community Readiness Model is to apply the assessment results to the intervention strategy in order to create change in the level of readiness. Thus, the community experts must hold the assessment capacity to use the prevention tools in order for them to continually implement programs and strategies even if researchers and external funding are not present (Plested, Jumper Thurman, Edwards, & Oetting, 1998). The approach of the Community Readiness Model that encourages community-led research to incorporate research findings as a tool for reflection and improvement is an evidence-based model to establish community leadership, capacity development, and community investment for adolescent health (Plested et al., 2006).

While Community Readiness stages are extremely relevant to intervention work, they are also integral to assessment. In fact, data collection by and with local key respondents is fundamental to determining the readiness level. Knowledge of community readiness stages can help guide the development of appropriate and effective research tools. For example, community members who feel that adolescent alcohol use does not occur in their community may be less likely to participate in surveys on this topic. Community readiness level can also help guide the type of questions included in surveys or interviews so that they are more likely to match the reality of how the issue is perceived by the community at large. By acknowledging the current stage of the community health priorities and current norms on adolescent alcohol use and the associated prevention efforts, research efforts are more likely to be successful and to benefit the community.

The leadership role of community members in assessment is partially derived from the fact that many community-based programs have encountered local community members who perceive outsiders to be out of touch with local issues. Consequently, community members are more likely to be cautious and critical of research lead by outsiders; moreover, they are less likely to cooperate with research activities. The Community Readiness Model recommends that rather than relying on large-scale data, as many prevention projects do, the focus with Community Readiness is to obtain local community data that are personalized and community specific. However, lower income communities often have lower levels of education and less experience and exposure with research; moreover, they often have high levels of distrust of research and researchers. These are challenges that we discuss in the South Tucson Prevention Coalition (STPC) project and we discuss how community-led research strategies changed over time (also see Chap. 9).

2.5 Defining Community and Their Involvement

Community involvement and recognition of community assets is essential to the Community Readiness Model. Community here is defined by where residents experience society and culture, in this manner of definition it can be a professional group or a community of interest (Kelly et al., 2003). Typically cities are considered too large to be a "community"; however, in our project we focus on the entire city as the community, because it is clearly defined by geographic boundaries of 1 mile by 1 mile square. In most large cities, a location of this size might be considered a neighborhood. In many ways the City of South Tucson is a "community of place" in that the residents share a geographic location as a social context for activities (Edwards et al., 2000), and this is one reason why ecological place-based strategies are appropriate for alcohol prevention because it is a socially based health behavior. The identification of key stakeholders for a specific health issue is one of the first steps in community readiness; it is the key stakeholders that help begin, lead, and sustain the prevention strategies (Donnermeyer, Plested, Edwards, Oetting, & Littlethunder, 1997). The city boundaries helped to limit our definition of key stakeholders. We also included stakeholders who were not only knowledgeable, but also directly affected by adolescent alcohol use, which included youth, parents, CBO leaders, police, local government, and outside agencies with a focus on adolescent prevention.

At a minimum community membership was considered to be residence in the City of South Tucson; however not all residents are eligible to participate in city-level decision-making that primarily takes place through voting for city council members (Donnermeyer et al., 1997). For example, immigrants and adolescents cannot vote; however, there are other ways in which immigrants and teens can effectively participate as active members of their community to influence decision-making. Specifically, relevant and meaningful activities include volunteering, attending council meetings, speaking publicly, and creating/signing petitions (Watts & Flanagan, 2007). Previous to STPC most youth did not actively participate in community decisions or express their views at a community government level. This means it is critical to acknowledge the traditional role of political gatekeepers and the current processes of public decision-making conducted by adults. However, in order to influence significant community change, it is also critical to include youth as equals in the coalition's collaborative work and decision-making.

Creating the community involvement that was necessary for effective prevention of adolescent alcohol use was challenging. In part, because it is not typical for community members to be included as equal members in prevention program planning, grant planning or the development of externally funded strategies. Even when individuals are included, they are often left out of budgeting discussions and decisions for funded projects. It is more likely that community members, especially adolescents, are primarily included through their participation in after-school prevention programs or formal standardized surveys. At times youth may also be asked to help recruit other youth to participate. It is especially uncommon for youth perspectives to be included in the planning or development of health promotion or health intervention programs. Including youth as equals in the planning process is not easy, and there are few guidelines that exist to support the creation of coalitions that include participation of both youth and adults (Ginwright & James, 2002). In service of the practical application of these activities, we describe some of the pitfalls and challenges as the STPC worked to develop inclusivity of youth and adults as equal partners (see Chaps. 8, 10 and 11).

2.6 Readiness Stages of South Tucson Prevention Coalition

The nine stages of readiness and six dimensions of assessment guide our summary and analysis of changes led by STPC over 8 years. The dimensions are described at each stage and then describe how intervention strategies and research strategies were approached at each stage. The six dimensions for assessment of readiness include: existing community efforts, community knowledge of efforts, leadership, community climate, community knowledge about issues, and resources for prevention. Descriptions of how STPC Phase 1 was in the earlier stages of readiness, and how it focused primarily on youth and youth allies who were ready for in-depth training for alcohol prevention. Quotes from interviews with STPC coalition members are integrated in this chapter and further elaborated on in other chapters. Some of the interviews were conducted during 2007 while the coalition was first coming together (Sofia Blue, Library Associate, Andrea Romero, University Researcher), and some interviews were conducted in 2010–2014 as retrospective interviews (Gloria Hamelitz-Lopez, John Valenzuela Youth Center Executive Director, Michele Orduña, STPC Coordinator, Maricruz Ruiz, STPC Outreach Specialist, Josefina Ahumada, Social Worker). We discuss the transition from Phase 1 to Phase 2 where the coalition came together and how they moved the needle on community alcohol norms through community activities and community-led research. Finally, we discuss how the coalition and community worked to identify and change city-level policy with relevance for alcohol use. This chapter only provides an overview of the changes over time for STPC, the following chapters provide in-depth methods, results, and analysis. Utilizing this model we describe changes in adolescent alcohol use prevention over an 8-year span in one community that moves from Stage 1 to Stage 9 (see Table 2.1). The analysis we provide here and in later chapters is community level based; although, it is important to acknowledge that individuals or certain agencies may have been at different stages of readiness (Plested et al., 2006). There is a significant change over time in readiness level as reflected in the prevention intervention strategies and the integration of research evaluation in community decision-making.

2.6.1 *Early Stages 1–3: Tolerance, Denial, and Vague Awareness*

In the beginning, most community stakeholders could be classified as ***Stage 1 Tolerance or Stage 2 Denial or Stage 3 Vague Awareness***. Gloria Hamelitz-Lopez, who in a post-STPC interview (2010) describes not only tolerance, but normalcy of alcohol and drug use in their community before STPC: "*Drugs (were) a huge issue in our community. They are a big problem. Part of the problem is that it (was) so normal that people are not seeing it as a problem anymore. To see somebody passed out on the sidewalk because they are drunk (was) nothing. It is just the same as seeing a bird on a tree and that is really scary when something that devastating becomes so normal that people are not shocked by it anymore and it is really scary.*" Gloria brings up a good point that when alcoholism is perceived as normal, that is dangerous, because it is hard to find motivation to create change. This is a reminder of why community readiness strategies are effective, because if the community does not perceive adolescent alcohol use as a problem or risky, then they will not be motivated to engage in community change strategies. An example of tolerance is exhibited in this comment in a 2007 community readiness interview with Sofia Blue, librarian: "*It's a good effort to prevent any of those negative things that might happen, but I am also hesitant, because I also think that there is a certain amount, for*

Table 2.1 Community readiness stages linked to intervention and research

Year	Community readiness stage	Intervention activities	Goal of activity	Use of research
2001–2002	Stage 1, 2, 3: Community Tolerance Denial	Unstructured activities mainly aimed at youth in adjudication		None
2002–2003	Stage 3: Vague Awareness	Youth after-school substance use prevention program	Raise awareness among small groups of youth	Beginning of data collection with after-school program youth
2003–2004	Stage 4: Preplanning	Youth after-school substance use prevention program Community building with Youth Safe Haven leaders	Raise awareness with youth Review existing programs	Sharing national data and local data in small groups
2004–2005	Stage 5: Preparation	Planning for Coalition Development Youth Summer Leadership Conference Beginning of Youth-to-Youth (Y2Y) program	Reach out to broader group of key stakeholders in small group discussion	Sharing local data with new partners and at city level
2005–2005	Stage 6: Implementation	STPC and Y2Y regular meetings and community events	Raise awareness with community	Use of existing local data with coalition and presentations to City Council
2006–2006	Stage 6 Implementation	STPC & Y2Y regular meetings and community events organized together New external funding for community engagement	Community level engagement	Use of existing local data with coalition and presentations to City Council
2007–2007	Stage 7: Institutionalization	STPC and Y2Y regular meetings and events Community readiness training for coalition Media campaign radio PSA's led by Y2Y	Raise community awareness Community engagement	Use of existing data with coalition and presentations to City Council. Community Readiness interviews
2008–2008	Stage 7: Institutionalization	STPC and Y2Y regular meetings and events New external funding	Raise community awareness. Community engagement in events	Grant for Youth-led Participatory Action Research Alcohol Mapping
2009–2009	Stage 8: Confirmation and Expansion	STPC and Y2Y regular meetings and events Expansion of activities to neighborhood preservation	Community attempts to improve and change the physical environment. City level policy changes	Community-led research Sharing data with City Council
2010–2010	Stage 8 Confirmation and expansion	STPC and Y2Y regular meetings and events Expansion of activities to prevent new liquor licenses	Community successful efforts to limit alcohol advertising on businesses and prevention of new liquor licenses	Community led research and use of data at local and state-levels

under aged kids, of experimentation that is hard to get around. I think that they tend to be more curious and they are in that weird phase of between being teenagers or kids and adults. They are trying to feel that out, but I think that a lot of the community leaders are making efforts just to be positive about (what to do) and to offer alternatives." Sofia provides another honest example of how tolerance of adolescent experimentation with alcohol can also be a stopping point for engaging community adults in prevention strategies.

However, early focus group data [$N=20$ parents and their 20 adolescents (13–18 years) conducted at a local charter school] collected by Dr. Romero, STPC evaluator, indicated that youth and parents were at a vague awareness stage. Focus group results with youth and parents indicated that they felt substance use was a concern in the local community indicating that they are at Stage 3, Vague Awareness. However, at this time in the community, there were no existing community efforts through structured activities for youth alcohol prevention; there was also little community knowledge of efforts according to youth, parents, youth program leaders, and community-based organization leaders. There was at least one community service program for adjudicated youth, yet there was no structured curriculum. Some CBO (Community-Based Organization) youth leaders felt that initiating new programing would be overwhelming or impossible due to lack of sufficient funding and lack of existing resources for new prevention activities. In fact, the existing youth community organizations felt overextended in terms of staff time with their current programs that primarily focused on youth physical activity, such as basketball, volleyball, and dancing. Each of the CBOs including Project YES, House of Neighborly Service, and John Valenzuela Youth Center also provided tutoring, but they were constantly seeking volunteers to sustain the tutoring programs. It was clear that there were not sufficient existing resources for prevention issues at the community level.

In terms of community climate, there was some acknowledgement about the need for prevention through previously funded programs, such as Weed and Seed, which had strong police leadership, especially by the Police Chief at that time. In fact, Kimberly Sierra-Cajas indicates that the police community involvement was unique "*When I started working in South Tucson I noticed that the police department was heavily involved with the community and interacting with the Safe Havens. From my perspective this was very unusual from other communities, and the police were always sure to be present at the Safe Haven meetings, events, and even leading the effort in some community events.*" However, there were no specific structured programs targeting adolescent alcohol use. Furthermore, according to some community anecdotes, there was pushback from community members to deny issues such as adolescent risky sexual behavior associated with alcohol use because the community rejected previous HIV prevention programs. The variance in different community sectors awareness of adolescent alcohol use is indicated by Sofia Blue, as she comments: "*Well I was thinking that the fire department is at least like ten (highest level of perceiving underage drinking as a problem). But I think that most of the community members not having to face that everyday in their face, its lower (for) church leaders or people in other agencies.*" This anecdote suggests that community climate was not receptive to prevention programs with youth and this shaped the next steps for intervention strategies. Thus, it could be argued that while parents, youth, and some youth program leaders were at a stage of vague awareness, the larger segments of the community were at Stage 1 or Stage 2 in terms of tolerance or denial.

During 2001–2002, there was not coordinated structured intervention or coordinated use of research by community agencies. There was a deep-seated mistrust of university research; however, Dr. Romero was given entrée because she was introduced to CBO leaders by a local South Tucson community member who worked at the university. There was limited community involvement at this stage, when Dr. Romero began by conducting focus groups and then worked with youth and teachers to develop a prevention program. She delivered a pilot version of this program with a pretest and posttest survey that she developed with input from teachers and youth. The results of the data were then shared in small one-to-one settings with CBO leaders. These initial activities helped to begin establishing trust between the CBO leaders and Dr. Romero, because she demonstrated that she followed through with the delivery of the program for youth, she provided the incentives that she promised, and the program was popular and well received by the youth. Additionally, CBO leaders were interested in her positive and culturally based approach to research on youth; they often expressed concern that outsiders viewed South Tucson youth in a negative and stereotyped view that only focused on problems and overlooked the assets of the community. During Stage 1–3, the most effective method of changing the stage of readiness is through small group activities, and the pilot work and one-to-one meetings were factors that helped build relationships that could be built upon in the next stage.

2.6.2 *Stage 4: Preplanning*

Stage 4 Preplanning is when there is more awareness about the issue and some agreement that something needs to be done. The CBO leaders were now willing to admit to an outsider that there were problems; they saw firsthand how alcohol use and drugs were factors driving youth toward dropping out of school, getting pregnant, or entering the juvenile detention programs. The larger community climate and knowledge about the issue was unchanged at this stage. Thus, there was increased awareness among a small sector of youth and youth program leaders that alcohol and substances were an issue and that something should be done; however, there were still not sufficient resources.

Dr. Romero and the CBO leaders, such as Kimberly Sierra-Cajas and Gloria Hamelitz-Lopez, were willing to participate in gaining new funding to address these issues. However, in terms of community involvement, CBO leaders still saw their role as primarily opening their doors to outsiders to recruit and provide substance use prevention services. Ms. Hamelitz-Lopez put the grant writer at the City of South Tucson in touch with Dr. Romero. At this stage, youth were not involved, and the community had only minimal involvement in grant planning and budget planning. Dr. Romero began to engage in 1–1 meetings with CBO leaders and internal government grant writers about pursuing future funding. At this stage, she shared the national data of relevance to the topics of adolescent alcohol and substance use.

Dr. Romero also shared some of the local data from the focus groups and previous pre-/post-surveys that she had collected in South Tucson. The sharing of data and discussion of results became a more regular aspect of the small meetings, but it was not shared at a community level. There was only intervention in small group settings; yet, the extent of community partners was growing slowly, and the involvement of the local city government representative was a pivotal step toward future changes. All of this initial work was done before Phase 1 of STPC.

2.6.3 Stage 5: Preparation

It was in 2002 that ***Stage 5 Preparation*** began in earnest for STPC Phase 1. Preparation occurs when the community plans strategies based on information gathered and reaches out to a broader audience of stakeholders to work together and to take ownership of the preparations. This stage is indicated by the growth in resources for prevention, growth in community knowledge of the issue among some sectors, and growth in community climate, and development of youth and adult leader capacity for adolescent alcohol prevention. It was during Stage 5 that Dr. Romero and the representative from the City of South Tucson, along with Southern Arizona AIDS Foundation (SAAF), worked on submitting a federal grant. The grant was mainly written and submitted by Dr. Romero with small sections submitted by each partner and requests for budget.

Stage 5 really took off when the federal grant was approved, and prevention programming for integrated substance use/HIV prevention began in earnest. Michele Orduña (retrospective interview) reminds us of the low level of readiness in the community that had been persistent for a long time: "*(this grant) was first of its kind in the City of South Tucson for adults or youth for HIV prevention.*" This grant brought together for the first time the City of South Tucson, a local community-based health promotion agency SAAF, and the three local Youth Safe Havens (John Valenzuela Youth Center, House of Neighborly Service, and Project YES). Each of these groups received a portion of the subcontract to incentivize their participation. The three primary agencies, University of Arizona, Southern Arizona AIDS Foundation, and the City of South Tucson, received comparable funding amounts in order to nurture equitable relationships. However, the three Safe Haven partners received substantially less, and their funding was distributed by the City of South Tucson. The amount given to the Safe Havens was not a large sum, but it was enough to help leverage their participation in recruitment and planning meetings.

Now, there were more resources for prevention; there was funding to support structured community efforts to implement an after-school adolescent prevention program. However, there was still minimal community knowledge of these efforts, leadership was not very involved, and the overall community climate had not seemed to change. In fact, Chap. 4 discusses how the prevention program leaders felt community pressure to not share too much about the content of the program. However, during this time, the group began to meet regularly, including Dr. Romero, Ms. Michele

Orduña (STPC project coordinator), Luis Perales & Patty Valera (SAAF program leaders), and the City of South Tucson grant writer. Yet, the South Tucson community involvement continued to be limited, as Safe Haven Directors were primarily involved in the recruitment of youth and providing meeting space for the program. Chapter 4 provides more background on the development and implementation of STPC Phase 1, the Omeyocan YES (Youth, Empowerment, Sexuality) prevention program. This after-school 72-hour integrated substance use and HIV prevention program was implemented over a 2-year-time period and reached 125 youth in total.

At this stage youth completed quantitative surveys before and after the program was implemented, primarily as a way to evaluate the program outcomes of substance use and risky sexual behaviors. The majority of the measurements were mandated by the federal agency, and no modifications could be made to the federal set of measures. However, Dr. Romero and her research team added their own local measures; these measures were reviewed by the key leaders from the City of South Tucson and the health promoters. However, there was little to no involvement of youth or other community leaders. A thorough description of the program and the evaluation are provided in Chap. 4, but Omeyocan YES evaluator Michele Orduña summarizes: "*(the curriculum) was unique in that it gave the youth the historical context, what cultural things they carry with them, cultural assets and how that plays into mainstream society, and then it went into HIV prevention, substance use, and sexuality, in terms of this is the whole spectrum, you need all the information you can, you need to know the risk factors, or what risky behaviors are, at the end of the day it is your choice, you have to own your body, you need to own your choices. It was interesting in that the teenagers really felt validation, (it) really helped them make better sense of their world, sometimes you know where you come from, but you don't know the historical context of all of it. That really improved their self-esteem, self-worth, and resiliency.*"

However, it was during the final year of the grant that the participating groups really began to transition to a more involved level of participation that led to the next readiness stage, STPC Phase 2. Toward the end of the grant period (2005), the key stakeholders begin to meet regularly again, this time being more inclusive of the Safe Haven leaders. Michele recalls:

> "*What was happening, which is trending now, we were on the right path to begin with, was breaking down those silos, because that was the first time that those six agencies had ever worked together on such a large-scale project, where of course everyone got a piece of the pie, but you had to integrate all those six—and they all had very different missions, visions and agendas—but the fact that we were able to work well together for 3 years, and at the end of those 3 years, there was no reason why we wouldn't continue to work on something together. When we came across Drug-Free Communities grant. CoST became the grantee, the goal of the grant was to create and sustain a coalition for adolescent alcohol prevention environmental strategies. We had a diverse group to begin with, we just had to add on to our working group. We were on the stepping stone to take that next step.*"

The group began to call themselves South Tucson Prevention Collaborative. Now, all partners were more involved in decision-making, especially for budget decision-making during the final year of the grant.

In fact, it was their influence that funneled money into a summer youth leadership conference for the Omeyocan YES youth graduates that was pivotal to the creation of the local Youth-to-Youth (Y2Y)-led after-school program. The Y2Y became essential to the progression through the following stages because it was youth-led/adult-guided and housed at a local Safe Haven, John Valenzuela Youth Center. Youth Omeyocan YES graduates met with the South Tucson Prevention Collaborative in order to decide on the criteria for participation in the leadership conference. In the next several chapters (Chaps. 5–7), these transitions are discussed in more detail. Youth participation in these meetings was fundamental to developing trust in the leadership capabilities of the youth and also to the future involvement of youth in the decision-making. Josefina Ahumada, STPC coalition member and Social Worker, describes the change in her retrospective interview: "*One of the most critical outcomes for this project was that youth grew to have a sense of self-worth, sense of empowerment, different perspective on themselves and the role that they could have in the community. So there was this consciousness raising about what they could do, within themselves, as well as the assets within themselves, within their culture, and within the community.*"

It was also during the final year of the grant that Dr. Romero and other key stakeholders began to present their findings to the City of South Tucson City Council. It was assumed that the city representative had been regularly sharing updates and data, but this was not the case, and in fact the city council members were at earlier stages of readiness, such as tolerance, denial, or vague awareness. They were not familiar with the Omeyocan YES program, and in the first presentation to the city council, Dr. Romero and the project coordinator, Ms. Michele Orduña, summarized the study and the findings. This presentation was met with a flurry of questions and suspicions that the participants were not actually from the City of South Tucson. As a result, the research team returned to organize and analyze the zip codes of the participants. Dr. Romero and Ms. Orduña returned to another city council meeting to share the results of the zip code analysis, which demonstrated that approximately 85 % of the participants were from South Tucson. The city council members continued to have quite a lot of questions, and it was clear that there was confusion over what the HIV prevention component of the grant meant. For example, the grant was referred to casually within the city government as the "HIV grant" which the Safe Haven leaders tried regularly to correct because they were concerned that this may lead to assumptions that the youth participants were HIV positive.

Some of the lessons learned from these presentations to the city council that were essential to moving forward is that the city leadership should have been much more integrated, and perhaps one-to-one meetings or small group meetings would have been beneficial to move to the next level of readiness for preplanning or preparation. Another lesson was that effective communication between all stakeholders is a critical component of community-based research. Additionally, it was clear that the City Council did not entirely believe the data and the description from the outsiders of the community who lacked internal city credibility. Most of these suspicions were not specific to the current project, but were derived from the city's previous experiences with researchers and bad experiences with grants, subcontracts, and partners who were more "smoke and mirrors," or illusion of implementation, rather than actual implementation or provision of services to community members. Unfortunately, it is still too common that researchers conduct "helicopter research" where they fly in and collect data and then leave the community with few benefits from the research. However, it was an important reminder about the need for matching readiness with prevention approaches led by community members instead of outsiders. In many ways, the city council was acting in the best interests of the community, to serve as gatekeepers to ensure that their members benefited from programs. A lesson learned was the importance of including community partners and youth in the presentations about the program. City Council leaders were much more interested in hearing directly from the local youth that they knew in order to confirm their participation and their results.

2.6.4 Stage 6: Implementation

It was exactly these transitions and the lessons learned that lead to ***Stage 6 Implementation*** where the community really took the lead in developing and submitting (through the City of South Tucson) a federal grant for Drug-Free Communities. At this stage, it is clear that there was more community awareness of the lack of existing community efforts, more community knowledge about the issue of adolescent alcohol use, there is more leadership involvement by multiple sectors of the community (Safe Haven leaders, youth, and government), and there are more resources for prevention (such as financial, personnel, staff, space, and equipment.).

At this stage, the intervention was taken over by the community leaders in terms of development, active seeking of grants, receiving funding, and leading the implementation of the project. The executive directors at the local Safe Havens, Kimberly Sierra-Caja, and Gloria Hamelitz-Lopez organized and led meetings to reach consensus on the logic model and budget for the application for a Drug-Free Community grant that would be submitted by the City of South Tucson. These meetings included the City of South Tucson grant writer and Dr. Romero who both worked together to write the grant application. Each participating Safe Haven submitted a written section of the grant describing their agency and their existing activities. The coalition created a logic model that was submitted with the grant, and these community-based activities to raise awareness about adolescent alcohol use were then implemented by community members (see Fig. 2.3). The grant planning meetings were held at the police station, with regular representation from law enforcement officials. The Safe Haven leaders reached out to include all the required representative sectors for a Drug-Free Community (government, law enforcement, media, youth-serving organizations, health professionals, school, state, civic/volunteer group, parents, and youth) (see Table 2.2). Importantly, the group also changed the name of the South Tucson Prevention Collaborative to South Tucson Prevention *Coalition (STPC)* in order to be better aligned with the grant requirements. At this stage, the city was

Table 2.2 South Tucson prevention coalition: Members and organizations that represented drug-free community grant sectors

Member name	Organization	Sector represented
Gerald Porter	City of South Tucson	Local government
Mary Specio	COPE Behavioral Services	Behavioral Health professional
Sixto Molina & Sharon Hayes-Martinez	City of South Tucson Police	Law enforcement
Patty Ruiz	Clear Channel Media	Media
Gloria Hamelitz	John Valenzuela Youth Center	Youth serving organization
Kimberley Sierra-Cajas	House of Neighborly Service	Religious Organization
Andrea J. Romero	University of Arizona	Schools & State
Jan Daley & Jamie Arrieta	Southern Arizona AIDS Foundation	Healthcare Professional
Steven Kreamer	Private Consultant & STPC Coordinator	Civic and Volunteer Groups
Charles Monroe & Paul Lyons	Project YES	Youth-serving Organization
Georgianna Romero	South Tucson Explorers #327	Civic and Volunteer Groups
Mary Alfaro	Mary's Market	Business Community
Carmen Kemery	Wakefield Middle School	Schools
Sister Leonette Kochan	Santa Cruz Catholic School (k-8th)	Schools
Heidi Arranda	Ochoa Middle School	Schools
Patty Mentz	Mission View Elementary School	Schools
Neal Cash	Community Partnership of Southern Arizona	State
Veronica Madueno	Parent	Parent and Volunteer in Native American Youth Program
Stephanie Sierra	Youth and Omeyocan YES graduate	Youth
Matthew Monsisvais	Youth and Omeyocan YES graduate	Youth
Maria Mora	Parent	Parent
Dr. Antonio Estrada, director	Mexican American Studies & Research Center	School & State
Dr. Sally Stevens, director	Southwest Institute for Research on Women	School & State

centrally involved and when the grant was approved, they had several press releases to announce the grant (see Fig. 2.2). This signifies a major shift in the centrality of community involvement.

However, once again during this period of rapid growth and outreach to broader segments of the community, it was clear that community readiness mattered, and not everyone was on the same level. Since the South Tucson Prevention Coalition was still active and regularly meeting, they quickly moved into expanding the coalition to include more sectors of the community. One of the early meetings had up to

EXECUTIVE OFFICE OF THE PRESIDENT

OFFICE OF NATIONAL DRUG CONTROL POLICY

Washington, DC 20503

FOR IMMEDIATE R
Wednesday, Septe

2-395-6618

ANNOUNCES $100,000 ANTI-DRUG COALITION GRANT FOR_CITY OF SOUTH TUCSON _

(Washington, D.C.) –The Office of National Drug Control Policy today announced that the City of South Tucson will receive a $_100,000_ Drug-Free Communities matching grant for the South Tucson Prevention Collaborative. The grant was one of 176 new grants totaling $17.1 million awarded today to community anti-drug coalitions across the country. The goal of the 711 local coalitions is to work together to prevent and reduce drug, alcohol, and tobacco abuse among youth. Coalitions are comprised of diverse groups of people, including community leaders, parents, youth, teachers, religious and fraternal organizations, health care and business professionals, law enforcement, and the media.

"This is great news for the anti-drug efforts of City of South Tucson and local community." said Mr. Castro, City Manger. "The Drug-Free Communities Program and other drug prevention efforts are important elements of a balanced national drug control strategy. STPC is doing crucial drug prevention work in our community and this additional influx of Federal money will help them expand their efforts and reach more of South Tucson's children."

John Walters, Director of National Drug Control Policy and President Bush's "Drug Czar," said, "As a nation, we have made significant progress in protecting our young people from the dangers of substance abuse, with a 17 percent reduction in drug use over the last three years. This grant will help the dedicated citizens of_City of South Tucson to contribute even more to this effort and will help build on the important progress being made to keep our children healthy and drug-free."

We are pleased to be working with ONDCP to administer the Drug-Free Communities Program," said Charles Curie, Administrator, Substance Abuse and Mental Health Services Administration. "Some of the most important work to reduce drug use comes from our Nation's grass-roots community coalitions. These coalitions, teamed up with our Strategic Prevention Framework Grants to the states, create a powerful force that can continue to drive down the numbers of young people using illicit drugs."

The Drug-Free Communities Program provides grants of up to $500,000 over five years to community organizations that serve as catalysts for citizen participation in local drug prevention efforts. The 176 new grantees were selected from 411 applicants through a

Fig. 2.2 City of South Tucson drug-free community press release

competitive peer review process. To qualify for matching grants, all awardees must have at least a six-month history of working together on substance abuse reduction initiatives, develop a long-term plan to reduce substance abuse, and participate in a national evaluation of the Drug-Free Communities Program.

Created under the Drug-Free Communities Act of 1997, the Drug-Free Communities Program has earned strong bipartisan support from Congress. In December of 2001, Congress passed and the President signed into law a five-year extension of the Drug-Free Communities Act, authorizing $399 million in funds through FY 2007.

In addition to the 176 new grants awarded today, another $54 million will support continuation grants to 535 existing community coalition projects operating in all 50 states, the District of Columbia, and Puerto Rico. Since 1997, eight competitions have awarded $320 million in grants to more than 1000 community anti-drug coalitions. ONDCP administers the Drug-Free Communities Program in conjunction with the Substance Abuse and Mental Health Services Administration.

More information about the Drug-Free Communities Program is available at: www.whitehousedrugpolicy.gov, and http://drugfreecommunities.samhsa.gov/

-30-

Fig. 2.2 (continued)

30 people, which had grown from a solid 7–10 members. At this early meeting, the goals and mission of the coalition were discussed, and it lead to some honest and open comments by youth and community leaders that was perhaps too early because many of the new members were still at earlier stages of community readiness, such as tolerance, denial, or vague awareness. There were surprised responses and some denial from adults when they heard that youth were drinking alcohol and had access to alcohol in the community, through local stores and at family parties. At this early stage dialogue, procedures and equality among members had not been established, and there was a need to develop trust among members. Chapter 11 describes the process of coalition trust and organization that ultimately led to success with community-led strategies. After some of these initial challenges, the group began to stabilize in membership and developed a specific focus on preventing underage drinking through raising awareness about alcohol norms and alcohol availability.

Michele also describes how the environmental strategies were first hard to organize around: "*When it came to figuring out environmental strategies, that took us years to figure out because the grant we had just finished was all about individual direct service, but environmental strategy was "How do you change the landscape by adding or removing something? How do you impact underage drinking on an environment strategy, not an individual strategy?" CoST was heavy in service agencies, so it was hard to wrap our heads around. There were questions like, Why*

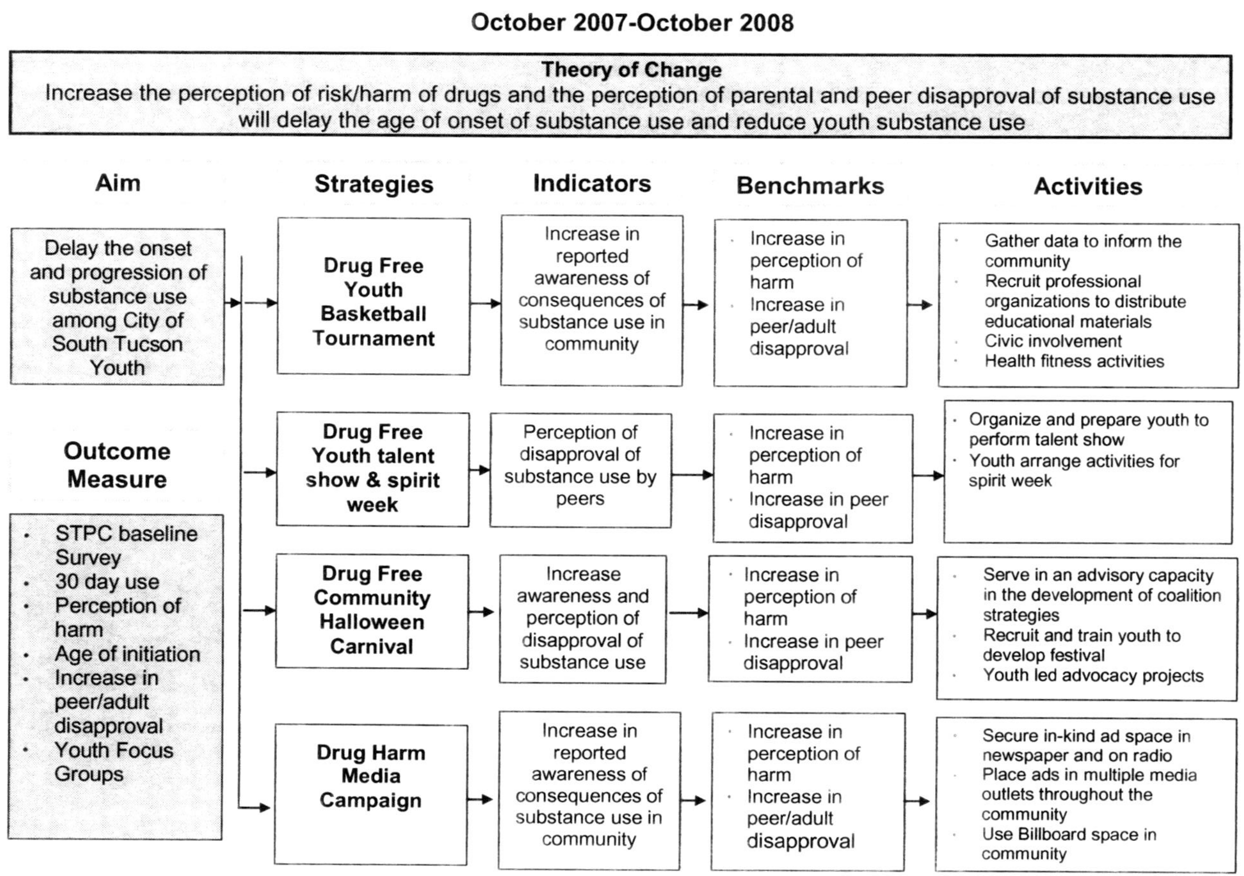

Fig. 2.3 STPC coalition logic model October 2007–2008

can't we initiate this program?" At an early meeting, there was debate about planned activities and the use of anecdotes and the relevance of research findings. The police representatives were eager to host an event where they would show an existing video about a drunk driving accident in the South Tucson community with teenagers that resulted in more than one death. They described the horrific nature of the negative outcomes of drunk driving accidents. They felt that this was something that was important for young people to be made aware of and to remember as a form of prevention. At first, personal anecdotes were favored, and the data shared by Dr. Romero was often dismissed as not relevant to the community, consistent with early stages of community readiness. Dr. Romero disagreed with the proposed video which used a classic "scare tactic" because public health research has shown that this often has a negative effect or only short-term effects on teen's behavior (O'Grady, 2006). This example also demonstrates how often agencies who focus on the same primary goal, youth alcohol prevention, can become silo-ed, separate, and take extremely different approaches to the same issue (Kania & Kramer, 2011). Yet, by working together, they are likely to both benefit from a more comprehensive view of adolescent alcohol use.

STPC agreed to host the police event; almost 30 youth attended and watched the graphic video. Afterward, the youth were shaken by the video partly because some of them knew the youth who were killed in the accident. Due to the unexpected response of the youth, the John Valenzuela Youth Center held small discussion groups afterward to help youth process the information. At the next coalition meeting, there was much reflection about the activity and how to move forward as a group; one lesson learned after this event is that despite disagreements neither the police nor Dr. Romero left the group, and both attended the event because of their dedication to the prevention of alcohol use. It is important to note that each agency has their own unique perspective about underage drinking, and specifically the police noted the serious nature of the police perspective that was focused on saving lives. Michele reminds us that *"Looking at the readiness to change mode, there are baby steps (such as), how ready are we to change (environmental strategies), denial, not recognizing problem, agreeing there is a problem, individuals and different agencies were in different paces/stages. We just took it slow for a couple of years."* Despite relatively slow progress in the first few years of the coalition, the following years between 2007 and 2010 moved rapidly through the higher levels of community readiness and with more consensus than ever before.

2.6.5 Stage 7: Institutionalization

It was during 2007 that the community moved into the ***Stage 7 Institutionalization and Stabilization***. The coalition met regularly with representation from the Safe Havens, City Government, police, food banks, churches, and schools. At this point there was greater community awareness about existing community efforts, more community knowledge about adolescent alcohol use, more resources for prevention, more leadership and integration of leadership, and an increasingly receptive community climate. Maricruz Ruiz, STPC Outreach Specialist, comments in her retrospective interview, "*Just by existing, the coalition galvanized the community to get involved. They brought lots of light to underage drinking, like with National Night Out events. We shed light on those challenges, and the community came a long way.*" Major factors that contributed to this progress through stages were some of the consistent community awareness raising events offered such as (1) National Night Out event in August, which was attended by 600 community members on average; (2) Shining Stars youth award event which was held in April with 8 awards provided to outstanding youth and attended by an average of 50 people including parents, family members, and community leaders; (3) Y2Y activities which were supported with a continual stream of new cohorts of youth who had attended the Voz after-school youth substance use prevention program offered by Southern Arizona AIDS Foundation during this time (Chaps. 6 and 7); (4) New local grants which were awarded to provide public service announcements for health promotion (see Chap. 8) and alcohol mapping (see Chap. 10); (5) STPC retreats which provided expert training in community readiness and assessment. At this time, there was also increasing acceptance and use of community collected data. The evolution toward community-led data collection is described further in Chap. 9.

2.6.6 Stage 8: Confirmation and Expansion

By 2008, STPC entered ***Stage 8 Confirmation and Expansion*** because of youth-led research. Josefina describes how useful the readiness to change model was, but also how the different segments of the community worked to push toward the next level: "*The readiness to change model helped us to take it slow. (The Youth Programs) were beneficial because when youth had access to knowledge and interpretation, they soaked it up, and then they were the ones who started noticing things and they started asking "I don't want to live in a community that does that.*" The coalition received another small local grant to fund youth-led alcohol mapping of their community. The youth worked closely with the city planners, community leaders, and university students to help them plan out and achieve a high quality research collection of community-level data that was translated into a city map by the city planners. Johnny Quevedo, Y2Y youth leader, comments in a retrospective interview "*The research was done by the youth.*" The results of the alcohol-mapping project clearly and tangibly indicated the locations of the current liquor licenses in the city in the context of locations where youth frequented, such as schools and community-based organizations with youth out of school activities. The youth presented their findings in a city town hall with many government employees in attendance; they also presented their findings at the University of Arizona and at a national conference. Josefina: "*We had to keep asking is the community ready for change. We discovered that the readiness came more from the* *youth than the adults.*" As a result of this highly integrated research and intervention, the community had achieved a significant shift in their understanding of community alcohol norms and alcohol availability. During Stage 8 there was a significant shift to more community-led assessment and utilization of research findings to create change in their community.

2.6.7 Stage 9: Professionalization

This lead to the next ***Stage 9 Professionalization*** and a high level of community ownership that led to the youth–community partnerships to create changes in city policy on issues of alcohol advertising and on new liquor licenses. Josefina describes how: "*The full range of community readiness existed in South Tucson, but with this campaign, that readiness got sparked and whatever pessimism that may have existed got turned around to optimism.*" This required a high level on all dimensions of community readiness and resulted in the success in policy changes. The STPC goal during the professionalization stage was to create policy that would be sustainable that would reach the greatest amount of people, youth as well as children and parents, and other adults in the community for what was truly a "community-level" intervention. Juan "Johnny" Quevedo, Y2Y youth leader, STPC coalition member, notes in a retrospective interview, "*We took things to a whole other level, now that I think about—It makes me really proud. First off, we forced the city council to deny the liquor license for Walgreens. We didn't want more alcohol, we had enough for one square mile city*" Thurman et al. (2003) argues that often political changes within community are reasons why efforts are not sustainable, in part because community members do not work with politicians to consider policy change. However, the success of the coalition building and regularly public reporting was integral to working with the local government agency. Additionally, once the STPC was able to move past the earlier stages of community readiness, which were some of the most challenging, they were able to make great strides through later stages. Their success demonstrates the utility and importance of considering community readiness stages and the need to match intervention and assessment strategies to the appropriate stage. Josefina sums it up "*We went from no awareness, and even pessimism, but with leadership of youth, they stood up and said, "Hey this affects us, and we can make a change." They led the community through this process.*"

2.7 Conclusion

In sum, this chapter demonstrates the utility and relevance of the Community Readiness Model for Change for community level change on the issue of adolescent alcohol prevention. The coalition was able to tackle ecologically based strategies to change community alcohol norms and alcohol related policies (e.g., alcohol advertising and new liquor licenses) through integrated youth and community partnerships. The goal of this chapter was to provide an overview of community changes as demonstrated and by the Community Readiness Model for Change. The theoretical structure behind the coalition building infrastructure demonstrates how communities may begin their own process of working toward community transformation for adolescent health. The Community Readiness Model was helpful to increase consciousness among coalition members about the diversity of perception of health issues and the complex dynamics of relationships within the community (Thurman et al., 2003). Moreover, it provides structure and insight into the importance of consensus in coalition decision-making that is much more likely to lead to collective action which will result in institutionalization and professionalization, the highest stages of community readiness (Plested et al., 2006).

References

Beal, G. M. (1964). Social action: Instigated social change in large social systems. In J. H. Copp (Ed.), *Our changing rural society: Perspectives and trends*. Ames, IA: Iowa State University Press (Chapter 7).

Bronfenbrenner, U. (1986). Ecology of the family as a context for human development: Research perspectives. *Developmental Psychology, 22*(6), 723.

Burrow-Sanchez, J. J. (2006). Understanding adolescent substance abuse: Prevalence, risk factors, and clinical implications. *Journal of Counseling and Development, 84*, 283–290.

Castro, F. G., Boyer, G. R., & Balcazar, H. G. (2000). Healthy adjustment in Mexican American and other Hispanic adolescents. In R. Montemayor, G. R. Adams, & T. P. Gullotta (Eds.), *Adolescent diversity in ethnic, economic, and cultural contexts*, (pp. 141–178). Thousand Oaks, CA: Sage.

Donnermeyer, J. F., Plested, B. A., Edwards, R. W., Oetting, G., & Littlethunder, L. (1997). Community Readiness and prevention programs. *Journal of Community Development Society, 28*(1), 65–83.

Edwards, R. W., Jumper-Thurman, P., Plested, B. A., Oetting, E. R., & Swanson, L. (2000). Community Readiness: research to practice. *Journal of Community Psychology, 28*(3), 291–307.

Ginwright, S., & James, T. (2002). From assets to agents of change: Social justice, organizing, and youth development. *New Directions for Youth Development, 2002*(95), 27–46.

Kania, J., & Kramer, M. (2011). Collective impact. *Stanford Social Innovation Review, Winter*, 36–41.

Kelly, K. J., Edwards, R. W., Comello, M. L. G., Plested, B. A., Thurman, P. J., & Slater, M. D. (2003). The community Readiness model: A complementary approach to social marketing. *Marketing Theory, 3*, 411–426.

Merves, M. L., Rodgers, C. R., Silver, E. J., Sclafane, J. H., & Bauman, L. J. (2015). Engaging and sustaining adolescents in community-based participatory research: Structuring a youth-friendly community-based participatory research environment. *Family & Community Health, 38*(1), 22–32.

Milam, A. J., Furr-Holden, C. D. M., Cooley-Strickland, M. C., Bradshaw, C. P., & Leaf, P. J. (2014). Risk for exposure to alcohol, tobacco, and other drugs on the route to and from school: The role of alcohol outlets. *Prevention Science, 15*(1), 12–21.

Minkler, M., & Wallerstein, N. (Eds.). (2011). *Community-based participatory research for health: From process to outcomes*. San Francisco, CA: Wiley.

O'Grady, M. (2006). Just inducing fear of HIV/AIDS is not just. *Journal of Health Communication, 11*(3), 261–262. doi:10.1080/10810730600628748.

Oetting, E. R., Donnermeyer, J. F., Plested, B. A., Edwards, R. W., Kelly, K., & Beauvais, F. (1995). Assessing community Readiness for prevention. *International Journal of the Addictions, 30*, 659–83.

Oetting, E. R., Jumper-Thurman, P., Plested, B., & Edwards, R. W. (2001). Community Readiness and health services. *Substance Use & Misuse, 36*(6 and 7), 825–843.

Pearson, A. L., Pearce, J., & Kingham, S. (2013). Deprived yet health: Neighborhood-level resilience in New Zealand. *Social Science & Medicine, 91*, 238–245.

Plested, B. A., Edwards, R. W., & Jumper-Thurman, P. (2006). *Community Readiness: A handbook for successful change*. Fort Collins, CO: Tri-Ethnic Center for Prevention Research.

Plested, B. A., Jumper Thurman, P., Edwards, R. W., & Oetting, E. R. (1998). Community Readiness: A tool for effective community-based prevention. *The Prevention Researcher, 5*(2), 5–7.

Prochaska, J. O., DiClemente, C. C., & Norcross, J. C. (1992). In search of how people change: Applications to addictive behaviors. *American Psychologist, 47*(9), 1102.

Rogers, E. M. (1983). *Diffusion of innovations* (3rd ed.). New York: Free Press.

Thurman, P. J., Plested, B. A., Edwards, R. W., Foley, R., & Burnside, M. (2003). Community Readiness: The journey to community healing. *Journal of Psychoactive Drugs, 35*(1), 27–31.

Trucco, E. M., Colder, C. R., Wieczorek, W. F., Lengua, L. J., & Hawk, L. W., Jr. (2014). Early adolescent alcohol use in context: how neighborhoods, parents, and peers impact youth. *Developmental Psychology, 26*(2), 425–36.

Walters, J. L., Canady, R., & Stein, T. (1994). Evaluating multicultural approaches in HIV/AIDS educational material. *AIDS Education and Prevention, 6*(5), 446–453.

Wandersman, A., & Nation, M. (1998). Urban neighborhoods and mental health: Psychological contributions to understanding toxicity, resilience and interventions. *American Psychologist, 53*(6), 647–656.

Watts, R. J., & Flanagan, C. (2007). Pushing the envelope on youth civic engagement: A developmental and liberation psychology perspective. *Journal of Community Psychology, 35*(6), 779–792.

Chapter 3
Integrating Research into Prevention Strategies Using Participatory Action Research

Andrea Romero, Juvenal Caporale, Robby Harris, Elisa Meza, Joel Muraco, and Jesi Post

Abstract This chapter describes the relevance of a participatory action research approach to working with marginalized communities because it emphasizes the equal involvement of community members in conceptualizing, conducting, and interpreting research. We describe the key principles of participatory action research that were implemented with South Tucson Prevention Coalition, including open dialogue, community-led research, and reflection linked to collective action. Given the importance of equal roles between researchers and community members, the university researchers who participated in South Tucson Prevention Coalition and the students who interviewed key stakeholders for purposes of this book provide their own subjective positionality statement to shed light on their own privileges, assumptions, and revelations gleaned from their work with South Tucson Prevention Coalition.

A. Romero, Ph.D. (✉)
Family Studies and Human Development, University of Arizona,
650 N. Park Avenue, Tucson, AZ 85719, USA
e-mail: romeroa@u.arizona.edu

J. Caporale, M.A.
Mexican American Studies, University of Arizona, Tucson, AZ, USA
e-mail: jcaporale@email.arizona.edu

R. Harris, M.S.
University of New York, New York, NY, USA
e-mail: robby.d.harris@gmail.com

E. Meza, M.S.W.
San Francisco Unified School District, San Francisco, CA, USA
e-mail: mezae520@gmail.com

J. Muraco, Ph.D.
Human Development and Women's and Gender Studies, University of Wisconsin-Green Bay,
2420 Nicolet Drive MAC C323, Green Bay, WI 54311, USA
e-mail: muracoj@uwgb.edu

J. Post, M.S.
Mel and Enid Zuckerman College of Public Health, University of Arizona,
3950 S. Country Club, Suite 330, Tucson, AZ, USA
e-mail: jhpost@email.arizona.edu

A.J. Romero (ed.), *Youth-Community Partnerships for Adolescent Alcohol Prevention*, DOI 10.1007/978-3-319-26030-3_3

Keywords Research • Prevention • Participatory action research • Adolescent alcohol use

As we noticed in Chap. 2, the Community Readiness Model for Change describes how effective and sustainable change happens over time at the community level. Specifically, it helps communities understand their own level of readiness in order to determine the most effective strategy to create change. While this model is incredibly useful, it is so focused on community-led approaches that it leaves little room for outsiders, such as university researchers. Additionally, the model primarily focuses on community-led research strategies on assessment to identify readiness, with few other guidelines for other types of research or evaluation. Thus, in this chapter, we also integrate principles from participatory action research (PAR) that helped South Tucson Prevention Coalition (STPC) develop strategies for (1) guiding equal participation of community members and researchers, (2) studying changes in alcohol norms through community-led and researcher supported research, and (3) linking research to action. Participatory Action Research principles helped South Tucson Prevention Coalition (STPC) to engage community members and researchers to work together toward a common goal as a collective, in order to use research to systematically address the community-identified adolescent alcohol use issues (Cammarota & Fine, 2008).

The STPC utilized a participatory action research approach (Cousins & Earl, 1992) in the development of their coalition and their integration of research and action. This method is particularly useful when researchers desire a balance between technical rigor and responsiveness to stakeholder needs, through the following methods (1) the researchers and community stakeholders jointly share the control of the research, (2) number of stakeholders is limited to those with a vital interest in the program, and (3) members of the collaborative effort are involved at all stages of the research including designing and preparing the project proposal, defining the design, selecting/developing instrumentation, collecting data, processing and analyzing data, and reporting and disseminating results. In Chap. 2, we described the 8-year evolution where community members began primarily as participants, then became advisory members as consultants and reviewers, and ultimately became the primarily leaders and researchers with only minimal counsel and support from researchers. Over time, the STPC members became directly involved in joint analysis and dissemination of findings. This chapter will provide more in-depth discussion as to the PAR techniques that helped guide this change over time in community involvement and coalition building. Some community-based participatory research (CBPR) approaches, such as the one proposed by Turnbull, Friesen, and Ramirez (1998), allow for variation in community participation, while others, such as the one proposed by O'Fallon and Dearry (2002), argue for a much more strict definition of participatory research that is only community-led. However, we found that a PAR-guided process helped to achieve a level of trust and capacity among community members and researchers that contributed to successful participation, research, and action.

3.1 Place-Based Approaches and PAR with Minority Communities

By taking a place-based approach with STPC that focused on the City of South Tucson, we can specifically identify the current and historical economic, political, and social contexts of adolescent alcohol use. Community readiness and PAR both remind us of the importance of community involvement, and in this case, we also consider youth as equal community members. Ginwright and Cammarota (2006) argue that PAR with youth is most effective when the following factors are considered: (1) youth experiences are best understood within their economic, political, and social contexts, (2) youth positive development is seen as the answer to current marginalization of all youth, (3) youth have agency to create change; they are not only subjects that need to be changed, and (4) adolescents have basic human rights. Rodríguez and Brown (2009) agree with many of these principles, particularly that the work needs to be situated within the unique place-based context of the youth. Additionally, any sort of program or pedagogy needs to be participatory and rooted in the problem-posing framework of Freire (1968), that is inquiry-based and oriented toward action to change the existing status quo. We follow these key principles in much of our work with youth–community partnerships as a way to consider the broader societal context of coalition building and collective action (Ginwright & Cammarota, 2006). Place-based PAR techniques empower local community members through reflection and awareness of the health issues in their own community combined with practical application of research and action to improve health outcomes (Grekul, 2011).

These are a few of the reasons why place-based PAR strategies with the primarily Native American and Mexican American community of South Tucson are particularly relevant and effective. The tragedies over the past 500 years for Native Americans and Mexican Americans have resulted in blaming current alcohol and substance use on the breakdown of tribal systems, families, cultures, and traditions, while overlooking any positive sources of resilience and maintenance of culture (Rodríguez, 2014; Walters & Simoni, 2002). It is the continued prejudice in public spaces that reminds us of the importance of the work done by STPC to fully engage youth and adults in their community in a positive manner. In many ways, the historical denial of access to resources and the continued silencing of ethnic minority voices highlight the radicalness of youth and community partnerships that can lead to changes in the system to ultimately promote health and provide access to supportive resources for healthy minority youth development (Torre & Fine, 2006).

PAR is a meaningful way to conduct research that helps reject deficit models and allows space to listen and reflect on sources of resiliency among marginalized groups (Rodríguez & Brown, 2009). These approaches are described as facilitating the re-membering of an oppressed and silenced history through a process of unveiling privilege and power (Cahill, Rios-Moore, & Threatts, 2008; Fine & Torre, 2004). PAR principles remind us that research needs to build on the positive aspects of the community that contribute to strengths, resources, and relationships because this approach will help bring benefits to all participating partners (Ramey et al., 2014). Place-based and PAR strategies also help to avoid stereotypes and expectations of universality by focusing on community-specific knowledge, resources, and strengths. For example, among Latinos or American Indians, there are many ethnic subgroups with a wide range of language and cultural norms; even so among those of Mexican descent, there is a wide range of diversity. In the local South Tucson community, there are two primary American Indian groups, the Tohono O'odham and the Pascua Yaqui, each one has their own distinct history and cultural worldviews. Unfortunately, the research on these groups continues to be sparse in alcohol prevention and in PAR. This only further emphasizes the need for community-led and place-based strategies for these communities.

3.1.1 Participatory Action Research Principles

Action research has been utilized for many decades among many fields of social research (Adelman, 1993), and it has many variants including Community-Based Participatory Research (CBPR) (Minkler & Wallerstein, 2008), Participatory Action Research (PAR) (McIntyre, 2008) or Youth Participatory Research (YPAR) (Cammarota & Fine, 2008), action research (Adelman, 1993), or application of developmental science (Lerner, Fisher, & Weinberg, 2000). In general, it is a methodological and philosophical orientation to research that integrates dialogue, research, and action into a cyclical process (see Fig. 3.1; Minkler & Wallerstein, 2008; Rodríguez & Brown, 2009). The cyclical spiral moves among five central components over and over, including (1) question, (2) investigate, (3) action plan, (4) implement, and (5) reflect/investigate.

Participatory Action Research (PAR) relies heavily on cooperation between partners and equal participation between community members and researchers (Minkler & Wallerstein, 2008). According to McIntyre (2008), participatory means that there is equal respect for all voices who are participating in discussion, and that each person is viewed as contributing unique expertise to the group. Action is the purpose of research for both the researcher and the community and may include prevention/intervention programs or collective action for policy. Research indicates that something is systematic, generalizable, and derived from existing knowledge and methods (Rodríguez & Brown, 2009). The overarching approach is one that connects researchers to the community, beginning as early as during the planning of research goals, and continuing through the progressive stages of the research process, including data collection and analysis (Rodríguez & Brown, 2009). Regardless of the approach taken, or the degree adhered to, all PAR approaches emphasize a collaborative approach that equally involves the community in the research process and recognizes and utilizes the strengths the community brings (Minkler & Wallerstein, 2008).

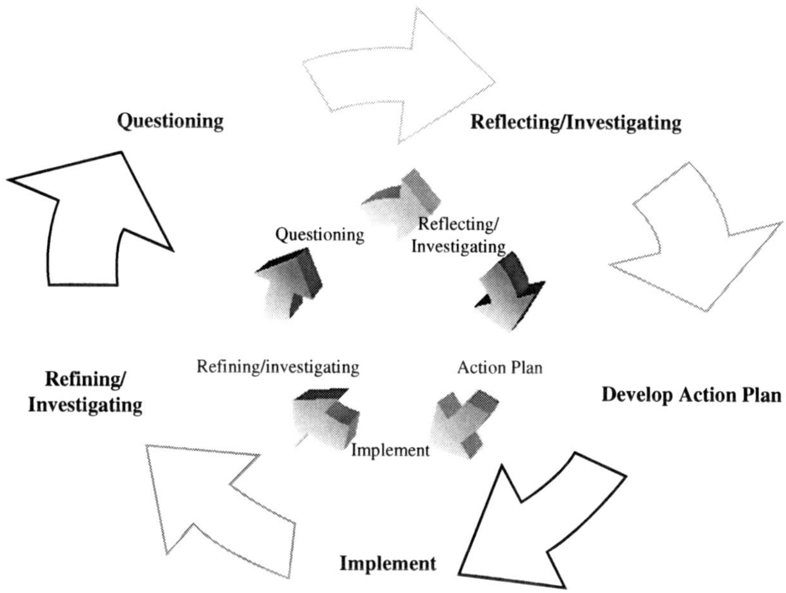

Fig. 3.1 Cyclical processes involved in participatory action research and similar methodologies

3.2 Participation Via Dialogue for Coalition Building

Participation is at the center of PAR projects and is based on dialogue among members. Creating equality among participants and effective dialogue can be challenging, particularly given existing negative stereotypes and differences in power privilege among youth, adults, and researchers. Fundamental to effective dialogue is that everyone participates as equals in discussion and decision-making no matter their age, socioeconomic status, or title within the community. Equality is based on all individuals participating as co-learners with the common goal of creating social knowledge together through the process of dialogue, reflection, and action. Effective dialogue procedures can be developed when they are rooted in the following participation components: (1) collective commitment to the issue, (2) self and collective reflection to gain clarity on the issue, (3) joint decision-making to engage in action that will lead to a useful decision that benefits people involved, (4) building of alliances between researchers and participants in planning, implementation, and dissemination of research, and (5) balance between technical rigor and stakeholder needs (Cousins & Earl, 1992; McIntyre, 2008). Essential to effective dialogue methods is engagement of problem-posing techniques, in a manner that discussion remains community-driven and place-based (Freire, 1968; McIntyre, 2008). Utilizing the

Freire's three-stage methodology for problem posing helps to focus on the conversation by listening to understand the felt issues or themes of the community, engaging in participatory dialogue from all members, and identifying action or positive changes that participants envision.

This method of dialogue through problem-posing facilitates raising awareness about the health issue rather than didactic methods that state problems and solutions as if they are predetermined by experts. Problems are posed in a manner that participants work together to uncover the root causes of the issue within their own community. Problem posing also helps participants to consider the socioeconomic, political, cultural, and historical aspects of the problem context that can also shed light on unfair social systems. The development of group critical thinking processes helps to link prevention/intervention strategies for community level change. The process of awakening to critical consciousness is what Freire (1968) termed *concientización*, where individuals come to view themselves as active participants in society with the capacity to change existing structures. This process of open dialogue and problem posing can be difficult because it requires conscious acknowledgement of health problems and conscious discussion of both negative and positive factors within the community. However, critical consciousness resituates perspective such that blame is no longer placed on the culture as with the cultural-deficit model; instead, participants begin to become critically conscious of the broader ecological context of health behaviors and the potential for community-led solutions (Romero et al., 2008).

3.3 Praxis: Reflection and Action in PAR

The Freirian approach to STPC's work in the coalition and with youth prevention programming created new ways to understand adolescent alcohol use in terms of how environment shapes youth behaviors (Freire, 1968; Ginwright & Cammarota, 2006; Watts & Guessous, 2006). Freire's (1968) work is based on the concept of praxis which represents an integration of critical awareness of societal inequities with action to create change (Cammarota & Fine, 2008). These two factors of reflection and action are central to praxis and are also elemental to the process of PAR. The critical awareness and analysis that considers privilege and power is essential to engaging minority communities because it acknowledges their current situation while allowing for opportunities to create knowledge and change. In one study, Watts and Guessous (2006) found that youth who reported more civic involvement were those who engaged in more critical analysis to understand societal inequities and those who were also committed to collective action approaches. It is this focus on social justice through analysis that contributes to the development of critical consciousness and is one reason why PAR is relevant and effective with marginalized minority communities (Freire, 1968; Ginwright & Cammarota, 2002).

3.4 Integrating Research and Researchers

Woven throughout the PAR process is the integration of research to help guide identification of local issues and to evaluate action strategies. However, there is often a general distrust of university researchers within minority communities due to previous negative experiences. Perhaps this distrust also stems from lack of involvement in the educational system when working with lower income communities who have low education rates, as in South Tucson. Specifically, community representatives in South Tucson shared anecdotes that indicated that previous portrayals of the city were one-sided and only supported existing stereotypes of the high crime and alcohol/drug use.

3.4.1 Assumptions of Traditional Research and PAR

The assumptions of traditional research often place barriers for researchers to actively and equally participate in community-based research. For example, research and science have long been assumed to be objective, universal, and value neutral (Ramirez, 1998). However, many scholars, particularly within cultural studies, have questioned these assumptions and identified contradictory aspects that point to the undermining of these original assumptions in a way that opens the door for PAR techniques. For example, in his classic writings, Rosaldo (1993) discusses the Myth of Detachment, which debunks the myth that any individual, particularly a researcher, can be fully detached from their surroundings or fully detached from their own worldview that has been shaped by their personal experiences. Thus, he and several other scholars argue for the need to not try to attain an unrealistic ideal of detachment, but rather one of clarifying one's subjectivity within the context. Thus, by making one's own worldview conscious and public, then the research is more likely to be more accurate, and the readers can then understand the personal framework from which the researcher is using for their research approach and interpretation (Delgado-Bernal, 1998). This perspective also addresses universality, or the assumption that all groups have the same worldview, as well as value neutrality. By acknowledging one's worldview, there is clarity in how it may differ or be similar from the group that is participating in the study. This further destabilizes any inherent ethnocentrism that may introduce cultural bias into the research.

Furthermore, utilizing PAR to reflect on researcher's own personal worldview can improve research in a manner that increases ethical, valid, and reliable research with underrepresented populations. Some researchers have argued that there is epistemological racism in the nature, status, and production of knowledge that is based on preexisting societal norms that diminish ethnic minority group culture and norms (Delgado-Bernal, 1998; Ramirez, 1998). Too often the traditional methodologies only reflect and further reinforce the social history of the dominant cultural group and at worst overlook or negatively portray ethnic minority groups. PAR has the potential to be not only a research method but also a form of restorative justice that can help to establish trust with communities who have suffered historical trauma or detrimental effects from working with researchers in the past (McIntyre, 2008). However, there is a need for researchers to gain critical consciousness about their own privileges and perspectives in order to achieve PAR success. Previous studies have utilized CBPR practices for alcohol and suicide prevention in an Alaskan Native community (Allen, Mohatt, Beehler, & Rowe, 2014) with success. In this study, they effectively integrated cultural values into a prevention program through community members and university researchers working together. They describe how the forced history of assimilation and history of distrust of outsiders shaped their prevention approach and use of CBPR, so that the community retained local control over the infusion of their cultural values and over the final version of the program.

3.5 South Tucson Prevention Coalition and Research Integration

For several years, the STPC worked closely with Dr. Romero from the University of Arizona, to jointly conduct regular evaluation activities and to collect and organize new qualitative and quantitative data to help mobilize the community around specific prevention issues. As you may recall, a key step of the Community Readiness Model for Change is to train local community members to conduct interviews and to assess the community readiness level in order to develop strategies (Plested, Edwards, & Jumper-Thurman, 2006). However, in the practice of these activities, it was found that analyzing and calculating scores were often a stopping point for community members. University researchers could assist with transcription and calculation of scores. Final decisions on scoring and interpretation were done through discussion and consensus with coalition members. It was in these ways that the collaboration with a university professor and graduate students served as a complementary aspect of the community readiness approach and assessment.

One of STPC's long-standing policies was to create a collaborative environment such that each member of the coalition had a stake in the work (see Chap. 10 for coalition building). Using a participatory action research approach, a cycle of research and feedback was utilized ensuring that all members were equal participants in decision-making. Data was gathered from a variety of sources to ensure that STPC members had the information needed to understand the current realities facing of the community (see Chap. 9 for details on data collection). However, the purposeful approach to integrating research through PAR is central to success of research with ethnic minority communities. PAR allows research to evolve over time within a real societal context that is more likely to lead to solving contemporary social issues, yet this is unlikely to be accomplished with only one research project. Rather multiple studies may piece together as part of a larger puzzle that is shaped by community influence over time. Yet, PAR is not only about "doing good," it is about producing quality research, because ultimately high quality research and rigorous testing of interventions can provide better quality results to inform communities about their health.

In reality, PAR research may not always be mutually beneficial to each partner, rather at times it may be more meaningful to community members and at other times more meaningful to researchers (Rog et al., 2004). Often there is a tension for researchers who still have pressure to work on publishable research projects judged by traditional scientific criteria, yet who desire to work with community partners in a manner consistent with PAR that emphasizes community-driven projects. Few researchers have spare time to devote to community projects that will not produce any sort of academic approved outcomes such as grants or publications. Additionally, many graduate students have not had experience or exposure to ethnic minority communities. This can be a difficult barrier to include student researchers in an equitable manner in PAR projects.

There were tensions faced by Dr. Romero and student researchers as part of this process with STPC. Before students participated in the project, they had all taken a course with Dr. Romero where they learned about participatory action research. They received human subjects training certification and also additional training from Dr. Romero. Dr. Romero emphasized the community cultural strengths of the community when training students. She also took each student on a tour of the City of South Tucson prior to beginning data collection; this tour emphasized the local community resources. During this tour, they also stopped and spoke with local community leaders about their work and their insights into the community. During and after the tour, students would write down their observations and reflect on their own privilege and their own perspectives. In the following section, graduate (Robby, Joel, Juvenal) and undergraduate student (Elisa) researchers who collected data with STPC members provide subjective positionality statements to describe their own views of their participation, and how it impacted them as individuals. This commentary on critical consciousness and privilege by several graduate student researchers and Dr. Romero who collected interviews with STPC members provides a very honest and insightful view into some of the challenges for students and researchers.

3.5.1 Robby

I entered the Tucson community identifying as a graduate student without any understanding of the social or political contexts in which Tucson existed. In my mind, I was going to complete my degree in family studies and human development and then move back to New York, where I was from. Although I did not explicitly think or understand this in the moment, the narrative in my mind existed exclusively within the confines of the university setting. I did not have any desires to explore the world outside of my life as a graduate student and was "successful" in this plan for the first year that I lived in Arizona. I spent each day on the university campus and each night with graduate students. When I began the second year in the program, I enrolled in Dr. Romero's Participatory Action Research course after hearing her explain the opportunity to engage with community members. In my undergraduate studies, I was a part of several community-based research projects and therefore was drawn to the idea of engaging in similar processes in Tucson. However, I could not have imagined how transformative this experience would have been.

The idea of not only involving but equally valuing community member participation in the formation and execution of research in order to elicit change was novel to me but immediately made sense. In fact, once being introduced to the idea of PAR, any alternative method of research no longer made sense. As Dr. Romero's class continued on and she presented the idea of our becoming involved with STPC, I was initially hesitant. Still comfortably residing in my bubble of academia, my only exposure to South Tucson was hearing stories about the violence and poverty present in the area. In fact, whenever I drove near South Tucson, I closed my car windows out of ignorant fear. Despite the fact that I moved to Tucson from New York City and was overwhelmingly frustrated by individuals who feared "bad parts" of New York even though they had never visited the neighborhood themselves, I fell into the same trap of criminalizing an entire community based upon inaccurate perceptions and fear of the unknown.

My first visit to the city of South Tucson took place almost a year and a half after I moved to Arizona. I remember that Dr. Romero drove our group of graduate students to a meeting of the STPC, and I immediately felt welcomed and at home. The passion for youth was profound, and I had never been in a room with so many individuals who each clearly cared so strongly about youth. However, perhaps more importantly was the distinct equitable nature of the meeting. Each member of the coalition held every other member in a similar regard and I, as a brand new member of the team, felt just as valued. This memory remains a beautiful image in my mind years later. With grace, passion, and agency, these individuals were enacting change in big ways, and it was my honor to witness these efforts.

Throughout my tenure in higher education, the moments of true collaboration and dialogue have been, unfortunately, rare. I know, as reflected by the title of this book, that a key component of why this youth-directed, community-facilitated change was possible lies in the very notion of cooperative collaboration. Now, as a school psychologist, this value guides my daily practice; I am committed to being a practitioner embedded in the communities in which I function. My experiences in working with the STPC and interviewing community members who serve the youth of Tucson have informed the way that I approach my role and I am forever grateful for that. As a school psychologist, it can be easy to fall into the trap of community- and context-reduced decision making. However, I choose to serve the youth and families with which I work from the position of empowerment and agency—just as I learned from the South Tucson community.

3.5.2 Joel

Currently, I am an Assistant Professor of Human Development at the University of Wisconsin—Green Bay. Originally from Tucson, Arizona, I attended the University of Arizona for all of my post-secondary education, culminating with the completion of my doctorate in Family Studies and Human Development. I first came to learn about CBPR as a graduate student. In what follows, I describe some of the lessons I learned from integrating CBPR techniques into my research.

One of the most difficult aspects of conducing CBPR is making and sustaining contact. In terms of making initial contact, it can be difficult to connect with the right person, especially given many individuals are not connected to their emails the way many academics are. For community members who are connected to their email, they are often swamped and have little time to sit in front of their computers and answer emails from strangers asking about research. But is it this initial contact that is vital to the success of the research as often it is specific community members who will gain you access to your community of interest. If you can work with these gatekeepers and gain their trust, you can gain tremendous insight into the lives of those you wish to study.

To initiate contact with Oscar, youth participant and youth outreach specialist, I went to the JVYC and attended a STPC meeting. Although he was not at that particular meeting, I was able to meet with him after and discuss my ideas for my project. He was eager to help me in the process, and we were able to, right there on the spot, schedule our next meeting. I learned that the best way for him and me to work together was to meet at the JVYC as it ensured we both designated time out of our busy schedules to continue the project. Meeting in person, at the center, also conveyed my dedication to the work and informally acknowledged to Oscar that I valued his time and the work that he does. This is in stark opposition to many researchers who ask community members to meet them on their college and university campuses.

Had I merely emailed Oscar, it would have been much more difficult to convey the details of my project, let alone sync our schedules. This experience has prompted me, as I continue with my research on gay and lesbian youth, to go to local nonprofits and ask to speak with the site directors instead of sending emails. It is much easier to dismiss or forget about an email than it is to dismiss a person standing in front of you. Further, the extra effort upfront, in my experience, yields much better results than an initial email ever has.

Another lesson I learned was the added complexity of bringing another member to the research team when the dynamic of the group has already been established. On the day I met with Oscar to interview him, I had a videographer join me, with the hopes that having a video record could add to the audio recording I was taking. What I had failed to recognize was the added component a third person would bring to the relationship I had built with Oscar. Bringing in a stranger with a camcorder, from my perspective, hindered the interview process, not only because of the person behind the lens, but because of the stipulations the recoding placed on me and Oscar as interviewer and interviewee, respectively. For instance, and unbeknownst to me prior, for ease of editing certain precautions were instituted that involved leaving pauses after each person spoke, which was difficult for me as I am a fast speaker, and repeating what had been asked when responding, appeared difficult for Oscar who was more focused on answering the questions in a natural and sincere way.

Despite the added complexities a videographer added to the interview process, I would still recommend videotaping your interviews if the opportunity presents itself. Based on my experience, two courses of action seem most evident: learn to videotape so you can be the one who sets up the camcorder and conducts the interview or be sure to include the videographer from the onset and ensure they can attend the meetings leading up to the interview so that they too begin to develop a relationship with both you and the interviewee. Lastly, and this is perhaps most important if you plan to videotape your interviews, be sure to discuss how the interview process will be structured because of the video recording. For instance, regardless of how you opt to have the interview recorded, be sure to talk with the interviewee ahead of time about how gaps between speaking as well as repeating the question as you answer help with editing. This way, the interviewee will have time to consider how to incorporate such structure into their responses.

Ultimately, my interview with Oscar was the culmination of my first experience with a community member in a research capacity utilizing CBPR. Since the interview I have been doing a lot of reflecting on the experience: what I learned, how I incorporated tenets of CBPR in the process, and what more I could have done to include even more CBPR relevant tenets. I have come to the realization that this whole experience was a learning process, and that while I did not do everything perfectly, I did much more than the average social scientist and that my research is all the better because of it.

3.5.3 *Elisa*

I am an alumni of Tucson Unified School District, raised in Barrio Centro, and was a community youth organizer while also pursuing a Bachelor's Degree in English at the University of Arizona. Working with Michal and Alejandro, along with several other youth that attend the JVYC, two colleagues and I first inquired about what they wanted to learn more about, utilizing the resources we had available to us. Based on the Youth 2 Youth's desire to know more about college, I discovered that my own experiences at the University of Arizona could be assets for their development. My experience as a student in college was a resource for encouraging the youth's consideration of higher education. I had even graduated from the same high school as most of the youth, which made me even more dedicated to providing what information I could articulate. This ***bidirectional learning*** model provided not only the youth with insight into what college would be like for them (dorm life, eating healthy, studying habits), but also provided us with the realization that we represented assets to their space. By being present in their community center, we were helping to build a bridge between community involvement and higher education.

When asked about the experience attending the college focus-group nights, Alejandro states:

> It's helped me a lot more because it motivates you to do better in school, 'cause my freshman and sophomore year, I did OK, but I got some bad grades here and there, but this year when we started doing this college night uh, I guess helped me a lot 'cause I'm receiving a lot of letters from different colleges and it's helping me like look into what I need to look for like, for the scholarships, helping me a lot with the requirements. I know it's my junior year, but it's something I won't really have to worry about next year because I'm starting to do that now.

Being able to assist Alejandro in considering college after high school has helped him sustain his focus now while he's still in school. His emphasis on wanting to remain focused illustrates the resiliency he has accumulated from his development as a community leader and someone who strives to want to do the best he possibly can, as soon as he is given the opportunity to prove that commitment. He knows that there is a community around him that appreciates his commitment and involvement, as he shows a lot of passion in expressing his appreciation for the bonds he has with the other youth in the JVYC. Without prompting more questions related to specific research prompts, when asked if he had anything else to add to the interview, Alejandro stated:

> Uh...(very long pause)...I just really like how UA students are coming down and helping us out and like getting to know what they do also, what types of things they do while they're going to school and stuff like that ... we went walking around campus with the iPads and we were asking questions to students around campus. Like we went into the little shop, the store, where the library is, and we went in there and asked the workers there like different questions about how they're going through school and work at the same time and like different questions so just we know what to expect and I think that was really fun. It's really fun you guys coming down here, using our resources to help us.

Being exposed to college students that come from similar backgrounds as himself helped Alejandro realize the reality of life in college as a student from a low-income family. But because my colleagues and I had also been from low-income backgrounds, it seemed that the connections we were able to build with students like Alejandro also helped us to understand how to better help with understanding college. While being proactive in his community, he was given an opportunity to see the college atmosphere firsthand. Being engaged in those two contexts resulted in his commitment to positive productivity in his studies in high school.

3.5.4 Jesi

I am currently a Research Specialist in Public Health at the University of Arizona. I became involved in this project as a graduate student in Family Studies and Human Development during a semester when I took a PAR course with Dr. Romero. Reading Freire's *Pedagogy of the Oppressed* during that course was something that changed my way of thinking forever. Prior to encountering the principles of PAR, I had been conceptualizing research as a method of questioning that could be conducted in order to gain knowledge, with which I hoped I would be able to use to affect individuals and communities for the better. It wasn't entirely clear to me what would need to happen in order for that change to occur; however, but that mysterious something was a component that I intuitively thought would need to be incorporated into my research in order to actually help improve the well-being of individuals and communities. Freire suggested that it was as simple as giving power and voice to the people who needed change.

Before enrolling in graduate school I had worked in education and human services and was passionate about helping to provide others with tools that could enable them improve their lives. Learning about the approach that PAR uses was enlightening and inspiring, to say the least. I had not yet then been formally exposed to such ideas before meeting Dr. Romero, but the principles fell right in line with my inner desires to actively empower others, help them be heard, and support processes that raise awareness of inequalities and make diverse experiences visible in order to promote positive change. In my past work, when taking on a role of an advocate, I frequently hung on to the notion "nothing about me without me," especially when it came to efforts that would directly impact an individual whom I or my team were intending to help. The PAR principles aligned very well with that same mindset—that the best way to help make change for an individual (and a community) is to involve them in that effort. This means including, not excluding, them from information, communications, and decision-making.

After reading Freire and talking about PAR with my classmates, research without the involvement of the people it is intended to affect seemed entirely misguided. I could not turn back to thinking about research as effective unless it actually incorporated this. Through Dr. Romero's encouragement to learn more about the STPC's community leaders and their role in the process of community change, I was given the opportunity to meet the Executive Directors of the community centers House of Neighborly Services and John Valenzuela Youth Center. It was an exciting and scary process for me because, to be honest, I was intimidated to start a conversation with these women whom I had heard so much about—I was just being introduced to the incredible power of PAR, and they were way ahead of me! Clearly they had learned much that I was just now beginning to understand. But the experience was inspiring. Talking with Gloria and Kimberly was an incredibly moving experience—their passion for youth and the communities they had been working within was tangible. Hearing their stories helped me to better understand the complex processes that occurred along the way; as it turns out, it wasn't any one thing that led to (seemingly magical) community change, but a long process that involved countless players, ongoing efforts, sometimes difficult changes and growing pains, and—really—a lot of faith in giving something new a try.

3.5.5 Juvenal

As a second year Ph.D. student in the Mexican American Studies Department at the University of Arizona, I have learned that Participatory Action Research (PAR) is hinged on researchers, educators, leaders, and/or activists serving and working with diverse populations. Despite possessing 17 years of experience working with government, nonprofit, and for-profit institutions who serve distinct communities of all ages, ethnic, and socioeconomic backgrounds, it was not until I worked in Tucson, Arizona, that I really understood the impact that PAR had on communities and vice versa.

When Dr. Romero took our research team on a ride along to see the City of South Tucson and meet leaders from the different organizations which comprise the South Tucson Prevention Coalition (STPC), I realized that the City of South Tucson closely resembled the inner-city San Diego community where I grew up. The City of South Tucson reminded me a lot of my community and I felt that I understood firsthand some of the social issues (i.e., underage drinking, high school drop-out rates, and teen pregnancy) affecting this community. In this ride along, I learned that it is essential that researchers and community leaders maintain an ongoing relationship which is based on trust, mutual respect, and dialogue. Becoming a researcher and working closely with Dr. Romero and her research teams gave me the opportunity to explore the dynamics of PAR, from an insider and outsider perspectives. If researchers are to help ameliorate the social conditions of any community, they must first understand the issues affecting that community and learn the perspectives of the members who make up and live in such community. In order to build a cohesive collaboration between different partners who dedicate their services assisting any community, it is my belief that researchers and leaders must embody an authentic care for the populations being served. Only then will a community's voice be heard and the possibility to create social change really take place.

While researching the Omeyocan Youth Empowerment and Sexuality (Omeyocan YES) project which was part of the STPC (see Chap. 4), Patty shared a story with me about a youth that made me think about my own adolescent experience and the many community leaders and teachers that had a positive impact in my life. I could relate to this youth because I too was raised by a widowed grandmother who came to this country from Mexico with only a third grade education. Having had an upbringing in different neighborhoods throughout the inner city of San Diego, I too felt that I was losing my "*hoping mechanism (see Chap. 4).*" Indeed, one-on-one and group conversations helped shaped me become the adult that I am today, and all the community leaders that I worked with operated under the motto that "it takes a village to raise a child." Having been adopted myself, arrested, and a former high school dropout, I openly shared my personal experiences with youth and they listened. Because I am sincere and I genuinely care for their future, most of them gave me an ear and were honest with me. When I was growing up, I remember being taken to San Diego State University (SDSU) while being court ordered to participate in a program that helped youth finish probation successfully, the San Diego CHOICE Program. Prior to this experience, I did not know that colleges existed and much less what they looked like. My Youth Service Worker (YSW) took a group of us CHOICE participants to get tutored by criminal justice students because I was failing my classes. It was not until my YSW told me that you too can come here that a seed to pursue a higher education was planted in me. Ultimately, without the assistance and intervention of community leaders who adhere to the principles of PAR, I feel that I never would have written this piece.

3.5.6 Dr. Andrea Romero

I am a full professor at the University of Arizona, and I conducted this work as an assistant and associate professor at the University of Arizona. My background is Mexican American, and I grew up in a several cities throughout the southwest that were similar to South Tucson with high rates of poverty and high rates of ethnic minorities of Mexican American and Native American descent, where English and Spanish were common languages. Although, I felt that South Tucson was familiar, I also realized that my position as a professor at the local university and my educational background were also aspects that might make others feel that I was an outsider to their community, as well as the fact that I had not grown up in South Tucson. I had already worked for 5 years in similar Texas and California communities with Mexican American and Vietnamese American low-income communities for data collection and health program interventions.

When I first began my job at the university, a staff member with the Chicano/Hispano Student Affairs office offered to take me to his neighborhood to meet some of the nonprofit leaders and others working with adolescents. This was my gateway to learn about and begin working in South Tucson. I spent the first year volunteering at one of the agencies with an after-school youth program. I then started with focus groups to learn more about the issues of the youth and parents in the community. This led to what is now 15 years of partnerships in the community. There were certainly missteps along the way and moments when community partners put up barriers to my involvement because of lack of trust. However, I always told them that it was wise to ask a lot of questions to researchers and to be clear about their research and intentions before beginning partnerships. I also felt that over time after demonstrating that I was true to my intentions and promises that several community members developed a deep sense of trust in working with me, and it is this trust and those relationships that has kept me committed to helping youth of South Tucson.

3.6 Conclusion

PAR is an effective method for community level change. In this chapter, we describe how the PAR cycle that is built on participation, action, and research was fundamental to the coalition building activities of South Tucson Prevention Coalition and to the success. The description of the importance and the process of dialogue in this chapter demonstrates how relationships and trust were built over time among coalition members. Most importantly, PAR offered a road map for the inclusion of researchers in the coalition as equal members. We discuss some of the unique challenges that researchers have when working with historically oppressed minority groups. The subjective positionality statements of all researchers who write or cowrite chapters in this book provide their personal insight into the meaning of PAR for their own personal transformation and lessons for others to follow.

References

Adelman, C. (1993). Kurt Lewin and the origins of action research. *Educational Action Research, 1*(1), 7–24.

Allen, J., Mohatt, G. V., Beehler, S., & Rowe, H. L. (2014). People awakening: Collaborative research to develop cultural strategies for prevention in community intervention. *American Journal of Community Psychology, 54*(1–2), 100–111.

Cahill, C., Rios-Moore, I., & Threatts, T. (2008). Different eyes/open eyes: Community-based participatory action research. In J. Cammarota & M. Fine (Eds.), *Revolutionizing education: Youth participatory action research in motion* (pp. 89–124). New York: Routledge.

Cammarota, J., & Fine, M. (2008). *Revolutionizing education: Youth participatory action research in motion*. New York: Routledge.

Cousins, J. B., & Earl, L. M. (1992). The case for participatory evaluation. *Educational Evaluation and Policy Analysis, 14*(4), 397–418.

Delgado-Bernal, D. (1998). Using a Chicana feminist epistemology in educational research. *Harvard Educational Review, 68*(4), 555–583.

Fine, M., & Torre, M. E. (2004). Re-membering exclusions: Participatory action research in public institutions. *Qualitative Research in Psychology, 1*(1), 15–37.

Freire, P. (1968). *Pedagogy of the oppressed*. New York: Seabury.

Ginwright, S., & Cammarota, J. (2002). New terrain in youth development: The promise of a social justice approach. *Social Justice, 29*(4), 82–95.

Ginwright, S., & Cammarota, J. (2006). Introduction. In S. Ginwright, P. Noguera, & J. Cammarota (Eds.), *Beyond Resistance!: Youth Activism and Community Change: New democratic possibilities for practice and policy for America's youth* (pp. xii–xxii). New York: Routledge.

Grekul, J. (2011). Building collective efficacy and sustainability into a community collaborative: Community solution to gang violence. *Journal of Gang Research, 18*(2), 23–45.

Lerner, R. M., Fisher, C. B., & Weinberg, R. A. (2000). Toward a science for and of the people: Promoting civil society through the application of developmental science. *Child Development, 71*(1), 11–20.

McIntyre, A. (2008). *Participatory action research*. Thousand Oaks, CA: Sage.

Minkler, M., & Wallerstein, N. (2008). Introduction to community-based participatory research. In M. Minkler & N. Wallerstein (Eds.), *Community-based participatory research for health: From process to outcomes* (pp. 5–19). San Francisco, CA: Jossey-Bass.

O'Fallon, L. R., & Dearry, A. (2002). Community-based participatory research as a tool to advance environmental health sciences. *Environmental Health Perspectives, 110*(2), 155–159.

Plested, B. A., Edwards, R. W., & Jumper-Thurman, P. (2006). *Community Readiness: A handbook for successful change*. Fort Collins, CO: Tri-Ethnic Center for Prevention Research.

Ramey, S. L., Schafer, P., DeClerque, J. L., Lanzi, R. G., Hobel, C., Shalowitz, M., … & Raju, T. N. (2014). The preconception stress and resiliency pathways model: A multi-level framework on maternal, paternal, and child health disparities derived by community-based participatory research. *Maternal and Child Health Journal, 19*(4), 707–719.

Ramirez, M., III. (1998). *Multicultural/multiracial psychology: Mestizo perspectives in personality and mental health*. New York: Jason Aronson.

Rodríguez, R. C. (2014). *Our sacred maiz is our mother: Indigeneity and belonging in the Americas*. Tucson, AZ: The University of Arizona Press.

Rodríguez, L. F., & Brown, T. M. (2009). From voice to agency: Guiding principles for participatory action research with youth. In T. M. Brown & L. F. Rodríguez (Eds.), *New directions for youth development: Youth in participatory action research* (pp. 19–34). San Francisco, CA: Jossey-Bass.

Rog, D., Boback, N., Barton-Villagrana, H., Marrone-Bennett, P., Cardwell, J., Hawdon, J., … & Reischl, T. (2004). Sustaining collaboratives: A cross-site analysis of the National Funding Collaborative on Violence Prevention. *Evaluation and Program Planning, 27*(3), 249–261.

Romero, A., Cammarota, J., Dominguez, K., Valdez, L., Ramirez, G., & Hernandez, L. (2008). "The opportunity if not the right to see": Social justice education project. In J. Cammarota & M. Fine (Eds.), *Revolutionizing education: Youth participatory action research in motion* (pp. 131–151). New York, NY: Routledge.

Rosaldo, R. (1993). *Culture & truth: The remaking of social analysis: With a new introduction*. Boston, MA: Beacon.

Torre, M., & Fine, M. (2006). Researching and resisting: Democratic policy research by and for youth. In S. Ginwright, P. Noguera, & J. Cammarota (Eds.), *Beyond Resistance!: Youth Activism and Community Change: New democratic possibilities for practice and policy for America's youth* (pp. 269–285). New York: Routledge.

Turnbull, A. P., Friesen, B. J., & Ramirez, C. (1998). Participatory action research as a model for conducting family research. *Research and Practice for Persons with Severe Disabilities, 23*(3), 178–188.

Walters, K. L., & Simoni, J. M. (2002). Reconceptualizing Native women's health: An "indigenist" stress-coping model. *American Journal of Public Health, 92*(4), 520–524.

Watts, R. J., & Guessous, O. (2006). Sociopolitical development: The missing link in research and policy on adolescents. In S. Ginwright, P. Noguera, & J. Cammarota (Eds.), *Beyond Resistance!: Youth Activism and Community Change: New democratic possibilities for practice and policy for America's youth* (pp. 59–80). New York: Routledge.

Chapter 4
After-school Youth Substance Use Prevention to Develop Youth Leadership Capacity: South Tucson Prevention Coalition Phase 1

Juvenal Caporale, Andrea Romero, Ana Fonseca, Luis Perales, and Patty Valera

Abstract This chapter is about South Tucson Prevention Coalition (STPC) Phase 1, which was an after-school prevention program for teens. In a low-income barrio where issues of substance abuse, underage drinking, and high teen-pregnancy were prevalent, insiders of this community created the Omeyocan Youth Empowerment and Sexuality (YES) program. Omeyocan YES was a dual-gendered adolescent project based on Paulo Freire's critical pedagogy model. The Omeyocan YES project was progressive, and was effective in meeting the socio-political interests and needs of the urban Latino/a Chicano/a youth of this community. The 13–17-year-old youth who participated in the program became critically conscious of the issues affecting their community, and afterward many became activists and led their own community transformation projects. The Omeyocan YES project is a reminder that leaders and youth, using a critical curriculum and revolutionary pedagogy, can transform themselves. The results of Omeyocan YES built the foundation for STPC Phase 2, which focused on community transformational resilience.

Keywords After school • Prevention • Critical pedagogy • Critical curriculum

---

This research was supported by a grant awarded to Dr. Romero, PI, from the Substance Abuse and Mental Health Services Agency (Grant No: 10318). Correspondence concerning this chapter should be sent to Juvenal Caporale at Email: jcaporale@email.arizona.edu

J. Caporale, M.A. (✉) • L. Perales, M.S.
Mexican American Studies, University of Arizona, Tucson, AZ, USA
e-mail: jcaporale@email.arizona.edu; perales@email.arizona.edu

A. Romero, Ph.D. • A. Fonseca, M.A.
Family Studies and Human Development, University of Arizona, 650 N. Park Avenue, Tucson, AZ 85719, USA
e-mail: romeroa@u.arizona.edu; anafonseca@email.arizona.edu

P. Valera, L.M.S.W.
Department of Veteran's Affairs, Tucson, AZ, USA
e-mail: Valera.patty@gmail.com

A.J. Romero (ed.), *Youth-Community Partnerships for Adolescent Alcohol Prevention*, DOI 10.1007/978-3-319-26030-3_4

The Omeyocan Youth Empowerment and Sexuality (Omeyocan YES) project was an integrated substance use and HIV prevention program designed to holistically address Chicano/a male and female adolescents' mental, emotional, spiritual, and physical well-being. Guided by Freire's (1968) pedagogical model, the program leaders created a revolutionary curriculum that was hinged in critical education, collective leadership, and ongoing dialogue between adults and youth. The program was revolutionary because it was created by members of the City of South Tucson who sought to bring fundamental social justice-based changes at the grass-roots level to prevent or reduce risk of substance abuse and HIV within their own community. The youth of the Omeyocan YES project learned how to critically assess and approach different forms of "oppression" (i.e., substance abuse, teen pregnancy, dropout rates, etc.) affecting their communities. Youth also learned to become social justice agents for health disparities change that they later put into use in Phase 2: South Tucson Prevention Coalition. In this chapter we triangulate the results of the program with the following three aspects (1) summary of the perspectives of the Omeyocan YES program leaders about the creation of the program, implementation of the program, effect of the program on the youth, effect of the program on themselves, (2) the pre- and posttest quantitative survey results from 105 youth surveys, and (3) summary of the open-ended responses of the youth.

4.1 Omeyocan YES Description

Omeyocan Youth Empowerment and Sexuality (Omeyocan YES), is a holistic prevention project designed to prevent or reduce risk of substance use and HIV among both male and female. Omeyocan is a nahuatl word that indicates balance created by dual opposing forces (such as male/female). The focus of the program was on positive development, particularly, on the optimal health of mind, body, spirit, and community with a focus on social justice awareness and leadership training. The Omeyocan program leaders designed and facilitated a comprehensive formal sexuality education curriculum that reinforces Chicana/o and indigenous cultural norms that provide the basis for balanced sexual health. A federal grant awarded to Dr. Romero at the University of Arizona brought together the University of Arizona with Southern Arizona AIDS Foundation and the City of South Tucson to implement an integrated substance use and HIV prevention curriculum at local charter schools and after-school programs. This grant and the Omeyocan YES program are considered Phase 1 because it was the impetus to bring together these diverse entities that had not previously collaborated, and it was the first time that any HIV prevention programs had been implemented in the City of South Tucson. The primary goals of the Omeyocan YES project were: (1) prevent or reduce substance use and (2) increase condom use or abstinence.

The Omeyocan YES project and its leaders from the City of South Tucson cannot be understood without understanding Freire's pedagogical framework, which is vital for community-based participatory research. In the *Pedagogy of the Oppressed*, Freire (1968) maintained that re-humanization and liberation are not only the tasks of the oppressed but that "educational projects" ought to be used as a means of organizing them (Freire, 1968). According to Freire, "*The correct method for a revolutionary leadership…lies in dialogue. The conviction of the oppressed that they must fight for their liberation is not a gift bestowed by the revolutionary leadership, but the result of their own conscientizacão*" (1968, p. 67). Putting both of Freire's concepts together, "revolutionary" leadership use educational projects based on the method of dialogue to help oppressed people achieve liberation through critical consciousness. From this perspective, the current project focused primarily on health and educational oppression. Oppression was described in terms of health disparities, lack of knowledge, lack of access to knowledge and care, and not having voice or access for decision making. It is through dialogue that one develops a critical consciousness about the existing inequalities in society and one's own community; critical consciousness is the foundation for empowerment to create change in one's society that changes the existing status quo that is based on societal inequalities. In this sense, the curriculum was considered "revolutionary," in that it sought to change the existing health status quo by changing existing norms and behaviors in order to lead to empowerment of marginalized groups, such as minority adolescents who could then lead community level changes. This is the root of the program's focus on social justice.

4.1.1 Existing Evidence-Based After-School Prevention Programs

This program is also revolutionary when considered within the context of existing evidence-based prevention programs because it has key unique elements of social justice and community level awareness to target for future change to promote adolescent health. To date, most face-to-face and individual-level HIV interventions have been designed with a cognitive-behavioral focus (e.g., Theory of Reasoned Action/Theory of Planned Behavior, social cognitive theory, or the Health Belief Model) to change individual-level adolescent behavior (Bandura, 1986; Peterson & DiClemente, 2000). Most of these interventions share common characteristics: They integrate risk reduction with exercises to promote positive attitudes toward safer sex, they encourage individuals to reduce their current high-risk sexual behavior, they teach behavioral risk reduction skills (such as condom use and sexual negotiation), and they reinforce behavior change attempts. The most effective HIV prevention programs for women and youth include community-based programs with cognitive-behavioral theories and strategies, such as safe sex education and behavioral skills (Amaro, Blake, Schwartz, & Flinchbaugh, 2001a; Villarruel, Gallegos, & Cherry, 2003). However, important contextual factors for minority youth, such as community, are typically not taken into consideration in the majority of these prevention programs (Amaro, Raj, Vega, Mangione, & Perez, 2001b); given the strong influence of collectivism for Latino adolescents, this may be an important consideration. Although the foundation of social cognitive theory is the interaction between the persons, their environment, and their behavior, the majority of research has solely focused on the individual's self-efficacy, belief in one's ability to exert control over one's sexual behavior, which is still considered one of the best predictors of sexual risk-taking, particularly among minority adolescents and MSM (Bandura, 1986, 1994; Misir, 1997; Seal, Kelly, Bloom, Stevenson Coley et al., 2000; Villarruel, Jemmot, & Jemmot, 2004).

Examples of current evidence-based after-school adolescent prevention programs include "Say it Straight" and "Keepin' it Real." The "Say it Straight" program has integrated both substance use and HIV prevention and is designed for school-based delivery with a focus on wellness, empowerment, self-efficacy, self-esteem, positive relationship, strength in roots, and diversity (Delgado Bernal, 2002; Englander-Golden et al., 2007). Results indicate reductions in early sexual behavior and fewer suspensions in school due to substance abuse (Edwards & Maxson, 1994; Englander-Golden, Elconin & Miller, 1985; Englander-Golden, Elconin, Miller & Schwartzkopf, 1986; Englander-Golden & Shwarzkopf, 1986; Morton, 1990). The "Keepin' it Real" is culturally grounded in Mexican American ethnic values that focus on resiliency (Hecht et al., 2003; Hecht, Graham, & Elek, 2006; Kulis et al., 2005, 2007; Marsiglia, Kulis, Hecht, & Sills 2004; Warren et al., 2006). This is a school-based curriculum (10 lessons of 45 min with boosters and can be teacher-led, Spanish version available). This program includes outcomes (1) alcohol, cigarette, and marijuana use; (2) anti-substance use attitudes; (3) normative beliefs; and (4) substance use resistance. The focus is on helping assess risk, making decisions, increasing resistance strategies, and changing normative beliefs. However, none of these programs included social justice or critical dialogue as central aspects of their program.

4.2 Omeyocan YES Curriculum Implementation: Sample Description

Youth who participated in the Omeyocan YES project were recruited from City of South Tucson Safe Havens, including the John Valenzuela Youth Center (JVYC), Project YES (PYES), and House of Neighborly Services (HNS). From the 180 youth who were recruited by the Safe Havens, 125 youth entered and 104 completed the program and filled out posttest surveys. The final sample size ($N = 104$) included 52 males and 53 females between 13 and 18 years of age. The majority of youth were of Mexican heritage at 80 %, followed by Native American heritage at 12 %, and other ethnicity at 8 %. Youth born outside of the USA comprised 26 % of the sample. Lastly, the majority of youth reported residing in the City of South Tucson (58 %); the other youth were from nearby areas in the southwest areas of Tucson.

The Omeyocan YES program was a 2-month, 72 h after-school program with 32 lessons. On average, the youth attended 43 h of the program, with a range from 0 to 71 h. However, 53 % attended 75 % or more of the lessons. This program had a strong cultural base to the overall content as well as specific sections of the curriculum. In this manner, the curriculum had both surface and deep structure to the culturally based content (Allen et al., 2014; Resnicow et al., 1999). Cultural appropriate programs need to include deep structural changes (e.g., etiological factors and values) as well as surface structure (e.g., language) changes (Allen et al., 2014; Resnicow et al., 1999). Thus, cultural appropriateness will have more meaning to the cultural group in terms of their traditions, norms, and values that extend beyond their language preference (Resnicow et al., 1999). At a surface level, the program was delivered in English, Spanish, and bilingually (both languages at the same time). This was an important aspect of accessibility of the program for all youth in the local community, where at least 26 % were immigrants from Mexico where their first language was Spanish.

The deep structure cultural content of the program was rooted in historical context of oppression, civil rights movement, and a focus on developing a positive ethnic identity based on indigenous and Chicano/a history and cultural roots. This aspect is essential to the development of Freirian critical consciousness. A positive ethnic identity that is based on historical knowledge of one's ethnic group has been found to be associated with better mental well-being (Phinney, 1992; Roberts et al., 1999; Romero & Roberts 2003a, 2003b) and is amenable to intervention (Cherry et al., 1998; Ghee et al., 1998; Lee, 2000; Marmarosh and Corazzini, 1997). The program also had a theoretical foundation in Social Cognitive Theory (Bandura, 1986, 1994) which guided the sections on self-efficacy for refusal of substances or risky sexual behavior. This theory also guided the social modeling aspect of the program, based on a peer opinion leader model, where youth were taught to develop their own skills as social models for others in their community context. The curriculum was based on 5 workshops with the following breakdown:

- Workshop 1: Ethnic identity and Cultural History
- Workshop 2: Sexuality
- Workshop 3: Substance Use/Violence
- Workshop 4: Community Organizing
- Workshop 5: Life Skills Handbook

4.3 Background and Training of Omeyocan YES Leaders

Understanding the background and training of the Omeyocan YES program leaders is important to understanding how they developed the content of the curriculum and how they delivered it to the youth. When the opportunities for the Omeyocan YES Health Educator positions presented themselves to Luis Perales and Patty Valera, they had an outsider and insider perspective to the community of South Tucson. Whereas Luis lived and worked in the City of South Tucson, Patty emigrated from Mexico and had been living in the USA for the past 7 years at that time and worked in the city. They were insiders in the sense that they currently lived in the community. They were outsiders because they did not grow up in South Tucson and also because they felt that having a college education was not common in the community. However, they both felt that aspects of their own cultural background and communities in which they were raised gave them insider insight into the local issues experienced by youth. Embodying the words of Freire, both Health Leaders believed that everyone is important and that people ought to possess critical thinking skills so that they could understand themselves and ameliorate the issues affecting their community.

Prior to their involvement in the Omeyocan YES project, Luis and Patty shared training and experience in community activism. Having a background in community organizing and working with youth in Mexico, Patty was aware of the social injustices surrounding the border when she became a health educator with the Omeyocan YES project. Patty believed that education is linked to identity and that people with knowledge have a responsibility to improve the lives of other people. Like Patty, Luis also had work experience with activism in the City of South Tucson doing grassroots community organizing and is now the director of a charter school. Beginning as an intern with the group, *Chicanos Por La Causa* (Chicanos for the Cause or CPLC), Luis first started as an education specialist and then moved toward curriculum design and program implementation. Additionally, he has a passion to his community because he not only works in South Tucson but currently owns several properties there as well. He believes in being an active member in one's community through extra-curricular activities and being involved politically.

Patty mentioned that her upbringing on both sides of the border prepared her to become an Omeyocan YES leader. She states, "*Growing up, it was normal to talk about coyotes (term for people who guide undocumented individuals across the border for a fee)… we fed people who were about to cross the border, fed them a little because we had a little.*" At an early age, Patty was taught by her mother to make the best of any situation and be an advocate for people who had less than her. Becoming an Omeyocan YES Health Educator was very natural for Patty because she believed in giving back to her new community by serving it. To leaders like Patty who possess a history in community activism on both sides of the US/Mexico border, critical thinking does not only entail questioning tangible economic factors such as where clothes are made, the brands that are in style, worker's rights, or the quality of restaurants, but also intangible factors such as being respectful to one's elders from his/her community. With such critical consciousness, her pedagogy varied from teaching youth about self-esteem and self-care to critical thinking, such as questioning the conditions of the workers who make clothes (i.e., sweat shops or maquiladoras). The Omeyocan YES project was personal to Patty because her father was killed while living homeless because of his alcoholism. From these challenging experiences that took place in Patty's life, she was taught to be strong, kind, and to take control of her life. Patty described alcoholism as an illness in the same way doctors describe diabetes. She stated, "*When you see a person with Diabetes, we are not disrespectful.*" Consequently, Patty believed that we need to treat alcoholism as an illness because there are other social and economic factors at work here and, thus, taking a compassionate approach is necessary.

4.4 Origins of the Omeyocan YES Curriculum

A crucial aspect of any Freirian educational project is engaging in an ongoing critical dialogue between the members of that group. According to Luis, the Omeyocan YES project was first conceptualized by Latina women who were members of the

Latina Leadership Project Southern Arizona AIDS Foundation. The progressive views of these women along with those of their female youth participants must be highlighted. While the women from the Latina Youth Leadership Project created a curriculum strictly aimed toward youth female empowerment, a male component was later added because the female youth raised concern when they interacted with their male counterparts in the community. As youth female participants were becoming more conscience of the issues affecting their community, they encountered a negative response with male youth. Luis states, "*The male component of Omeyocan YES project was added in 2001. The young women were becoming liberated and then they [the female youth] said that we have become empowered, but they [the male youth] don't care. They are treating us like we are crazy...It does not do any good to just liberate women and it is not going to work if we don't also include the men.*" The dialogue that took place between the women and young females of the Omeyocan YES project demonstrate the nuances and process that take place with educational projects as maintained by Freire (1968). The female youth participants realized that that their liberation would not be complete unless they also included their male counterparts. When the female youth participants realized that change in their behavior was being hindered because the program did not include the male youth who are part of their own community, they decided that it was necessary to include men in order for both genders to become liberated. Omeyocan YES was developed based on the female-led project and was entitled Omeyocan to indicate that it was inclusive of both men and women. Freire (1968) is correct that dialogue between the leadership and the participants must be ongoing so that a collective and cohesive liberation toward achieving a more just social order takes place, or in this case a more comprehensive and effective prevention program.

4.5 Social Justice Oriented Curriculum Content

According to Luis, the Omeyocan YES project used Freire's (1968) popular education model. Taking a critical stance on those issues which directly affected the community of South Tucson, the group explored issues of "*Colonization, imperialism, consciousness building, Iraq, prison, war, and school to prison and education pipeline.*" Additionally, as an Omeyocan YES educator, Luis urged his students to explore the root causes, as well as "*symptoms*" and to apply them to their own experiences and how they themselves had contact or came to know these systems of oppression. Exploring topics that were relevant to the youth, such as the criminal justice, education, and welfare systems, resonated with them because many of them had direct lived experience with these systems. All of them were in school, some of them had been incarcerated or knew someone who had, and others received welfare assistance. Discussing these systems in the open compelled youth to think critically not just about the issues that were associated with these systems but how they too were part or were affected by them.

As some of the youth were already engaging in risky behaviors, the program urged them to think critically as to why they were getting arrested and who benefits from this unequal process, why they were on welfare, and why the South Tucson community had high dropout rates. In other words, the Omeyocan YES leaders and youth were exploring how these theoretical models were relevant, and how they could be seen and applied in their everyday world. Thus, part of this critical consciousness process is being able to see how social issues affect an individual, but also the impact that it has on his or her larger community.

Similar to Luis, Patty maintained that issues of social justice must be addressed on an individual and social level. Considering the larger societal infrastructure of income inequity in the United States and how that shapes the experiences of youth living in poverty with single or teen parents, she described how discussions which youth initiated centered on issues of social justice. She stated, "*A conversation about social justice is a must when you come and talk about issues such as single parenting or becoming young parents…substance abuse, drugs, the pressure by the media for young people to buy expensive brands, is that fair?*" For example, once the group went on a field trip to an organic grocery store that catered to upper class clientele to learn about healthy eating; thus, they learned how health access is associated with socioeconomic class and race. A holistic approach was taken to considering health that did not only focus on telling youth to stop or to not engage in risky behaviors, but an approach that also encouraged and identified healthy behaviors for a holistic approach to body, mind, and spirit.

The issue of social justice was addressed by the students and leaders of the Omeyocan YES program critically and directly through the curriculum. According to Luis, the Omeyocan YES program addressed the topic of social justice using popular and political education. He says, "*We talked directly about it. We named oppression and injustice. Heterosexism, homophobia, white supremacy, racism, prejudice, and different systems of oppression.*" It is important to highlight how the program addressed issues of social justice through the concept of "*naming*." By directly addressing different systems of oppression, these issues were no longer discussed in an abstract manner, but more concretely. The intention of the Omeyocan YES curriculum was to also show the external oppressions in relation to healthy life in order to address other forms of "*internal oppressions,*" said Luis. The program sought to connect social injustices not just on a community level but also on a personal level, addressing issues of well-being. The youth who participated in the Omeyocan YES program addressed the topic of social justice both on a personal and communal level.

Patty mentioned that she would do close readings with youth on the subject of US history when she was a leader in the program. She claims that the program sought to give youth as many real-life examples. She states, "*We were doing what I understand as critical thinking. We studied the history of Rosa Parks and Cesar Chavez… I was learning with them in a nontraditional setting. We studied the history and origin of the term Chicano, Latino, Hispanic and their identities.*" It is important to reiterate that Patty considered herself an activist and maintained that the study of one's history is crucial to any transformation. Consistent with Freire's perspective that liberation could only come from the oppressed themselves, both Patty and Luis maintained that critical pedagogy is necessary with individuals who want to escape their own oppression, and in this case they situated substance use and HIV prevention within a broader context of oppression for youth.

4.6 Omeyocan YES Impact on Youth and Program Leaders

As youth became more knowledgeable in the areas of sexuality and empowerment, this change became evident to Luis and Patty through their observations of the youth behavior and through their critical consciousness. Patty describes how youth began to feel more open to share dialogue and the evolution of topics, "*Their topics varied from social justice to public health. They would talk about their parent's busy work schedule; they talked about condoms and issues regarding sexuality. It became a safe place to talk about prevention.*" Patty maintained that the youth did not know about many of these issues before the program, and Omeyocan YES became a safe place to talk about sexual health prevention. Additionally, Patty mentions that the change that occurred while youth participated in the project was inspiring because of their young age group. She says, "*They changed and you follow their transformations...They inspired me.*" In this case, witnessing the transformation with these youth take place has a lot do with spending time within a pedagogical setting, both teaching and learning from each other. Patty also discussed the change that she saw in the critical thinking engagement that took place with youth in relation to their community. Witnessing youth become more critical in their thinking, Luis and Patty also saw the youth want to be involved in their community and desire to create positive community-level change. When youth discussed the working conditions of their parents, this demonstrated the evolution of their critical thinking to consider socioeconomic context and societal level factors that impinge on their access to health resources and healthy role models.

Considering that South Tucson is a working class community with a high level of poverty, youth were better able to understand their own socioeconomic standing. The fact that youth in the Omeyocan YES project discussed issues of social change demonstrated that youth were not only being critical of the economic disparities that existed in Arizona in relation to their community but also that youth wanted to change these injustices and thus many became activists themselves. Considering that the U.S./Mexico International Border is in relative short proximity to the City of South Tucson, the Omeyocan YES program youth were also thinking in a transnational scale. As youth dug deeper in their own pedagogy critically, discussing issues of the border and the immigrant deaths that result when human beings cross them should not have been far from their discussions. In the age of Neoliberalism, youth discussed how globalization affected their own community.

Similar to Patty, Luis also noticed a big change with youth while they participated in the Omeyocan YES program, especially in their "*knowledge awareness.*" He stated, "*They know, they understood the contemporary issues. We use the cultural knowledge and popular culture education as a vehicle on how to use condoms…We used a simple platform and made it relevant to youth.*" The platform that Luis is referring has to do with being able to use popular culture and mainstream language to make issues relevant to youth. Rather than using an esoteric model or even an academic one, youth were educated through ideas that were familiar with to them. Part of this framework that Luis discusses has to do with meeting youth were they are at as opposed to expecting youth to put becoming self-educated. This platform is hinged on the idea of support and trust. It is important to highlight an interesting dynamic that took place with the Omeyocan YES youth as they progressed in the program. Luis stated that in the beginning of the program, youth were not engaging in risky behavior. But then they started to report having more sex, getting high with marijuana, and getting into more trouble. When the Omeyocan YES leaders asked the youth why they were engaging in more risky behavior despite becoming more educated about safe sex, the dangers of drugs, and not getting into trouble, Luis stated that youth informed the Omeyocan YES leaders that, "*We [now] like you and trust you.*" In other words, as youth became more comfortable and felt that they could trust the program leaders, they also became more honest about discussing their risky behaviors, previously they had not felt open to share.

A key reason why the Omeyocan YES program was effective in the City of South Tucson was because it embodied Freire's (1968) concept of creating dialogue between the leaders and those being educated. Whereas some youth shared more information in a one-on-one, others did so in a group setting. In order to be effective in community-based research projects, it is necessary to utilize both methods to reach adolescents which help youth open up. Patty discussed the experience of a student who was on probation and living with his grandmother. Though he never mentioned this to anyone before, it was not until this youth was given the opportunity to speak in a group setting that he shared his experience with them. According to Patty, "*His hoping mechanism was getting in trouble. We were teaching him that there was more. He deserved more and had the capacity to succeed.*" This young person was beginning to give up hope, and the program was teaching him not only that there was promise in his future, but also how he could achieve it. When community leaders who engage in community-based research genuinely engage and care for youth and their community, they will connect and have positive responses. This is what took place with the Omeyocan YES health education project.

4.7 Navigating Community Context for Advocacy and Caution

Both community activists maintained that the group was successful in accomplishing its goals because it provided the youth with tools in both how to critically understand their communities and how to enact changes from within. Consistent with Freire's model of revolutionary leaders organizing and creating pedagogical dialogue in their spaces, the project focused on youth ages 13–18 years that represented different subcultures within the communities. Patty stated, "*I think they accomplished a positive change and consequently, they shared their new acquired knowledge with their peers.*" Some of the people who voluntarily involved and helped in the project were artists, poets, and activists. Patty further stated that youth received all this information, and they took it to their communities and shared it with their peers. Similar to Patty, Luis strongly believes in praxis and distinguishes between theory and practice. Being a firm believer of political education, Luis maintained that learning local, transnational, and global issues is good for youth's educational experiences and the community. Luis strongly believed in community-based participatory research and using pedagogy as a means of taking action in order to change a community issue. According to Luis, civic engagement initially looked like advocacy because the program covered broad issues, but then moved toward a more personal level. From advocacy, the program then advanced toward organizing, but not in terms of rallies or marches "*but more like events, conversations, and representing in conferences.*" Luis takes community activism very serious and maintains that he was activist when he served as an Omeyocan YES leader, but that he now sees himself as an organizer and community developer. He stated that his role was simply to point kids in the right direction and to have a "*valuable place*" where they could share their experiences. Luis states that youth did not considered themselves activists when they started the program and it was not until completing the project that some of them became activists.

However, there was also tension and caution in how the program leaders navigated political and community contexts while implementing a youth program on controversial topics. It was the first HIV prevention program in the community, Luis mentioned that:

> The program operated under the radar because it was controversial for some staff in the City of South Tucson, not for the university or the program itself. They saw it as a good program, but the fear was having a government structure blowback. The debate centered on whether to take an abstinence/prevention or harm reduction approach. We decided that we are going to meet the youth where they are. We are not just going to do prevention and we took the reduction approach, and it was controversial... We were afraid that decision makers would believe we were encouraging youth to engage in risky behaviors... There was never any blowback, but there was a perception. The question became, if they are already engaging in risky behavior, how can you cut that down? We started with prevention but then it turned to intervention. We started engaging the youth in dialogue and many then said, this is what my friends are doing and this is what we need.

In other words, the program received funding to empower and teach youth about issues of sexuality, and the funders left latitude as to the precise manner in which the curriculum would be taught. As some of the leaders received training in Mexican–American Studies or Chicano/a Studies and ethnic studies, they incorporated the work of critical theorists in their pedagogy. Moreover, through the Omeyocan YES educational project, both leaders and students did not refrain from discussing issues that were deemed taboo or contentious. Consequently, the leaders felt that some of the discussion content which resulted from the program should be kept on a low key because the leaders did not want to spark negative attention to the critical educational space that was created with the youth. Luis says:

> We kept to ourselves for fear that we were talking about sex, drugs, race, class, gender, and sexuality… We were conscious that people of authority. Adults in our communities did not want to talk about it. What we said in public versus what we were talking to the youth about…We had to be careful from those who thought 'we know what it is best, you have to do it this way.' It was not in a negative way… the official stance was 'please don't create waves.' The unofficial stance was 'do what you have to do to help the community.' It all falls in the realm of politics…

Thus, while they were educating youth to speak out and be advocates for health, the program leaders often felt tension among adults and the community about the reality of adolescent health issues. He also mentioned that adults did not want to critically engage these issues with other members of their community at that time. The community organizations also felt this tension, and that they were often not included into the messages that the programs were developing. These tensions were part of what led to the next steps in the South Tucson Prevention Coalition partnership model. This perhaps is a sharp reminder about the level of community readiness during Phase 1, which was often at a level of denial among many adults. While this made it difficult, it also clarified the importance of moving Phase 2 toward more inclusivity of the broader community into dialogue and collaboration. So often youth are trained in these sort of safe youth spaces with youth allies, but are left with no infrastructure or resources in low income communities to continue their struggle for health advocacy.

It is important to highlight the role that the word *critical* plays in this discussion because it is what made this project a revolutionary one. It is one thing to theorize and talk about social change; it is another thing to organize, mobilize, and be politically active in one's community and take an intervention approach *versus* a prevention one. The Omeyocan YES project was unique because it created youth leaders who were ready to create change. The decision to stay under the radar by the leaders of the Omeyocan YES program they felt was necessary just to begin to get the information out to youth since there were no other programs in existence.

The topics that the Omeyocan YES program addressed must be explored by every community both to create awareness and as a form of safety prevention or in this case an intervention. Aside from the Omeyocan YES program's effectiveness in raising the consciousness awareness of the youth from their community, Luis mentioned that the group did not want to be mislabeled for being too "*critical, radical, or militant*" for taking an intervention approach to ameliorate community issues. Thus, despite being a progressive program, the leaders feared being stigmatized because members of the Chicano/a and Latino/a community have historically been labeled, especially when struggling to uplift the social conditions of their communities and navigating prevention and intervention approaches as it was in this case. Given that Arizona in just a few years later would enact new laws to limit ethnic studies in k-12 public schools and to expand immigration enforcement, perhaps it was judicious of the leaders to consider the political climate when deciding how to handle external relations (O'Leary, Romero, Cabrera, & RAscon, 2012). Youth, and their adult allies, were both navigating different cultural and social norms and such is the case with any educational project that seeks to bring about social change. It highlights the challenges that were ahead to integrating youth and adults who were assumed or perceived to not be allies. It also emphasizes the need for breaking down barriers between youth and adults when working on collaborative community projects.

4.8 Youth Leaders Carry the Message Forward

A key aspect in creating dialogue between the leadership and students in this case is making sure that the former makes itself accessible to the other body. Patty stated, "*Being a program in the barrio, bringing the program to their homes and making it easier for them to go. They just go there. It was a really good move. The staff was doing recruitment at one point. Our role was to go and teach one cohort and then they would go tell their friends and cousins about them.*" It is evident that the program was effective in its methods of recruitment because these leaders made themselves visible to the community of South Tucson. Through word of mouth and material incentives (i.e., stipends, books, gift cards, etc.), youth heard and learned more about the project and informed their friends and relatives about it. Consequently, it is important for adolescents like those who live in the City of South Tucson to get exposed to positive things and institutions, so that they could slowly break the cycle of poverty and oppression. Patty mentioned that they took the youth to the University of Arizona not only to motivate them to go there but to expand their thinking and make youth feel that they belong to a much larger community, the State of Arizona.

Both Patty and Luis maintained that the Omeyocan YES program was a huge success and an important step in their personal and professional developments. Patty believes that the program was a success because youth made a connection between social justice and their community. She stated, "*Social justice exists. It empowers and gives the community the tools to take action… Social Justice is una espada de dos filos [a doubled-edged sword] because it focused on prevention. Has two components. That was the best program because it gave me my foundation.*"

Patty's conceptualization of social justice precisely that it is a two-edged sword that both empowers and serves as prevention to youth. Additionally, the background of the leaders of the Omeyocan YES project is very important because their beliefs and past experiences helped not only guide the young men and women that they served but also empowered them to take a critical social justice stance to substance use prevention. Patty mentioned that she often saw herself in the youth and understood them very well because she too came from a struggling background. It is safe to assume that this outlook or perspective was reciprocal or else this project would not have been successful. In other words, whereas it is important for service providers to understand and see themselves in community-based participatory research, it is also as important for those receiving the service to see and understand those who are providing the service. Patty knew that using her past experiences in her pedagogy allowed her to teach her students that despite their community hardships and personal struggles, they could either become victims or agents of social change. Rather than being victimizing oneself individually or socially, it was best to have a proactive attitude and take control of one's destiny and the future of one's community.

4.9 Youth Quantitative Survey Data Results

All youth who participated in the program were asked to complete self-report questionnaires at two different time points (pre and post). Youth were asked questions about their attitudes and behaviors related to alcohol, drugs, and other health items at three time points (pretest and posttest).

4.10 Risky Behaviors Prior to Omeyocan YES

On average, youth began using alcohol at 13 ½ years old. Youth indicated that 17 % had never using alcohol in their lifetime, 55 % reported not using alcohol in the past 30 days and 75 % reported not being drunk in the past 30 days. Alcohol was the substance that is was most often used by the majority of the youth. Prior to beginning the Omeyocan YES program 77 % of youth reported *NOT* being involved in previous drug and alcohol use preventing programs. The majority of youth had never had sexual intercourse, 56 %, 57 % had not had sex in the past 30 days. Of those who reported having sex in the past 30 days, 63 % reported using a condom, 16 % reported drinking alcohol or using drugs before sexual intercourse, and 18 % reported being high or drunk before sex in the past 3 months.

4.10.1 Statistically Significant Changes from Pretest to Posttest

Youth reported significant changes in attitudes and behaviors from before the Omeyocan YES program compared to after the program. There was a significant decrease in frequency of drinking alcoholic beverages in the *last 30 days* from pretest ($M=1.95$, SD$=1.37$) to posttest ($M=1.65$, SD$=1.03$); $t(101)=2.24$, $p<0.03$. The difference from pre to post in binge drinking was not significant, but was trending toward decrease ($M=1.48$, SD$=0.98$) to posttest ($M=1.30$, SD$=0.63$); $t(101)=1.75$, $p=0.08$.

There were statistically significant increases from pre to posttest in youth comfort in speaking about (A), saying no to alcohol (pre $M=2.84$, SD$=1.12$; post $M=3.13$, SD$=1.01$; $t=-2.08$, $p<0.04$) (B), about family members using alcohol or drugs (pre $M=2.55$, SD$=1.18$; post $M=2.81$, SD$=2.81$, SD$=1.12$; $t=1.99$, $p<0.05$) (C), how using alcohol/drugs can make a person vulnerable to unwanted sexual advances (pretest $M=2.59$, SD$=1.14$; posttest $M=2.86$, SD$=1.06$; $t=-2.08$,

$p<0.04$). However, there were no significant changes in how often the youth spoke about these topics.

Youth also learned about HIV prevention in the Omeyocan YES program, and results indicate that youth demonstrated a significant increase in their HIV knowledge. Whereas youth had on average 3.63 (SD = 1.07) items correct out of 5 possible at pretest they had 4.05 (SD = 1.16) answers right at posttest ($t=-2.99$, $p<0.001$).

At posttest, after the end of Omeyocan YES, youth were significantly more likely to report feeling more self-efficacy to refuse alcohol from a friend (pre: $M=3.00$, SD = 1.03; post: $M=3.27$, SD = 0.82; $t(101)=-2.50$, $p<0.05$).

Youth also significantly increased their critical ethnic consciousness from pretest to posttest (pre: $M=3.16$, SD = 0.54; post: $M=3.30$, SD = 0.46; $t(104)=-3.01$, $p<0.01$). They also significantly increased their self-esteem from pretest to posttest (pretest: $M=3.76$, SD = 0.71; posttest $M=3.91$, SD = 0.78; $t(104)=-2.28$, $p<0.05$).

Lastly, there was a significant increase of youth participation at local Safe Havens where the Omeyocan YES program was offered. There was a significant increase in the frequency of their participation from an average of 2 days at pre-test ($M=2.33$, SD = 1.99) to an average of 3 days at posttest ($M=3.10$, SD = 2.14) ($t=-3.58$, $p<0.001$) This is a key factor for the transition to STPC Phase 2 where youth worked more directly with the adults in the local community centers.

4.10.2 *Qualitative Evaluation: Youth in Their Own Words…*

The experiences of the Chicano/a Latino/a youth who participated in the Omeyocan YES project sheds light on the complexity of how a revolutionary leadership helps create educational liberation (Freire, 1968). Freire (1968) states, "*The correct method…in the task of liberation is, therefore, not 'libertarian propaganda.' Nor can the leadership merely 'implant' in the oppressed a belief in freedom, thus thinking to win their trust. The correct method lies in dialogue*." It is clear that the leadership of the Omeyocan YES program neither created a *propaganda* project nor *implanted* the youth a belief of freedom because the youth derived their own conclusions of *liberation* through ongoing *dialogue*. This notion is corroborated by the youth who responded to open-ended questions at the end of the posttest survey. What follows are some of their comments regarding what they learned while participating in the Omeyocan YES program.

4.10.3 *What Youth Learned About Health from Omeyocan YES*

Youth were asked what they learned that was new about drugs or alcohol in the program. Responses included: "*That the amount of alcohol is not always the same in every beverage*," "*That drugs could get you into serious problems*," "*Drugs mess up your mind,*" "*I learn that I will never do those things because there is consequences.*" As mentioned earlier, one of the main goals of the Omeyocan YES program was to dispel the myths associated with drugs and alcohol by providing youth with the facts and realities that are scientifically proven regarding these issues. **From the Youth who completed the program**, responses included, "*That some of the drugs are really bad,*" "*I didn't know that just because of injection you could get your arm cut off,*" "*Everything,*" "*Don't abuse the use of drugs and alcohol,*" "*Es peligroso yo lo hago porque (illegible) pero si quisiera ahorita lo dejaba ahorita*" (*It is dangerous and I do it because (illegible) but if I wanted to right now, I would leave it right now], and "When you do cocaine that you are not hungry a lot.*" **From the Youth who did not complete the program**, responses included: "*nada" (nothing), "That they can do a lot of harm," and "Que son las consequencias que pasa" (What are the consequences that happen).* Clearly, youth in the program learned more specifics about how drugs work and why to avoid them given the short-term and long-term effects that they have on the human body.

Youth were asked what they learned that was new about sex or condoms. Responses included: "*How to put a condom and how to really say no to sex if you don't want to,*" "*How to use one,*" "*I don't know a lot of things,*" "*You could get pregnant even with a condom,*" "*That only sometimes your condoms would work,*" "*Always use condoms,*" and "*Condoms can break if you don't put them on right.*" Aside from learning safe practices when engaging in sex, youth also learned about the realities of it and how to assert their power if or when having sexual intercourse. Only one youth responded, "*Nothing I didn't know.*" **From the Youth who completed the program**, responses included, "*I learned how to properly put one on,*" "*Well everything was new to me except for the obvious things,*" "*Everything,*" "*That condoms had a certain way to be put on,*" "*muchas, cómo usarlas y protejerme" (many, how to use them and protect myself), "Hay muchas enfermedades y es mucho mejor usarlo plactiar bien es mejor la absiencia" (there are a lot diseases and is much better to use (illegible) good abstinence is better), "That you can get HIV with no condom,*" "*That sex should be enjoyable,*" and "*blue balls don't exist.*" Youth learned about the dangers associated with sex and condoms and about safe sexual practices. Whereas youth learned about abstinence being the safest and best method when it comes to sex, youth also learned about the different forms of STDs, especially about HIV. At minimum, the Omeyocan YES program helped achieved its goals of spreading awareness of the facts associated with sex and using condoms and dispelling the myths associated with these issues.

With regard to some of the things that youth learned about Sexual Transmitted Diseases (STDs), one youth responded, "*That if you don't protect yourself there are a lot of diseases that it is better to protect yourself.*" It is evident that the response of this youth touches on the issue of safety and encompasses the different sort of STDs that he/she learned while being in the program. He or she states why it necessary to protect oneself from STDs because they could be acquired through different ways and some symptoms could take time to become visible. As HIV was a main focus of the Omeyocan YES curriculum, this statement demonstrates that youth learned about the diseases which could take up to 10 years to show themselves; thus, "*It is better to protect yourself.*" Whereas this youth implicitly alluded to STDs like HIV, another youth made his/her statement more explicitly, when he/she stated, "*You can get AIDS if you don't use proper safety.*"

4.10.4 Did You Like the Program and Why?

In response to what part of the program they liked the most, many youth responded that they liked all of it. Some specifically said that they liked "*Learning things that I didn't know*." Several youth indicated that they liked the retreats and field trips. Other youth reported that they liked the content of the sex talks, STIs, and sexuality. They also liked learning about the world, culture, and discussing beer ads. Additionally, some youth reported that they liked the messages and attitude of the program. Youth also learned about Chicano/a Latino/a history and culture. One youth stated that he/she enjoyed, "*Learning about my culture and more*." As noted by Patty, youth not only learned about US history from a Chicano/a perspective, but also about health, how to think critically, and how to organize and become activists in their community. Indeed, a key theme of educational projects is the concept of pedagogy itself and the power that it has to influence and change the life of people through the way in which curriculum is carried out.

From those who **completed the program**, many stated that they really liked the retreats. Others indicated: "*Sobre sexo, los derechos de los jovenes, el primer retiro y las placticas sobre anuncios de cerveza" (About sex, the rights of youth, the first retreat and the discussions over beer ads), and "La explicación, mensajes, viajes, la actidud, todo menos estar 8 horas sentadas" (The, explanations, messages, trips, the attitude, everything except sitting down for eight hours).* Hence, some youth indicated that they like everything about the program with the exception of being in a classroom for 8 h a day at the retreats.

Whereas some youth enjoyed almost all aspects of the program, some youth did not share the same views. The **Youth who did not complete the program** commented about the money. One other youth said the lessons were not fun because they were really serious. However, most youth responded that they had fun with the lessons "*Because we learned new things*" and "*Because we were told things that we wouldn't hear from other people*." Indeed, community-based programs are significant because they can thoroughly explore concepts and subjects which are not addressed in school curricula. Another advantage of these programs is that youth do not have to adhere to the standards of formality associated with the school system and can feel more comfortable when learning. For example, **Youth who completed program** responded: "*They were fun because we had fun stuff like saying your thoughts," "There was days that were fun like hands on stuff," and "Because we laugh a lot*." However, youth who did not complete the program responded that: "*No podría decir" (I would not be able to tell), "Yes because they interacted with us," and "Sex because we made jokes of it*." Being completely voluntary, youth participated in the Omeyocan YES project because they found it interesting, comfortable, and fun.

Youth were asked if the Omeyocan YES staff made them feel comfortable. Twelve youth wrote "yes." With regard to how they felt around staff and what they liked about them, some added "*Because they were friendly," "Because they helped me out," "Because they were really nice, helpful," and "Because they were like people you could talk to about anything*." The Omeyocan YES program provided an inclusive space where youth felt they could share anything and be transparent about their experiences with adult allies. What is important to highlight here is that the youth actively took part in the creation of this collaborative process. However, there were two refusals and one blank. Additionally, from the **Youth who completed program**, seven responded "yes" and added: "*Because they were cool and they always listened to your every word,*" "*Because they would ask me questions to make me understand,*" "*Because they understood everything,*" "*Because they understand me,*" "*Porque son divertidos lo cual puedes relajarte y aprender major,*" *(because they are fun of which I can relax and learn major), "Mucha confinaza, deberían durar más tiempo no sólo 3 años" (lots of trust, should last more time not just three years), and "Because he was cool.*" Luis' general assertion of *meeting youth where they are* and engaging them in critical and theoretical analyses is one of the main reasons why the Omeyocan YES project curriculum resonated with youth, and they felt their interests were met. Educational projects are pedagogically effective because they address the sociopolitical and economic relations that surround individuals and their communities, and through ongoing dialogue, youth are able to explore, critique, contextualize, and formulate solutions or plan as to how they can change or alleviate social issues.

Freire's (1968) concept of creating dialogue highlights the importance of why leaders need to create a fun, productive, and healthy space that is based on trust. Once this trust is established, youth are then able to connect with adult leaders on a personal level and feel comfortable and valued. Two responded *yes* and added: "*Because they were part of my race" and "Because we would talk about lots of stuff very often.*" Indeed, the experiences of the youth from the Omeyocan YES program were enhanced by them seeing leaders from their own ethnic background because they were able to see themselves in these leaders and could relate to them on a cultural level. Although this is not a necessary condition in any educational project, doing so often makes a difference in the dialogue process. Understanding a person's language, culture, and traditional ways firsthand can make youth feel more comfortable.

4.10.5 What Youth Would Tell Other Youth about Omeyocan YES

One of the best ways to learn about the impact that a community-based program has on a community is to measure the effects that a project has on youth, their friends, and their relatives. A question asked if youths would tell their friends about this program and what would they tell them. Six youths wrote "yes" and added things such as, "*They should go because you learn everything you had always question yourself for,*" "*Because it's important and you can protect yourself from diseases and other things,*" "*You learn about stuff they don't teach in school,*" "*It's very interesting and it makes you think twice before you go out and do something,*" and "*That the program is fun.*"

Some of the goals of the Omeyocan YES project were not just to educate youth on matters of sexuality and empowerment but also for them to pass this information to their family and peers as well. From the **Youth who completed program**, three responded "*Tell them about it.*" Other responses were varied and included: "*I would just spread the word,*" "*Placticarles sobre las cosas interesantes que nos placticaron" (Talk to them about the interesting things that they talked to us about), "Jugar basquetbol, más juegos" (Play basketball, more games.), and "To talk with them.*" Other *responses included: "I would tell them that there is a lot of important stuff to do." "I would tell them what we studied about and tell them it was really fun!", "Everything," "I would say to join it or else they will regret not joining." "Que pueden asistir este programa porque es importante informales"* (That they can attend this program because it is important to inform them.), "*Les dije estuvieron interesados pero no pudieron asistir*" (I told them, they were interested, but could not attend), "*Yes, would tell them it's fun*" and "*Yes.*" As noted, many youth saw the positive impact that the program had on them, and they shared this information with others. As youth became educated and empowered with the information that they learned about health, youth saw the value of educating members of their own community as well. Indeed, part of the empowerment process is to also empower their family and friends. From the **Youth who did not complete program**, *one youth left the question blank and other responses included "Que te dan dinero por hacer las pruebas"* (that they give you money for doing the tests) and "*When I see them.*"

One of the goals of the Omeyocan YES project was not just to educate youth about the issues of sexuality, drugs, etc. but also to dispel myths associated with these subjects by teaching youth correct methods, especially with safe sex and contraceptives. Consequently, youth were asked about what they knew about these issues, and educators then, using the dialogue method, facilitated discussion around these issues. Elaborating on whether they would tell a relative or friend about the program, other responses included "*To go because they show you stuff you might not know," "That this is a great program for your future," and "Instead of doing nothing you could do this program and actually learn something.*" Youth corroborate why programs like Omeyocan YES serve as useful and personal learning experiences, and they are so valuable in the community.

4.11 Conclusion

Using a revolutionary curriculum that was inspired by Paulo Freire's pedagogical model, the leaders and educators of the Omeyocan YES project created a safe learning space for Chicano/a Latino/a youth that resulted in reductions in alcohol use, increases in self-efficacy to refuse alcohol, comfort in talking about alcohol, increases in critical consciousness of ethnic identity, and linkages to local community-based organizations. The Omeyocan YES project was successful in the development of youth leaders in a youth allied space that would be fundamental to Phase 2 South Tucson Prevention Coalition with youth working in the larger community with adults. Omeyocan YES gave youth the tools to seek social justice-based changes in their own community after they graduated from the program. In the following chapters, we will further discuss the key components that facilitated the collaborations and community changes. Additionally, this educational project allowed for bidirectional dialogue and learning to take place between leaders like Luis and Patty and youth that led to the capacity to ameliorate the issues of alcohol, drugs, and risky sexual behavior in their own community. The Omeyocan YES program demonstrates that critical pedagogy to prevent and reduce substance use and HIV can raise the critical consciousness of youth about how to see themselves in society and how to understand their ethnic background. To have youth positively engage in critical analysis of their community and world around them, it is absolutely necessary for them to see themselves as active members of it and to understand the potential role that each one plays as an individual and as a group.

References

Allen, J., Mohatt, G. V., Beehler, S., & Rowe, H. L. (2014). People awakening: Collaborative research to develop cultural strategies for prevention in community intervention. *American Journal of Community Psychology, 54*, 100–111.

Amaro, H., Blake, S. M., Schwartz, P. M., & Flinchbaugh, L. J. (2001a). Developing theory-based substance abuse prevention programs for young adolescent girls. *Journal of Early Adolescence (Special Issue: Substance Abuse Prevention Among Young Female Adolescents), 21*(3), 256–293.

Amaro, H., Raj, A., Vega, R. R., Mangione, T. W., & Perez, L. N. (2001b). Racial/ethnic disparities in the HIV and substance use epidemics: Communities responding to the need. *Public Health Reports, 116*(5), 434–448.

Bandura, A. (1986). *Social foundations of thought and action: A social cognitive theory*. Englewood Cliffs, NJ: Prentice-Hall.

Bandura, A. (1994). Social cognitive theory and exercise of control over HIV infection. In R. J. DiClemente & J. L. Peterson (Eds.), *Preventing AIDS: Theories and methods of behavioral interventions* (pp. 25–59). New York: Plenum Press.

Bernal, D. D. (2002). Critical race theory, Latino critical theory, and critical raced-gendered epistemologies: Recognizing students of color as holders and creators of knowledge. *Qualitative inquiry, 8*(1), 105–126.

Cherry, V. R., Belgrave, F. Z., Jones, W., Kennon, D. K., Gray, F. S., & Phillips, F. (1998). NTU: An Africentric approach to substance abuse prevention among African American youth. *Journal of Primary Prevention, 18*(3), 319–339.

Englander-Golden, P., Elconin, J., Miller, K. J., & Schwarzkopf, A. B. (1986). Brief SAY IT STRAIGHT training and follow-up in adolescent substance abuse prevention. *Journal of Primary Prevention, 6*(4), 219–230.

Freire, P. (1968). *Pedagogy of the oppressed*. New York, NY: Seabury Press.

Ghee, K. L., Walker, J., & Younger, A. C. (1998). The RAAMUS Academy: Evaluation of an educultural intervention for young African-American males. *Journal of Prevention & Intervention in the Community, 16*(1–2), 87–102.

Hecht, M. L., Graham, J. W., & Elek, E. (2006). The drug resistance strategies intervention: Program effects on substance use. *Health Communication, 20*(3), 267–276.

Hecht, M. L., Marsiglia, F. F., Elek, E., Wagstaff, D. A., Kulis, S., Dustman, P., & Miller-Day, M. (2003). Culturally grounded substance use prevention: An evaluation of the keepin' it real curriculum. *Prevention Science, 4*, 233–248.

Kulis, S., Marsiglia, F. F., Elek, E., Dustman, P., Wagstaff, D. A., & Hecht, M. L. (2005). Mexican/Mexican American adolescents and keepin'it REAL: An evidence-based substance use prevention program. *Children and Schools, 27*(3), 133–145.

Kulis, S., Nieri, T., Yabiku, S., Stromwall, L. K., & Marsiglia, F. F. (2007). Promoting reduced and discontinued substance use among adolescent substance users: Effectiveness of a universal prevention program. *Prevention Science, 8*(1), 35–49.

Marmarosh, C. L., & Corazzini, J. G. (1997). Putting the group in your pocket: Using collective identity to enhance personal and collective self-esteem. *Group Dynamics: Theory, Research, and Practice, 1*(1), 65.

Marsiglia, F. F., Kulis, S., Hecht, M. L., & Sills, S. (2004). Ethnicity and ethnic identity as predictors of drug norms and drug use among preadolescents in the US southwest. *Substance Use & Misuse, 39*(7), 1061–1094.

Misir, P. (1997). Behavioral interventions for black and Latino men who have sex with men. *AIDS Patient Care and STDs, 11*, 6–8.

O'Leary AO, Romero AJ, Cabrera NL, Rascón M, 2012. Assault on ethnic studies. Santa Anna O, González de Bustamante C, Eds. In: *Arizona firestorm: Global realities, national media and provincial politics*. Rowman & Littlefield, Lanham, MD, pp. 97–120.

Peterson, J. L., & DiClemente, R. J. (2000). *Handbook of HIV prevention*. London: Taylor & Francis.

Phinney, J. (1992). The multigroup ethnic identity measure: A new scale for use with diverse groups. *Journal of Adolescent Research, 7*, 156–176.

Resnicow, K., Baranowski, T., Ahluwalia, J. S., & Braithwaite, R. L. (1999). Cultural sensitivity in public health: Defined and demystified. *Ethnicity and Disease, 9*(1), 10–21.

Roberts, R. E., Phinney, J. S., Masse, L. C., Chen, Y. R., Roberts, C. R., & Romero, A. (1999). The structure of ethnic identity of young adolescents from diverse ethnocultural groups. *The Journal of Early Adolescence, 19*(3), 301–322.

Romero, A. J., & Roberts, R. E. (2003a). The impact of multiple dimensions of ethnic identity on discrimination and adolescents? Self-esteem. *Journal of Applied Social Psychology, 33*(11), 2288–2305.

Romero, A. J., & Roberts, R. E. (2003b). Stress within a bicultural context for adolescents of Mexican descent. *Cultural Diversity and Ethnic Minority Psychology, 9*(2), 171–184.

Seal, D. W., Kelly, J. A., Bloom, F. R., Stevenson, L. Y., Coley, B. I., & Broyles, L. A. (2000). HIV prevention with young men who have sex with men: What young men themselves say is needed. *AIDS Care, 12*, 5–26.

Villarruel, A., Gallegos, E., & Cherry, C. (2003). La uniendo de fronteras: Collaboration to develop HIV prevention strategies for Mexican and Latino youth. *Journal of Transcultural Nursing, 14*(3), 193–206.

Villarruel, A., Jemmot, J., & Jemmot, L. (2004). Predictors of sexual intercourse and condom use intentions among Spanish-dominant Latino youth. *Nursing Research, 53*(3), 172–181.

Warren, J. R., Hecht, M. L., Wagstaff, D. A., Elek, E., Ndlaye, K., Dustman, P., & Marsiglia, F. (2006). Communicating prevention: the effects of the keepin' it real classroom videotapes and televised PSAs on middle school student's substance use. *Journal of Applied Communication Research, 34*(2), 209–227.

Chapter 5
Breaking Down Silos Between Community-Based Organizations: Coalition Development

Jesi Post, Gloria Hamelitz-Lopez, Kimberly Sierra-Cajas, and Andrea Romero

Abstract This chapter explores how community-based organizations broke down silos to work together and to form the South Tucson Prevention Coalition (STPC), whose goals were to prevent and decrease underage drinking in the City of South Tucson. Through the development of the STPC, distinct community groups were brought together toward a common cause. This led to significant changes in the way that community agencies and leaders saw their role within the larger community. It also involved organized collective efforts from numerous community members. This included long-term relationship- and trust building with a university researcher, sharing of resources by community agencies, the initiation of a shared funding source through a community-focused grant, and the dedication of all parties to the betterment of youth and the community at large. To understand the processes behind the events, we bring stories from leaders of the community-based organizations House of Neighborly Services (HNS) and the John Valenzuela Youth Center (JVYC). We explore how these organizations evolved from operating as independent silos to community partners. Through their stories, they demonstrate how critical consciousness contributed to the important breaking down of these silos so that they could work together toward a common cause.

J. Post, M.S. (✉)
Mel and Enid Zuckerman College of Public Health, University of Arizona,
3950 S. Country Club, Suite 330, Tucson, AZ, USA
e-mail: jhpost@email.arizona.edu

G. Hamelitz-Lopez
John Valenzuela Youth Center, Tucson, AZ, USA
e-mail: gloriahamelitz@hotmail.com

K. Sierra-Cajas
Office of Undergraduate Research, College of Science, University of Arizona,
Tucson, AZ, USA
e-mail: kjsc@email.arizona.edu

A. Romero, Ph.D.
Family Studies and Human Development, University of Arizona,
650 N. Park Avenue, Tucson, AZ 85719, USA
e-mail: romeroa@u.arizona.edu

A.J. Romero (ed.), *Youth-Community Partnerships for Adolescent Alcohol Prevention*, DOI 10.1007/978-3-319-26030-3_5

Keywords STPC • Coalition • Coalition building • Silos • Building trust • Relationship building • Community readiness • Community involvement • Critical consciousness • Community grant writing

The South Tucson Prevention Coalition (STPC) was a coalition that served the City of South Tucson. ***The mission of the Coalition was to prevent substance use among adolescents (age 9–15 years) in the City of South Tucson. The long-term goals were (1) to expand and strengthen collaboration among Coalition members to support prevention and reduction of youth alcohol use; (2) to prevent or delay adolescent first use of alcohol through perception of risk and harm from drugs and disapproval of drug use by peers and family; (3) promote data driven prevention services for alcohol use among youth.*** The Coalition's plan to reduce underage drinking focused on: (1) past 30-day use frequency and (2) perception of disapproval of use by peers and adults. The coalition participated in coalition building activities, which promoted a community-level readiness for change (see Chap. 2). STPC coalition members were strongly engaged in efforts to prevent or delay youth alcohol use as a method of achieving community empowerment. They were also strongly engaged in transforming the resilience of their own community to promote the healthy development of adolescents.

The creation and development of STPC was essential to creating community-level change. However, this was not an easy process given that the participating groups were originally doing little to no work on adolescent alcohol prevention. While there were several Safe Havens and services groups in South Tucson, they were working in silos, such that they were not sharing information, were not sharing resources, and were not working together on projects. Breaking down these silos within a low-income community was challenging given that they often felt they were competing with each other for grants and community participation. This chapter will provide more insight into a case study of the process of coalition building based on historical documents and the retrospective perspective of in-depth interviews with key community leaders from the local community-based organizations that led South Tucson Prevention Coalition.

5.1 History of the Coalition Development

The Omeyocan YES program (described in Chap. 4) led to the development of a collaborative among agencies and individuals who were involved in recruiting youth at the locations where the program was offered. The organization of the representatives from each of the participating agencies came to be named South Tucson Prevention Collaborative, which included John Valenzuela Youth Center, House of Neighborly Service, Project YES, Dr. Romero from Mexican American Studies at the University of Arizona, Southern Arizona AIDS Foundation, and City of South

Tucson. Over 3 years of the Omeyocan YES program, the community-based organization (CBO) representatives began meeting monthly to further collaboration, increase communication across agencies, and discuss current topics. Previously no substance abuse or HIV prevention programs were available at these locations; thus, CBOs demonstrated a significant increase in awareness and capacity to prevent substance use and HIV issues.

Capacity building activities began by including an annual 1-day retreat for all coalition members. This was an opportunity to discuss progress, review the future goals of the grant, share experiences from the past year, and enhance communication and understanding among all collaborators. During the retreats, each agency led a workshop session, including evaluators, Safe Havens, City of South Tucson, Youth Graduate Peer Educators, SAAF, and local community members who were HIV positive. Participatory action research principles were the guiding model for interactions and community; for example, the majority of decisions were made collectively during regular meetings, and suggestions were always solicited from representatives of all collaborators. Additionally, research findings from the ongoing evaluation of the Omeyocan YES program were shared; however, at this stage community members were not involved in creating or conducting research. While the collective decision making was challenging to implement, it was a fruitful method of enhancing collaborative efforts. Annual retreats provided opportunities to increase capacity on substance use topics, as well as prevention techniques, culturally appropriate prevention techniques, and local prevention/intervention resources. This work was the foundation for the development of a Drug-Free grant proposal in order to fund further development of the Collaborative into a Coalition.

At the end of the third year of funding for the Omeyocan YES project, the collaborative decided to take on new federal funding opportunities. The first federal grant development was led by one of the Collaborative's community-based organization executive directors, Kimberly Sierra-Cajas. Several meetings were held in the City of South Tucson government buildings with representatives from the government, police, local agencies, and university. The grant was best suited for submission through the City of South Tucson, although the previous grant for Omeyocan YES was led by Dr. Romero and submitted through the University. Discussions were held on all aspects of the grant development (see Fig. 5.1) from budget development to the project narrative. The grant was primarily co-written by the City grant writer, Dr. Romero of the University of Arizona, Kimberly Sierra-Cajas, Executive Director of the House of Neighborly Services, and Gloria Hamelitz-Lopez, Executive Director of the John Valenzuela Youth Center.

The proposed goal of the Coalition was to educate and mobilize individuals and the community at-large to address substance abuse prevention through a campaign of activities to promote opportunities for working toward positive change within the community. Community prevention programs that aim to reach populations in multiple settings, schools, clubs, faith-based organizations, and the media are most effective when they present consistent, community-wide messages in each setting (Chou et al., 1998). A central goal of the STPC was to increase community-level readiness for change by increasing community awareness of services

Memorandum

To: Fernando Castro- City Manager, Richard Salaz - Planning Director, Drug Free Community Coalition Members
From: Jennifer Dederich-Planner I
Subject: Meeting with Michele Orduna (UofA)
Date: February 23, 2005

On February 23, 2005, Gerald Porter and Jennifer Dederich met with Michel Orduna – U of A/STPC concerning the DFCC grant. The below checklist and priorities for the next meeting were developed.

Checklist for required material for the DFCC grant

- ❑ DUNS Bradstreet number for the City of South Tucson
- ❑ Abstract (no longer than 35 lines, see example 4)
- ❑ Table of Contents
- ❑ Budget form (SF424A see example)
- ❑ MOUs from all 12 coalition members (members cannot double up…i.e. youth organization and religious organization, yet multiple people can sign the same MOU)
- ❑ Project Narrative
    - o Demographics (Police/UoA)
    - o Literary Citations (UoA/Police)
    - o Budget justification - Narrative form (existing and other support)
    - o Biographic Sketches (job descriptions for each position created and existing positions)
    - o Confidentiality
    - o Participant Protection/Human Subjects (if the City administers the grant do we need to do this??)
- ❑ Appendices (listed p. 15)
- ❑ Intergovernmental Review (SPOC) ???
- ❑ Public Health System Impact ???
- ❑ Send application MARCH 10TH by 2pm

Cultural competence and overall criteria
**Use the six delineated headings and the 5 steps (p28)

Fig. 5.1 Memorandum of initial grant planning meetings

provided at local Safe Havens; these services had the potential to empower community members to address adolescent substance use (Donnermeyer, Plested, Edwards, Oetting, & Littlethunder, 1997; Oetting et al., 1995; Thurman, Plested, Edwards, Foley, & Burnside, 2003). The Coalition's agreed upon Logic Model was based on a theory of change that stated that the increased perception of risk/harm of drugs and the perception of parental and peer disapproval of substance use would delay the age of onset of substance use and reduce youth substance use (see Fig. 5.2). The proposed planned objectives to reach this goal were: (1) drug-free youth basketball tournament to increase awareness of consequences of substance use, (2) drug-free youth talent show and spirit week to increase the perception of disapproval of substance use among peers, and (3) drug-free Halloween Carnival to increase awareness and perception of parental and community disapproval of substance use. Each strategy was linked to outcome benchmarks that were measurable. These activities were designed to promote positive assets of the community while reducing risk factors; this focus is especially important in lower income communities that tend to have a balance of fewer positive resources and more than their share of risk factors.

This case study of the South Tucson Prevention Coalition (STPC) takes us to the intersection of research and the community, and we hope it enriches understanding of each of the influential forces in this process—without each of them, their positive outcomes may not have been possible. As you learn about how participatory action research led to individual and community transformation, we hope that you may find something useful in their stories that can be used to transform your own communities. We present here stories from two people who spent significant amount of time working to develop STPC through the community Safe Havens of South

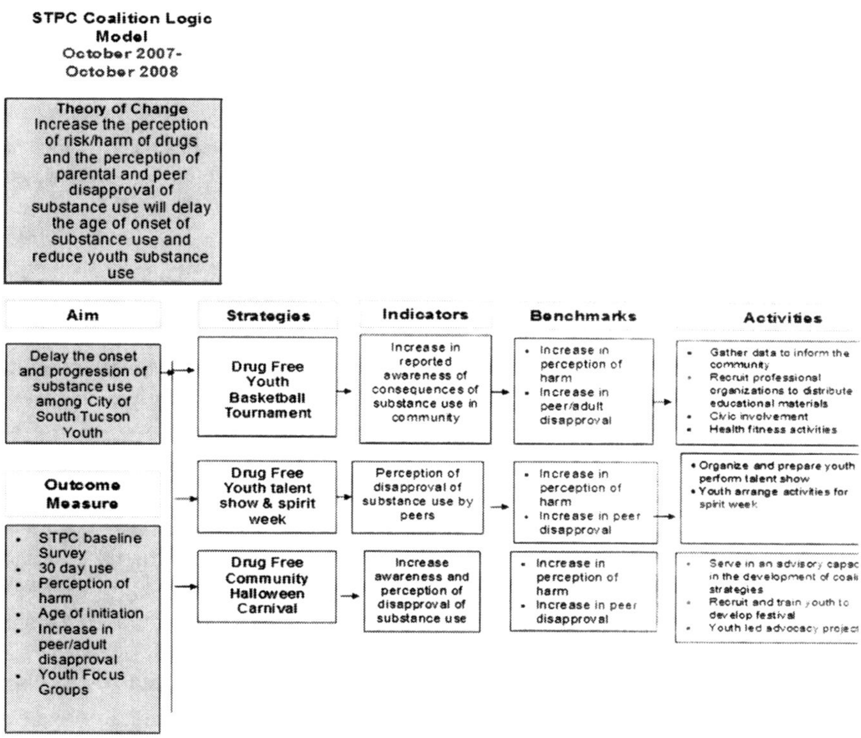

Fig. 5.2 Coalition logic model

Tucson. Through their stories, these individuals share insights about their experiences in breaking down silos and building allies through coalition development to prevent adolescent alcohol use. They discuss the nuances behind developing community connections that can lead to transforming their community to increase resilience of adolescents to risky behaviors.

5.2 Community Leaders: Kimberly Sierra-Cajas and Gloria Hamelitz-Lopez

Kimberly Sierra-Cajas worked as the Executive Director at House of Neighborly Service (HNS) from 2001 to 2007 and brings an inspiring story about the transformative things that can happen when community leaders choose to work collaboratively toward a common goal. HNS was an organization that had been around for more than 60 years. At the time that Kimberly was involved, HNS had eight programs serving the community. One program was a monthly brownbag program, where boxes of food were delivered to seniors. They also operated as a community food bank. They provided after school programs, which included tutoring and gang prevention programs. They had a tattoo removal program for ex-gang members who were rehabilitated or rehabilitating themselves. This included educational trainings in which people could go through the education program and have the option of having their tattoos removed at the completion of the program. HNS also offered a variety of activity programs: they ran a South Tucson basketball league, a double-dutch program in the schools, ballet folklorico, and a Native American youth program. Overall HNS was then serving about 400 youth per year, including the youth who were active in the double-dutch program; this total approximates to about 1000 youth per year.

Gloria Hamelitz-Lopez continues to work at the John Valenzuela Youth Center (JVYC) and tells the incredible story of the ways that small changes toward youth empowerment led to significant changes that affected the entire community. The involvement of various other community leaders is integrated throughout their stories, including the involvement and influence of the academic leaders from the University of Arizona, whose orientations to research included community-based approaches. Like HNS, JVYC provided a safe haven for neighborhood youth. The JVYC was dedicated to guiding and empowering youth and offered recreation, education, and drug and gang prevention. Their programs were extensive and include: day programs (crafts, cooking, games, sports leagues, fitness, and access to computers), after school programs, wellness programs (including financial planning, emergency clothing, health education), youth case management (provided through Pima County youth services, for youth ages 14–21 which included vocation training and career planning and support), community outreach (case managers and staff who provided community-based services), youth-to-youth (Y2Y) (youth-led workshops and recreational activities), special events (such as scrapbooking, cultural education, and sports tournaments), ESOL (a program partnership between JVYC and

Pima Community College, for adults who wanted to learn to speak and write English), and even a program called Girlz Nite which provided education, career development, and empowerment for girls ages 10–18 years old.

5.3 Competition and Community-Based Organization (CBO) Silos

In the city of South Tucson, there were three Safe Havens for youth: HNS, Project YES, and the John Valenzuela Youth Center (JVYC). Each of these programs offered a bit of something different to the community, and as Kimberly describes it, before the organizations came together under one large community grant, there was a clear separation between the youth who went to one Safe Haven or another. Like what was seen with the youth, Kimberly describes the atmosphere and relationships between community centers as clearly being divided as well: maybe they were resistant to collaborate because of competitiveness, or maybe it was because their programs' successes depended on retaining kids for the continuation of their grants. These are the some of the realities that community-based organizations face, which lead to silos or isolated storage of resources.

Whatever their reasons for resistance, all of that started to change, particularly through their involvement in a Weed and Seed grant (1998–2000). This grant, funded by the U.S. Department of Justice, provided $750,000 over 3 years to support the city of South Tucson in reducing violent crime, gang activity, and drug use in the community. The funding focused on a two-part approach to action: the "weeders" consisted of community law enforcement members whose focus was on reducing crime; the "seeders" consisted of social and service organizations that focused on fostering positive growth of the community's youth. Through the Weed and Seed grant in particular, all three Safe Havens were brought together. The grantees, including police and the youth centers, would have monthly meetings to plan events together. These meetings led groups to be aware of each other and to learn more about activities at the community level. The Weed and Seed grant and the birth of the South Tucson Prevention Coalition (STPC) were instrumental in bringing community groups together that otherwise were dissociated. South Tucson was recognized as a "Model Community," which demonstrated the City's experience with community-level prevention. South Tucson mobilized community members to fight crime, drugs, and gang activity by including various levels of government, nonprofit service agencies, faith-based organizations, and private business. This work with Weed and Seed certainly laid the groundwork for the further development of a coalition with STPC.

This was a critical turning point in the way that community groups began to interact with one another, eventually forging collaborative alliances, all for a unified cause of improving their community, and particularly providing more opportunities for the positive development of youth. While some social issues can be solved by individual community groups, others require larger-scale efforts that represent a collective combination of wisdom, people-power, and monetary support in order to achieve real change on the community level (Kania & Kramer, 2011). When a social organization faces a social problem alone, it can tend to operate as a silo, in other words, a storage house of information that isn't accessible to others. An organization may have learned ways of fund-raising and ways to structure events in order to impact the greatest number of youth primarily by working alone. This solo type of operation, however, can unintentionally shield valuable experiences and knowledge from like-minded others in the same community; on the other hand, becoming involved in collaborative endeavors is one way to bridge like-minded resources with one another in order to benefit a cause.

Like Kimberly, Gloria has been able to see many changes in the ways that the community centers have associated over the years she's been with JVYC. Her experiences also echoes Kimberly's acknowledgement that initiating collaboration can be a challenge between distinct community groups. This applied to community leaders as well as youth in South Tucson. To effectively collaborate, the community had to change the ways that leaders as well as youth were thinking about the organizations through which they had come to form their identities. Gloria explains,

> I think one of the things that had happened was that every social service agency was very competitive and that's partly because, you put a lot of work into developing your agency, promoting your agency, bragging about your agency, and, that's good, that's good in some sense, but it became very negative. We were trying to really involve all the kids from the different Safe Havens and our kids, each kid that went to those agencies, they love their agency, they were true to their agency. If you went to Project YES, there's no way in hell you'd come straight, hanging out at JVYC and if you were at JVYC you'd be like, 'oh, those are those Project YES kids' or HNS kids. You just wouldn't do it. And I was like, that's not really healthy because what we offer is going to be different from what they offer and we want to change that, HNS had some wonderful programs that we didn't and we're like, 'But our kids need those and they don't want to go over there because they're too proud' and, so, we really had to change some of that dynamic, and part of it had to do with the leadership, you know, you have to have the right leaders. At one point years ago we did have leaders that would instill that in the kids, 'Oh my god, what are you doing at HNS? You know you're supposed to be here,' and, like I said, that was part of that old style of thinking. You wanted to keep your numbers up, you wanted to keep your clientele, it's part of the business aspect.

Gloria also acknowledges how the Weed and Seed federally funded grant played a significant role in pulling these different community groups together.

> Part of that grant was really trying to build these coalitions; really getting the community to get together to talk. And, what happened was that the other Safe Havens that were in Tucson (which were Project YES and HNS) a lot of it really was geared towards getting the community together but especially the youth programs kind of trying to find some common ground eliminating that competitive—that unhealthy competitiveness, and really just getting us all to work together towards a better goal.

The conscious awareness that the societal infrastructure influences adolescent alcohol use was pivotal to the involvement of the key leaders in the coalition (Freire, 1968). Their understanding and acknowledgement of the larger origins of adolescent alcohol use were fundamental to their decisions for involvement and their decisions to work together. The fact that they could see the benefits of their collaboration for the youth in the community as a whole was an important building block to breaking down silos and building the coalition, because they understood that they could not achieve this goal alone (Kania & Kramer, 2011).

5.4 Benefits of Collaborating

For HNS, it seemed like a good fit for them to join forces with the STPC because they were already focused on prevention activities. Through collaboration, each of the centers found that they were able to share resources and distribute the burden of responsibilities amongst one another when planning large community events. Planning events together meant that one center could take on the primary leadership for the event, while at the same time having other organizations contribute ideas, resources, and organizational support throughout the process. This made it possible for the centers to host events together that were larger and reached more people than ever before, such as the Halloween Carnival and the National Night Out (see Chaps. 2 and 8 for more description and evaluation of these activities). And because each organization had its own venue, the hosting of events could be rotated between community centers, which made it possible to host more events collaboratively, than any of the organizations would have been able to do individually. These events were highly successful at bringing together the diverse sectors of the community while at the same time raising awareness about adolescent alcohol use and the need for prevention.

Alliances between community leaders had begun to form during their work under the Weed and Seed grant, but when the grant expired there was not any infrastructure to keep the Safe Havens working toward the community goals together. Collaboration, as Kimberly remembers it, revealed many more benefits than challenges: "*It was good for the kids to see us working together (some of the Safe Havens). By us eliminating some of the boundaries that existed between us, it helped eliminate some of the boundaries for them, so that they could cross (street boundaries).*" This is an important point to consider in terms of youth access to community resources, because while three Safe Havens were present and there was some degree of commonality in services, each one provided different opportunities and different access to health-promoting activities. Thus, by breaking down boundaries for youth to move between different agencies, it provided them access to as many resources as possible to help them in the greatest multitude of ways. Additionally, by the leaders setting examples of positive collaboration, it made it easier for youth to move between agencies and to be open to developing positive relationships with peers in their own community and to have access to more adult mentors and role models at each agency. Since the community was still at a preplanning level of community readiness (see Chap. 2), they had recognition of the problem of adolescent alcohol use and that something needed to be done, but they were not fully organized to work together on this issue (Oetting et al., 2001). At this stage, it was very effective to work in small groups of people who had some level of awareness. This helped to build trustful working alliances so that they could move to the next level of community readiness of preparation and initiation of implementing programs (Oetting et al., 2001). The small group environment allowed for open and honest discussion of disagreements about how to understand and change the issue of adolescent alcohol use.

The development of the South Tucson Prevention Coalition (STPC) was one way of maintaining these small group efforts toward coalition building. The benefits of sharing resources and ideas with one another proved to be one of the reasons that Gloria continued to stay involved in the STPC. Talking about why she became involved in STPC, and continued being a part of it, she explains:

> I had ideas and I didn't have money. And they had money, and we didn't have the resources. And, it's so difficult; it's difficult and impossible for one agency to change the community. It's ridiculous—if any one agency says they can do it, they're lying. It's impossible to do—and if they are doing it they aren't doing a good enough job. You have to be on board. We can't change this entire dynamic of the neighborhood all by ourselves, and, so, that was part of the draw was that, great, we can really collaborate. If any other group comes up with any awesome ideas, we're going to have some of the money behind it, so, that was part of it, being able to kind of fulfill those things.

It's evident from Gloria's framing of these events that her loyalty to providing positive experiences for the youth in her community was unwavering. It's clear that she was willing to make sacrifices, such as the advancement of her community center's reputation above all others, in order to have a bigger impact through collaboration, to help the youth and the community advance in positive ways. There's a sense that in any decisions she made, the foremost consideration would be whether a change has the community's best interest in mind. And what better way to provide the best support to them than through expanding resources? This is an example of critical consciousness from Gloria that is implicitly acknowledging the larger societal impact about the lack of infrastructure and resources among communities living in poverty, particularly over generations in poverty (Kania & Kramer, 2011). The social issues are much larger than any one agency can overcome, particularly nonprofit agencies in low income neighborhoods with few resources to begin with and little access to large donors or big fundraising events. Gloria is acknowledging that changing the effects of poverty in this community cannot be done alone—the job is too big. However, she is also acknowledging through her participation in South Tucson Prevention Coalition that decreasing adolescent alcohol use is one way to strategically improve the odds for the positive development of youth to stay in school and have healthier lifestyles by not getting involved in alcohol and the related risky behaviors, such as risky sexual behavior, violence, gangs, and drug trafficking.

5.4.1 Challenges and the Power of Dialogue

Collaborations among community members weren't entirely without adjustment over time. Gloria remembers challenges, such as differences in opinions about the approach that education programs should take, and the need to overcome competition between programs in order to begin to work cooperatively. For example, there were divergent opinions about what approaches to take for educational programming regarding underage drinking and driving. In the beginning, coalition members did not agree about which technique was best; for example, the police recommended using gruesome tactics of showing youth pictures of car wrecks or eliciting examples and personal experiences from the youth themselves to help them evaluate the impact of drinking and driving on possible outcomes. However, other coalition members, including Dr. Romero, did not agree with using what they termed "scare tactics" with youth. In working together through these challenges, though, they learned to manage differences and still maintain success toward their main goal: implementing community programs to enrich and improve the lives of the youth in their community. The coalition was guided by the Freirian (1968) model of dialogue and problem posing, which helped them maintain levels of respectful disagreement and discussion that was still oriented on finding action-oriented tactics to try to change the problem. And as their relationships were further developed, these advantages grew through the development of trust and positive relationships among coalition members. Additionally, the basic principles of participatory action research were utilized at the beginning of each meeting as reminder that all coalition members were equal and that participation of everyone was encouraged to engage in group decision making (McIntyre, 2008). The community grant that allowed them all to work together toward one main goal had fundamentally changed the way they approached community goals, for the better.

5.4.2 *Role of Research and Researchers: Trust*

Not only did HNS, Project YES, and YVYC begin to work together, but the grant also connected them with other key members of the community who had taken part in writing the grant, including City of South Tucson government representatives, City police department, local schools, churches, and other service agencies. One such person was Dr. Andrea Romero who was involved in research at the University of Arizona. Working with Dr. Romero was advantageous, as it presented the community with a facilitator who wasn't wrapped up in the same concerns as the nonprofits and who was able to bring an outsider perspective to making things more collaborative. Yet, Dr. Romero was also well-versed in adolescent alcohol prevention and community-based participatory research techniques. As Harper and Salina (2000) describe, the development of effective collaborative relationships between university researchers and community-based organizations (CBOs) should be based on reciprocal relationships that are nonexploitive.

Researchers may often bring financial support, research knowledge, and other resources that the community members don't have. As Wallerstein and Duran note, "*Although CBPR researchers expect that building collaborative relationship with community members will be sufficient to surmount any differences, power differentials can and often do remain substantial. Academic researchers almost always have greater access to resources, scientific knowledge, research assistants, and time than small community-based organizations do*" (2008, p. 30). Successful collaboration often recognizes and utilizes the strengths of all partners, especially community partners. As Minkler and Wallerstein point out, "*Community based participatory research can foster the conditions in which professionally trained researchers adopt the role of co-learner, rather than outside expert, and communities better recognize and build on their strengths and become full partners in gaining and creating knowledge and mobilizing for change*" (2008, p. 18). It's important for researchers to be aware of some of the differences that may exist as far as what resources are available, and how these differences can create discrepancies of power between partners (Harper & Salina, 2000). Partnerships where researchers are dedicated to identifying community strengths, build on those, and provide ways for the shared resources to enable the community to strengthen itself, prove most fruitful (McIntyre, 2008; Minkler & Wallerstein, 2008).

STPC was where Kimberly first met Dr. Andrea Romero, who was giving a presentation about an HIV/AIDS prevention program, called Omeyacon YES, at a local library to a small group of directors from local community-based organizations. Kimberly learned that the prevalence of HIV/AIDS was rising, and that drug and alcohol were big factors leading to Latino youth getting HIV/AIDS. The local data results Dr. Romero presented, however, showed the successes of the Omeyocan YES peer-to-peer intervention program. These results were very salient for the South Tucson community, and highlighted the importance of sharing this knowledge within the community. Kimberly acknowledges that her introduction to Dr. Romero greatly influenced the way she thought about how to approach the issues facing the community's youth. Having research that was based on data that was gathered within their own small community, and becoming knowledgeable about real issues facing their youth, such as HIV/AIDS rates and high rates of teen pregnancy in South Tucson, showed just how important the researcher's skills and expertise could be for their community. Without the information brought forth by these researchers, Kimberly explains, such as the neighborhood surveys the team conducted, the community centers wouldn't have been aware of the great community need for focused efforts on health issues facing their youth and families.

This brings up an important consideration that researchers interested in becoming involved in the community may benefit from also considering. Collaboration isn't only about finding others to work with. Rather, at the heart of successful alliances is a strong dedication to relationship building through personalismo (Alegría, Canino, & Pescosolido, 2009; Gallardo, 2013; Harper & Salina, 2000). The development of trusting and confiding relationships are essential in order to move forward to improve health; failed interventions have often been premised on a lack of community trust, poor interpersonal interactions, and limited access to providers (Alegría et al., 2009). Particularly for communities that have faced continued injustice and the associated inequities, it is likely that they have reasons to be distrustful of service providers and university researchers. This distrustfulness may manifest in resistance to commitment to involvement in partnership and resistance to supporting health programs that are perceived as originating outside of the local community (Gallardo, 2013).

For Gloria, part of what led to her willingness to collaborate with Dr. Andrea Romero and her student researchers came from an understanding that she could trust that they were dedicated to working with the community and had the community's best interest in mind. Thus, evidence of passion about prevention and investment in the local community helped Gloria to break down the silo between her agency and the university. Gloria explains how she began working with Andrea and her student researchers:

> I think part of the success was that, you know, we were approached with this grant by people that had already proven to be wonderful—not only role models for our kids—but they were really invested in our community. It wasn't this outside group that said 'Hey, I know you have these problems by I want to fix them,' it was somebody who was already here. Andrea had already started—not only with Omeyacon YES, but previously before that, there was another activity that she had done which was a Latin Hip-hop group, and you know, I think, that's part of the success, it's that trust, knowing, 'okay, great, I know you can back up what you say you're going to do,' you're reliable, I think this is going to be a wonderful project and I think that's part of the reason we were—we jumped right on board and we were so excited about it, because we had seen what Andrea could do, we'd seen what her team could do, her interns and all of her groups, so we were excited about it.

In essence, Andrea had been able to show, through other projects, that she possessed qualities that made her a successful community collaborator: she had demonstrated, in many ways, that she could be *trusted*. This foundation of trust of Andrea as a researcher and as a community participant laid the groundwork for future advances in youth-led and community-led research because it broke down uncertainty about the engagement with research. However, it had to be based on experience and evidence of following through on commitments. Breaking down of silos and learning to develop mutual trust was not driven by grant money, it was driven by personalismo. Through the development of trusting relationships, the integration of research and research findings were more welcome and came to be more regularly used in meetings and to help inform group decisions.

5.4.3 Involving Community Members

Not only were leaders of the community centers and researchers beginning to collaborate together, but other community members also began to get involved. This represented incremental changes in community readiness: once small groups had developed awareness, capacity, and experience working together, then they were ready to move to the next level of community readiness of implementation of activities (Edwards, Jumper-Thurman, Plested, Oetting, & Swanson, 2000; Oetting et al., 2001). This is such an important part of the community-based approach; individual engagement is a key element to influencing larger-scale community change. Kimberly explains,

> So many people look at the community as like, ohh, they need all this help and we are providing all of these great resources and stuff to them. Well, the community themselves can be empowered and they can take charge and they can have things the way they want it. So, we knew they could take more responsibility, or they could be more a part of the center.

> We also try to have more community members on our board. We just made a lot more effort to do that.

Reaching out to families and involving parents was another way they influenced and engaged members of the community. Kimberly continues:

> We had the big Christmas party, and so, we would have, parents were required to do volunteer hours to get Christmas presents and so then they got to pick out Christmas presents and wrap them themselves and give them to their kids. So, the parent earned it; the parent pretty much paid for their present themselves (with their volunteering), so it wasn't coming from us as a charity, it was coming from the parent.

These attitudes described by Kimberly were a major shift in the expectations of community members. The coalition members began to see the importance of including community members, particularly including youth. The following chapter will go more in depth to describe the evolution of the youth group that became leaders within South Tucson Prevention Coalition. However, these initial activities, described here by Kimberly and Gloria, were primary achievements that helped the adults work together more collaboratively and equally in order to be prepared to work with youth as equals. As the coalition worked to begin implementing the proposed activities they learned that involving community members also encouraged ownership of the community changes. Furthermore, it encouraged the internalization of prioritized issues, which were to change community alcohol norms through increased awareness of consequences, and to encourage the role of community and parental involvement. Some of the ways in which the STPC first began to reach out to community members is evidenced in their early invitations to meetings (see Figs. 5.3, 5.4, 5.5, 5.6). This set the tone for the intent and goals of the meeting. Even through these early efforts, the STPC was working on raising awareness about alcohol norms for adolescents.

5.5 Reflections and Concluding Remarks

The role of the community can vary in community-based participatory research (Minkler & Wallerstein, 2008). The range of "participation" by community members may indeed vary, as some participatory action methods devise systems that value community members' participation simply as respondents (Turnbull, Friesen, & Ramirez, 1998). These methodologies would perhaps request key community leaders and community members as participants in focus groups or interviews led by researchers or research assistants. Researchers then could perform analyses and perhaps make recommendations based on the research findings. Another more community-beneficial approach to community-based research would allow for a reversal of these roles, whereby community member participation is at the core of decision making about the research process as well as funding (Turnbull et al., 1998). This type of methodological approach would place community members in charge of efforts that affect them and researchers as supporting team members or

EXECUTIVE OFFICE OF THE PRESIDENT
OFFICE OF NATIONAL DRUG CONTROL POLICY
Washington, DC 20503

FOR IMMEDIATE RELEASE: Contact:
ONDCP
Wednesday, September 21, 2005 202-
395-6618

ANNOUNCES $100,000 ANTI-DRUG COALITION GRANT FOR_CITY OF SOUTH TUCSON _

(Washington, D.C.) –The Office of National Drug Control Policy today announced that the City of South Tucson will receive a $_100,000_ Drug-Free Communities matching grant for the South Tucson Prevention Collaborative. The grant was one of 176 new grants totaling $17.1 million awarded today to community anti-drug coalitions across the country. The goal of the 711 local coalitions is to work together to prevent and reduce drug, alcohol, and tobacco abuse among youth. Coalitions are comprised of diverse groups of people, including community leaders, parents, youth, teachers, religious and fraternal organizations, health care and business professionals, law enforcement, and the media.

"This is great news for the anti-drug efforts of City of South Tucson and local community." said Mr. Castro, City Manger. "The Drug-Free Communities Program and other drug prevention efforts are important elements of a balanced national drug control strategy. STPC is doing crucial drug prevention work in our community and this additional influx of Federal money will help them expand their efforts and reach more of South Tucson's children."

John Walters, Director of National Drug Control Policy and President Bush's "Drug Czar," said, "As a nation, we have made significant progress in protecting our young people from the dangers of substance abuse, with a 17 percent reduction in drug use over the last three years. This grant will help the dedicated citizens of_City of South Tucson to contribute even more to this effort and will help build on the important progress being made to keep our children healthy and drug-free."

We are pleased to be working with ONDCP to administer the Drug-Free Communities Program," said Charles Curie, Administrator, Substance Abuse and Mental Health Services Administration. "Some of the most important work to reduce drug use comes from our Nation's grass-roots community coalitions. These coalitions, teamed up with our Strategic Prevention Framework Grants to the states, create a powerful force that can continue to drive down the numbers of young people using illicit drugs."

The Drug-Free Communities Program provides grants of up to $500,000 over five years to community organizations that serve as catalysts for citizen participation in local drug prevention efforts. The 176 new grantees were selected from 411 applicants through a competitive peer review process. To qualify for matching grants, all awardees must have at least a six-month history of working together on substance abuse

Fig. 5.3 Press release of grant award by city

reduction initiatives, develop a long-term plan to reduce substance abuse, and participate in a national evaluation of the Drug-Free Communities Program.

Created under the Drug-Free Communities Act of 1997, the Drug-Free Communities Program has earned strong bipartisan support from Congress. In December of 2001, Congress passed and the President signed into law a five-year extension of the Drug-Free Communities Act, authorizing $399 million in funds through FY 2007.

In addition to the 176 new grants awarded today, another $54 million will support continuation grants to 535 existing community coalition projects operating in all 50 states, the District of Columbia, and Puerto Rico. Since 1997, eight competitions have awarded $320 million in grants to more than 1000 community anti-drug coalitions. ONDCP administers the Drug-Free Communities Program in conjunction with the Substance Abuse and Mental Health Services Administration.

More information about the Drug-Free Communities Program is available at:
www.whitehousedrugpolicy.gov, and http://drugfreecommunities.samhsa.gov/
-30-

Fig 5.3 (continued)

subcontractors to the community's efforts and is the best and most inclusive option for participatory action research (Wallerstein & Duran, 2008). Through the course of this book, we will discuss the evolution and change in level of community transformational resilience. We will also examine how that evolution occurred over time through the development of community based on trust, relationship building, and integrated use of research for collective decision making.

One of the strongest impressions from this community's story is that we can often benefit from examining the roles that each of us play in interactions and collaborations with others. As these stories illustrate, the sharing of experiences and resources, as well as the engagement of individuals involved in their communities, is essential to strengthening individuals and communities. The development of critical consciousness was essential in order for community leaders to begin work at breaking down silos. It is important to note that not all coalition members were at this same stage of critical consciousness or willingness as Gloria and Kimberly, but with these two individuals as key leaders and role models, they were able to set the tone for the type of collaboration that was possible. By witnessing the success of working together, more agencies and community leaders were invigorated to join STPC. Kania and Kramer (2011) would argue that the key to the success of STPC's collective impact was rooted in (1) the common agenda (to prevent underage drinking), (2) mutual reinforcement of activities, (3) continuous communication, and (4) a backbone of supporting organizations. Clearly HNS and JVYC made up part of the organizational backbone. The City of South Tucson was also instrumental through their willingness to host the grant, directly support efforts intended to benefit the community, and participate publicly in events. Furthermore, Dr. Romero's continuous involvement through the University of Arizona contributed to the

What is **STPC?** South Tucson Prevention Collaborative

What is Drug Free Communities?

- **GOAL:** to reduce substance use, like alcohol, tobacco and other drugs among youth
- **GOAL:** strengthen & work in the local community with

  -youth
  -parents
  -businesses
  -the media
  -schools
  -youth organizations
  -law enforcement
  -religious organizations
  -civic groups
  -health care professionals
  -state government
  -local government

How can I participate in STPC Drug Free Community?

- Sign up and come to our next meeting
- Let your voice be heard by STPC
- Help create a healthy positive community for our families & children

STPC was 1 of 176 NEW Drug Free Communities Grant recipients in October-2005!!!

Any questions or concerns please call Michele Orduña, Project Director, at 626.1442 or email at michelef@u.arizona.edu

Fig. 5.4 Bilingual coalition adult recruitment tools

Coalición Prentiva del Sur Tucson

Nuestra Meta

- Prevenir el uso de substancias, como alcohol, tabaco, marihuana, y otras drogas entre la juventud

Miembros

-Ciudad del Sur Tucson
-Policia y Cuerpo de Bomberos del Sur Tucson
-Fundación AIDS del Sur
-Universidad de Arizona
-Casa de Servicio a la buena Vecindad
-Proyecto YES-TUL
-Centro de la Juventud John Valenzuela
-Liderazgo de Joven a Joven
-COPE Comportamiento de Salud
-Y muchos más

Necesitamos nuevos miembros para la Coalición

-Jovenes
-La Prensa
-Policias y Bomberos
-Grupos Civiles
-Personas de Negocios
-Familiares
-Escuelas
-Organizaciones Religiosas
-Profesionales de la Salud
-Personas del Gobierno
-Organizaciones para Jóvenes

¿Que Puedo Hacer?

Asista a nuestra próxima junta, y firme
Las juntas se llevan a cabo el cuarto jueves de cada mes

Para cualquier pregunta o asunto comuníquese al teléfono 792-2424 con Michele Orduña, Directora del Proyecto o e-mail michelef@u.arizona.edu

Fig. 5.4 (continued)

COME JOIN US

<u>South Tucson Prevention Collaborative</u> is asking for your participation. Come give your input. Our motivation is the prevention of drug use among young people. We believe working together to reach community goals.

You are invited to take part in a community meeting on <u>January 24, 2006</u> at Sam Lena Library, 1607 S. Sixth Avenue, South Tucson, Tuesday at 6:00 p.m.

<u>Dinner will be served at the meeting</u>

Please RSVP by January 20, 2006
Michele Orduña 626-1442 or email
michelef@email.arizona.edu

The South Tucson Prevention Collaborative is supported by the City of South Tucson and a 2005 recipient of a Drug Free Communities grant funded by SAMHSA.

Fig. 5.5 Invitation to first meeting

capacity of the community to participate in shared measurement and to work to develop community leadership in research (Kania & Kramer, 2011).

The importance of tapping into the community's voice is highlighted in this story in two main ways: breaking down silos between community agencies and the development of successful partnerships between researchers and community leaders. In both of these stories, we see how awareness of the larger societal infrastructure was impacting this community in poverty and shaping the choices and opportunities for adolescents. However, the community leaders deconstructed their own decisions to participate in the larger coalition and how they viewed the possible benefits not so much for their own agency but for youth in the community as a whole.

5.6 Conclusion

The most significant element of community-based research that is highlighted in Kimberly's story is the enormous benefit that collaboration between community leaders, specifically the leaders of the South Tucson youth centers, had on the youth programs. Importantly, Kimberly shares the story of how she saw the association of the various community groups changes while she was involved with HNS.

Drug Free Communities Basics-

The mission of the Coalition is to prevent substance use among adolescents (age 9-15 years) in the City of South Tucson.

Our long-term goals are
1) prevention and reduction of youth substance use
2) to prevent or delay adolescent first use of alcohol, tobacco, marijuana, inhalants, and methamphetamines

Our first goal is to
- **creating a listserv of all members and sending an annual newsletter**
- **STPC Summits, Coalition members and community members at carne asadas (barbeques)**

The community level activities, including both family-oriented and youth-oriented activities.
- **a marketing campaign with drug free messages on billboards and public service announcements on local radio stations (in English & Spanish).**
- **provide a Drug Free family-oriented activity (Family Fitness Fun Day) event the risk and harm of drugs with fun games, activities, and food**
- **youth peer educators from our STPC project to assist with planning the annual Drug Free Youth-Led Activity (Halloween Haunted House)**
- **disapproval of drug use by peers and to provide drug free fun opportunities for youth during the summer (Talent Show & Spirit Week).**

Fig. 5.6 Coalition goals and objectives

The sharing of information, resources, and responsibilities is one way that community strength can be enhanced through collaboration. Each member's resources, approaches, and knowledge helped develop a path that none of the groups would have been able to lead alone. The collaborative effort that evolved from the STPC impacted not only the way that community centers were structured and dealt with one another but also greatly impacted the youth and the community at large.

For the coalition, engaging the community in conducting local research was just one way that it allowed the community to also become knowledgeable and invested in the issues facing one another, and it was one of many steps the researchers took toward building a trusting relationship with community members. In Gloria's experiences working with the youth, the implementation of peer-to-peer education and empowerment programs and youth-led events had a positive impact on the youth and on their community as a whole. These changes gave youth the power to become involved in the issues facing themselves and their peers. By taking on positive leadership roles, youth were able to help improve the lives of their peers and the community as a whole, leading to changes that were unlike anything that had been seen before.

References

Alegría, M., Canino, G., & Pescosolido, B. (2009). A socio-cultural framework for mental health and substance abuse service disparities. In B. J. Sadock, V. A. Sadock, & P. Ruiz (Eds.), *Comprehensive textbook of psychiatry* (9th ed.). Baltimore: Wolters Kluwer Health/Lippincott Williams & Wilkins.

Chou, C. P., Montgomery, S., Pentz, M. A., Rohrbach, L. A., Johnson, C. A., Flay, B. R., et al. (1998). Effects of a community-based prevention program on decreasing drug use in high-risk adolescents. *American Journal of Public Health, 88*(6), 944–948.

Donnermeyer, J. F., Plested, B. A., Edwards, R. W., Oetting, G., & Littlethunder, L. (1997). Community readiness and prevention programs. *Journal of Community Development Society, 28*(1), 65–83.

Edwards, R. W., Jumper-Thurman, P., Plested, B. A., Oetting, E. R., & Swanson, L. (2000). Community readiness: research to practice. *Journal of Community Psychology, 28*(3), 291–307.

Freire, P. (1968). *Pedagogy of the Oppressed.* New York, NY: Seabury Press.

Gallardo, M. (2013). Context and culture: The initial clinical interview with the Latina/o client. *Journal of Contemporary Psychology, 43*, 43–52.

Harper, G. W., & Salina, D. D. (2000). Building collaborative partnerships to improve community-based HIV prevention research: The university-CBO collaborative partnership (UCCP) model. *Journal of Prevention & Intervention in the Community, 19*(1), 1–20. doi:10.1300/J005v19n01_01.

Kania, J., & Kramer, M. (2011). *Collective Impact.* Stanford Social Innovation Review.

McIntyre, A. (2008). *Participatory action research.* Thousand Oaks, CA: Sage.

Minkler, M., & Wallerstein, N. (2008). In M. Minkler & N. Wallerstein (Eds.), *Community-based participatory research for health: From process to outcomes* (pp. 5–19). San Francisco: Jossey-Bass.

Oetting, E. R., Donnermeyer, J. F., Plested, B. A., Edwards, R. W., Kelly, K., & Beauvais, F. (1995). Assessing community readiness for prevention. *International Journal of the Addictions, 30*, 659–83.

Oetting, E.R., Jumper-Thurman, P., Plested, B., & Edwards, R.W. (2001). Community Readiness and health services. *Substance Use & Misuse, 36*(6 &7), 825–843.

Thurman, P. J., Plested, B. A., Edwards, R. W., Foley, R., & Burnside, M. (2003). Community readiness: The journey to community healing. *Journal of Psychoactive Drugs, 35*(1), 27–31.

Turnbull, A. P., Friesen, B. J., & Ramirez, C. (1998). Participatory action research as a model for conducting family research. *JASH, 23*(3), 178–188.

Wallerstein, N., & Duran, B. (2008). In M. Minkler & N. Wallerstein (Eds.), *Community-based participatory research for health: From process to outcomes* (pp. 25–46). San Francisco: Jossey-Bass.

Chapter 6
Adult Perspectives on Nurturing Youth Leadership and Coalition Participation

Robby Harris, Jesi Post, Jaime Arrieta, and Gloria Hamelitz-Lopez

Abstract The goal of this chapter is to describe how youth leadership and coalition participation were nurtured by after-school programs and community infrastructure. Key adult allies provide insight into their role in supporting youth-led programs. They describe the changes in youth participation that they witnessed over time. Importantly, they describe changes in their own perspectives on youth leadership and participation. Moreover, they discuss youth development and the steps that they took to move into leadership positions and a more fully realized participation in coalition activities.

Keywords Youth leadership • Adult allies • Youth participation • Youth agency • Respect • Dialogue

The youth component of the South Tucson Prevention Coalition (STPC) was the Youth-to-Youth program (Y2Y). The Y2Y program grew out of the positive youth development strategies that Dr. Romero, Gloria Hamelitz-Lopez, Jaime Arrieta, and the STPC enacted over several years through after-school and summer research-based prevention programs and participatory action research. Y2Y has been a formal organization since 2005, after a group of 7 youth attended an international conference with STPC funds. Over the past 8 years, the youth involved with Y2Y have

R. Harris, M.S. (✉)
City University of New York, New York, NY, USA
e-mail: robby.d.harris@gmail.com

J. Post, M.S.
Mel and Enid Zuckerman College of Public Health, University of Arizona, 3950 S. Country Club, Suite 330, Tucson, AZ, USA
e-mail: jhpost@email.arizona.edu

J. Arrieta, M.P.H., C.H.E.S.
Carondelet Health Network, Tucson, AZ, USA
e-mail: jarrieta1@carondelet.org

G. Hamelitz-Lopez
John Valenzuela Youth Center, Tucson, AZ, USA
e-mail: gloriahamelitz@hotmail.com

A.J. Romero (ed.), *Youth-Community Partnerships for Adolescent Alcohol Prevention*, DOI 10.1007/978-3-319-26030-3_6

continually developed into robust community leaders—driven to help their peers and serve as role models for younger children to lead empowered, drug free lives.

Through their own development of alcohol risk awareness and capacity to provide prevention activities, youth began to work with their peers to make smart choices, raise community awareness of the consequences of alcohol use, and community norms of availability to ultimately bring about positive youth development in the City of South Tucson. At least twice a year, Y2Y held an all-day youth retreat that they planned and led with adult guidance. Y2Y recruited new members each year, and they continued to build upon prior success in empowering youth and creating sustainable change for a healthy community. During this same time, adults were also beginning to form a coalition, South Tucson Prevention Coalition (STPC). Y2Y members regularly attended and participated in the STPC and served as key decision makers in the group through their research leadership, educational sessions, central participation in community activities, and participation in decision making (see Fig. 6.1 for an early recruitment flyer for youth).

However, it would be wrong and inappropriate to idealize or romanticize youth and their ability to create change. In fact, most individuals who work with youth on Youth Participatory Action Research (YPAR) would agree that there is need for adult participation, and this is usually in the form of adult allies or veteran activists (Noguera & Cannella, 2006). There, however, are few models for youth working on partnership with adults who do not already have critical consciousness about youth's role in society and their ability to be agentic and involved in positive change. In the South Tucson Prevention Coalition, youth worked with youth and adult allies in small settings to develop critical consciousness and to engage in YPAR activities; however, one of the things that made STPC unique was that youth were then integrated into an adult coalition. This was not an easy task, and certainly the youth development programs rooted in Freirian models were fundamental to develop critical consciousness and foster leadership among youth before and during their participation with adults.

At first, adults expected youth to carry out the adult decisions, or they expected that they would not participate in discussion or decision-making. Yet, it was the adults who were often surprised by the level of youth participation and by the youth's honesty in discussions about alcohol use. In fact, some of the initial meetings were challenging for all participants, youth and adults alike. In the beginning, youth were still seen as "the problem," due to negative stereotypes and low expectations, and adult privilege contributed to unequal relationships. However, the adults that continued to participate began to change their perspectives and their expectations of youth. They found that the youth voice added value to the conversation and to the planning of activities. They found that youth often had innovative contributions for ideas for strategies and solutions that had not been previously considered by adult leaders. Although the primary goal of the coalition was to focus on preventing underage drinking, a consequence of our YPAR approach was that adults gained critical consciousness about the humanity and equality of youth in their own community. The end result of STPC was community transformational resilience to create systemic changes to promote adolescent health in a sustainable manner. This was done in such a way to develop youth participation within the existing

South Tucson Prevention Collaboration
Teen Leadership development

The 3 safe havens in South Tucson, House of Neighborly Services, John Valenzuela Youth Center, & Project Yes, along with the U of A are in the process of forming the South Tucson Prevention Col aboration. . The goals of STPC are to offer positive activities to families and youth to combat the drug abuse problems our community faces.

The col aboration seeks to invite members from our community and it is crucial for the teens in south Tucson to have a voice in the decisions made. Teen leaders are being sought to serve as an active participant of STPC.

As a member you will assist STPC in forming decisions on developing programs, community events, education & training opportunities. Meeting generally will take place in the evening once a month. Meetings will begin in the fall of 2005.

STPC is offering training to interested teens to develop leadership skills through various activities such as trainings, mentorship's, volunteer opportunities and much more. To kick off the training we will be offering a training in California from July 9-July 15. 2005.

If you are interested plan on attending the informational workshop on June 2, 2005, 5:30-6:30 at JVYC (1550 S. 6th Ave). Parents are encouraged to attend.

Fig. 6.1 Teen leadership recruitment flyer

sociopolitical system. It was a form of disruption to the previous status quo, but executed in partnership with community leaders and adult allies.

An important element of the success of the Y2Y youth leadership program was the development of critical consciousness of the adults and their ability to facilitate and nurture youth leadership within the coalition. This chapter highlights interviews with two adult community leaders, Jaime Arrieta and Gloria Hamelitz-Lopez, who worked to provide space for youth to express their voice and to also empower youth to use their voice for good and specifically for prevention of underage drinking in their community. Gloria and Jaime both consistently framed their efforts within the larger efforts of the STPC to empower the youth of South Tucson. The sense that they were one small piece of a working organization pervaded our dialogue and is telling of one of the greatest strengths of the STPC and the larger South Tucson community. It becomes very clear in this chapter how crucial the role of continued youth leadership development was in bringing about the amazing community change that was achieved by STPC.

6.1 Gloria Hamelitz-Lopez: Youth Realities of Culture and Gender

Gloria Hamelitz-Lopez was the Executive Director of the John A. Valenzuela Youth Center (JVYC). Her story of how she observed the youth change over the years in South Tucson involves many of the same themes that are foundational to participatory action research and serves as a parallel to what had also been seen within the partnerships that developed in the South Tucson community at large. During her interview, Gloria explained how the youth programs evolved over time at JVYC from being predominantly led by adults to being more youth-led as the coordinators re-thought the way the programs were being carried out. In particular, the participatory action research approach used as part of the Omeyocan YES and Voz programs changed their thinking:

> Their main focus was the HIV prevention portion. But, what they did that was really different that I hadn't seen in other presentations or other classes was that they had this huge focus also on Mexican American studies. And, really getting our kids empowered to make positive choices. This wasn't a scare tactic like, "here, here's a genital wart, look at how gross. Be scared. Don't have sex" and, we know that those things are very short-lived, those kind of scare tactics don't really work, you know, they may work for a little while, but, that's about it.
>
> And, what we saw happening was that they really talked about culture and some of our kids had never been exposed to that, we were really focused on middle school kids and beginning high school kids and they hadn't yet been to La Raza studies classes and they just came up so empowered. They were really proud and they had seen how great all these Chicano leaders made all these differences and they stood up and they fought for all these issues in their community and they were looking around and they weren't seeing that in their community, you know, but, what was really cool is that they kind of felt they wanted to take over and that they wanted to do something different, so, starting with that, Our kids were really, they were motivated, they were ready to go and we were kind of unsure what to do with that energy, you know, great, okay, we have standard, you know, boring stuff, "great! Let's go clean the neighborhood"... and we wanted something different.

By making material more concretely rooted in actual lives and cultural understandings of the youth, Gloria explained that the programs became more impactful and began to spark the desire for action. It is important to note how this spark, in its small scale, was what eventually grew into the youth-led alcohol and substance use prevention program. This desire for action, as Gloria described, was the seed that eventually evolved into raising community awareness, increased youth involvement in research and action, and making presentations to the community and City Council in South Tucson in order to be civically engaged and to change city-level policy. In other words, this work created community transformational resilience by increasing positive community assets, aligning resources, and also reducing risk factors at the community level.

6.1.1 *Raising the Consciousness of Adult Allies*

As leaders at JVYC continued to create opportunities for youth to take on peer-to-peer leadership roles, an important moment for the youth and the adult leaders came when Gloria and others attended a Community Anti-Drug Coalition (CADCA) conference. She explained:

> Part of the grant also gave our staff some money to travel and we went to a national conference…the CADCA conference…We were able to kind of go and see what other programs [were] doing nation-wide, especially programs that [were] working and one that really stuck out to us was the international youth-to-youth program…We were looking around at the conference and we had seen a lot of kids, a lot of teenagers, and I was like, how didn't we bring teenagers to this, why didn't that occur to us? And the more we started looking at other programs and activities, it clicked, like, this is what we need to get our kids involved in. And everything just started to snowball from there, so, that's how the idea and premises of youth-to-youth came up.

The opportunity for national and international connections at this conference was critical and one that afforded the JVYC leaders exposure to diversity in approaches, programs, and activities which could best target the youth of South Tucson. Another important decision was for youth to attend the Y2Y international conference which was a collaborative effort among all three of the South Tucson youth centers (JVYC, HNS, and Project YES). A total of seven youth attended with the adult leaders who were excited, since they had seen how youth in other communities had been involved at the CADCA conference. The importance of seeing how other communities were working with and involving youth became clear from these experiences. These understandings were pivotal among JVYC leaders to evaluate how they were serving the youth of South Tucson and how they could do things differently and better.

6.1.2 *Gaining Perspective: From Negativity to Positivity*

Gloria explained what it was like the first time they attended the conference and highlighted how change did not occur "overnight" but rather was an adjustment for the youth and adult leaders alike:

> We ended up becoming a group of theirs (Y2Y), which I now think we're more successful than theirs which is really cool, but and then we were able to, with some of that extra money we had from South Tucson Prevention Collaborative: Omeyocan YES, we were able to take our kids to the youth-to-youth international conference which was in California, and that was just mind-blowing. And it was this huge week-long retreat that was focused on drugs, dating violence, on just about every issue that affects teenagers, and to see teenagers in charge of this was so surprising.
>
> We took 3 kids from YVYS, we took 2 from HNS and 2 from Project Yes, because, you know, we still wanted to keep that whole community vibe going. And, it was almost sad, you know, this whole environment was super positive, and people were jumping and they were clapping, and our kids had never seen anything like that! You know, they were just like, they were looking around like, 'what is this fool DOING? Why is he jumping? Why is he happy? Why is he clapping?' And that was disturbing to me, like, what do you mean, you should be happy! Why don't you have a happy childhood? And honestly, it actually ended up giving a couple of our kids a headache. It was just so difficult for them to process that kids were in charge, and they were happy and they were positive and they were making differences. It was just, it was too much for them, you know, and it took them a good day or two before they finally started to get into it, and they started to embrace it. And it was after that conference that they came back and they were like, 'That was really fun! We've never had anything like that, EVER, not even in Tucson,' so that kind of also started getting this whole notion started. They want to do something, they want to have healthy positive lives, and once we found out about this grant we were like, 'Let's do it! Let's go, let's see what we can accomplish with it.' So, we were really excited, and like I said, a lot of it had to do with the prior programs that came into it. I think if we didn't have any of that, I don't think this would have been so successful… it was this building up of lots of different things.

The initial unfamiliarity and confusion that the South Tucson youth experienced regarding their peers at the conference is quite powerful. This experience raised the awareness and raised the expectations of both youth and adults. But this process of becoming more aware was difficult; it required some awareness of what their own community was missing and being conscious about the low expectations and negative stereotypes of youth in their own community. As Gloria explained, it was "*difficult for them to process that kids were in charge" and were "happy, positive, and making differences*." The majority of youth and children (65 %) in South Tucson live in poverty, many at extreme poverty levels (U.S. Census Bureau, 2010), and this is typically associated with a range of other stressors (see Chap. 1 for a more completed description of the local community). However, many of the youth were embedded in their community and may have been accustomed to this lack of resources, lack of support, and even the negative stereotypes about youth from South Tucson. Even the youth who were previously involved in community organizations and attended this conference were taken aback by the Y2Y youth leaders. This internal stress and conflict over seeing this new vision of youth action and leadership was not only negotiated by the youth. It was also present for Gloria, who explained that her understandings of the identity of the youth and where they were coming from changed. Initially, she could not make sense of the South Tucson youth's confusion over their happy peers in leadership positions. However, she explained how rapidly South Tucson youth internalized this notion of action and leadership just over the course of the days they spent at the conference. This demonstrates how quickly critical consciousness and praxis can be stirred among adolescents when they are in the right conditions and particularly among other youth who are already engaged in action and taking on new roles that turn youth oppression upside down.

6.1.3 Shifting to Youth-Led Strategies

Putting youth in charge, and developing peer-to-peer opportunities at JVYC, was the next step to bringing youth-to-youth leadership home to their community. Thinking about the youth population in South Tucson in particular revealed an opportunity to put youth in action at JVYC:

> For many years we always did leadership classes—teaching kids to be leaders and, it was basically adult-guided. Adults were up there telling you, this is how you organize, this is how you rally, and a lot of this was really just this lecture-based thing, and then there was never any action or follow-up behind it and, part of it was, kids weren't really motivated. It was just like school: you go, you learn about something, in one ear, out the other, you took a test, and you move on. And we got tired of doing that. You know, everyone does leadership classes but we never see anything different happen.

This quote from Gloria highlights how youth leadership development may not always be nurtured in impoverished community settings, because often the infrastructure, opportunities, and expectations of leadership are missing (Rogalsky, 2009). It is exactly the missing infrastructure that Gloria and the youth became more aware of during the training and retreat sessions outside of their community. This new understanding empowered them to bring such an infrastructure to South Tucson and create structured, regular opportunities for youth to be leaders and to develop the next generation of youth leaders. Many scholars agree that didactic, lecture-based adult-led classes are not conducive to learning and certainly not conducive to internalizing leadership, civic engagement, or community change practices (Cammarota & Fine, 2008; Freire, 1968; Ginwright, Noguera, & Cammarota, 2006). Rather, engaging in participatory-based leadership was meaningful to the youth, particularly within a context in which they were supported and able to bring it back home through their activities at the JVYC (Ginwright et al., 2006).

This is another important reminder why after-school programs are often not sufficient to really create long-term change; the root of the risky behaviors is within societal infrastructure, particularly within impoverished communities, and attempts to only focus on individual responses to pervasive and constant messages and opportunities to engage in risky behavior are unsuccessful. This is exactly why community transformational resilience is necessary, particularly within low income communities with multiple layers of structural inequalities. There is a need to transform the environment in order to create more resilience promoting factors. Individual level resilience in a community with few resources and many risk factors is not likely to be enough to keep youth on a positive developmental trajectory. Furthermore, sustaining efforts to change the surrounding community is a daunting task that, for communities in poverty, has not been successful for generations—let alone something that adolescents could enact independently. They needed help from other youth and from adults who have developed a critical consciousness about the humanization and capacity of adolescent leaders.

It could have been easy for the JVYC youth to return home and perceive that the community problems were too big to change or that their own individual efforts were insufficient. And in fact, it was the critical combination of youth and adults working together that amounted to the change. With the desire to implement new techniques and to create city-level change through the support of more young people, those involved helped to grow the program into something much bigger than how it began. It was the commitment to creating change from youth and adults alike that, in the end, was transformative for the entire community's resilience. This program was different because it prompted something to change within the youth that they could carry back to change the harsh realities that they witnessed in their own neighborhoods.

6.1.4 Relationship Approach to Prevention

Gloria went on to explain how JVYC began to pay more attention to what the youth were already doing in their existing networks and reoriented their programming to match the strengths of the youth and consider the types of interactions that were meaningful to the youth in their own community. This rethinking by the JVYC adult staff was pivotal in the way they conducted all of their programming and ultimately in the result that it had on the youth.

> There were conversations, you know, we always talk to our kids, and we know everything that's going on in their lives, and one of the things we noticed was that if one of their friends had a problem, or even one of our kids had a problem, as much as they trusted us, they wouldn't come to us first for advice, they always went to their friends. And we started thinking about that, 'so why aren't we really educating the kids more' so they can give their friends educated answers, to a problem like, 'Hey, I think I may be pregnant,' they were giving crazy answers like 'Well, dude you should do jumping jacks' or 'drink this' or something.
>
> So a lot of it came from some of the one-on-one relationships we had with our kids here. We really push a relationship-based approach here. If we have a good relationship with our kids they're so likely to, do what we ask them, like 'Come on, join this class,' or 'Come on, join this, let's do this' so, it is a positive getting them to do really interesting things.

By contextualizing their programming in the existing social networks employed by the youth, Gloria explained that their efforts began to have more of an effective influence. In these ways, JVYC's approach was rooted in personalismo, in other words taking a personal relationships approach to adults working with youth and youth working with their peers. Through educating youth on issues such as pregnancy, in which much misinformation and "crazy answers" are shared among youth, Gloria and JVYC tapped into the strengths and needs of the community. The peer-to-peer model was also the foundation of the Omeyocan YES program which had been successful, particularly in increasing youth knowledge and comfort in talking about substance use and risky sexual behavior prevention among teens (see Chap. 4 for details).

6.1.5 Empowering Female Youth Leadership

Two youth in particular who attended programs at JVYC stood out in Gloria's mind when she thought about how the programs and the youth involved began to change. She explained how engaging two young women led to positive outcomes for the group. For the protection of these individuals, their names have been changed. Gloria highlighted the strengths of the youth and explained the changes that happened when they took on leadership roles:

> And about that same time we had two young ladies that were here, they came to the Center. One was named 'Yesenia' and one was named 'Angelina' and… during that time I had also been the case manager here for all of the kids, and those two girls had been coming to the center since they were in Kindergarten, and, part of our measures is that okay, great, if we've been working with a kid since Kindergarten and now these girls are supposed to be in 11th grade, that should be kind of a mark of if we're doing good and the problem with these girls was that they were awesome—they started off in our Girl Scouts, they were in Cross Country, they were in all these positive activities when they were in Elementary School. Middle School hit and we saw a decline. High School hit and it was a disaster. These girls had already since—for 3 years—had already been kicked out of about 12 schools, 12 different charter schools—some for drug use, some for fighting. And these girls were just, they were just, not doing well.

This anecdote is representative of national trends for Latina adolescents. For over 30 years, Latinas have had the highest rates of depressive symptoms and suicide attempts during adolescence (CDC, 2008; Eaton et al., 2008, 2011; Romero, Edwards, Bauman, & Ritter, 2013; Zayas, 2011). Depressive symptoms and suicide attempts are associated with risk factors that represent marginalization from school, peer isolation, and lack of belonging (Romero et al., 2013). While overall high school dropout rates have decreased for all groups and for Latinos specifically over the past 40 years, Latino male and female adolescents still have the highest rates of dropouts, 13.9 % and 11.3 % respectively (U.S. Census Bureau, 2013). Thus, Gloria's approach to further involve the young women and link them to something important, like improving their community, and being peer role models was in so many ways a revolutionary approach to responding to young women who were clearly getting pushed out of educational systems. Additionally, Gloria's approach demonstrated that she believed in the young women, and in fact, given her history with them, she had witnessed a positive and leadership side of the young women when they were younger. However, given the larger context of negative stereotypes of Latinas, and specifically Mexican American adolescent females from South Tucson, Gloria's belief in something good and worthwhile in the young women was an important pushback to the messages that they were receiving from the larger society and certainly from their local school settings.

She continued:

> Before I became their case worker I had worked with them on this program called, Girlz Nite, which was really a girl's empowerment program, and these girls were bright, and they had such aspirations, and it was so sad to me to see them decline.

> So, as a social worker, we really try to work at getting them back at school, kind of motivating them. We had gotten them back into Las Artes, which is a GED program here and, part of that program, as I said, we really did a lot of family involvement. It was really intensive case management. I was constantly supervising them.
>
> And, these girls actually managed to attend their GED classes for 4 months, and not ever be late, not ever get kicked out, which was a huge feat. One of the girls, Yesenia, she got her GED, and she was really excited. But Angelina failed her GED. And I was so ready—I was like, 'oh my god, this, she's gonna go back, she's gonna go back to her bad ways, I don't know what to do 'because she can't do this whole program again.' And I was just so pleasantly surprised when she said, 'you know what? I don't want my GED. I'm gonna go back to high school.' And she went back to [high school], she did the accelerated program summer school and she got her high school diploma.
>
> And that wasn't enough… these girls wanted to go to college now.

The stark difference between the young woman who dropped out of high school and the one who was resilient even in the face of adversity lies in the investment. Gloria's non-traditional investment in her positive development and, as a result, achievement flies in the face of all the odds that were against this young woman. Although several factors were certainly at play, the influence of youth leadership and positive programming in this young woman's life is unambiguous. Through her involvement in the JVYC and by having a positive adult mentor such as Gloria encouraging and expecting great outcomes, Angelina began to internalize the understanding that she was able to take ownership of her aspirations and achieve them, despite whatever obstacles stood in her path. Gloria continued on and described how the two young women eventually took on roles of youth leadership with the JVYC and began to inspire within their peers the changes that they had experienced. Thus, the young women became the solution instead of the problem.

> So they both decided, 'we're gonna go,' it was Tucson College I think at the time, they wanted to get their medical assistant degrees, and, I was just so excited, and part of the reason that I'm selecting these two girls was because, what I started seeing was that these girls were leaders, and they kept getting all the kids riled up. They wouldn't go and get high with themselves, they took five kids, they would come to our program, they would say 'come on, let's go,' and, you know, we're a drop-in program, we're like, 'Nooo! Don't leave!' and I started to see that but what I also started to see when they were doing good, they were telling the kids, they'd be like, 'Hey fool, you're not even in school, you should come to school with me,' and they must have gotten 20 kids enrolled in Las Artes that had already been dropped out, and it was just like, 'wow! They're listening to these girls! That's crazy, you know! Like, here I am, begging these kids, showing them all these things, doing a wonderful show, 'Please come back to school, do this.' I couldn't get them motivated and I was just like, 'it's the power of teens on teens'—that peer pressure, whether it's good or negative is so powerful!

Gloria's description of the young women here also demonstrates how intricately linked substance use and educational outcomes are, particularly in the community of South Tucson where 42 % of the adults did not have a high school diploma (U.S. Census Bureau, 2012).

> And, so, we had an idea. We're like, you know what, we had some extra money in our budget and we needed to hire a Rec Aid and I said, 'Why don't we hire those two? Look at them—if they can get all these kids in high school, I bet you if we start doing this class, they'll get all of them to join. If we start doing this… they'll get them all to join.' So, it really became about, let's get them all to do positive things and it just worked out amazing.

While Gloria saw that the youth were still engaging in some risky behaviors, she also noted that they were beginning to have a positive influence on youth educational achievement. This reflection is the essence of strengths-based programs, where Gloria chose to hire the young women and to build on the strengths that they had. Her decision was also strategic because it ensured that the young women had to stay in the building—they couldn't just "drop-in" and then leave and return again. This was much more likely to limit their opportunities to engage in substance use and thus limit the young women's access to taking other youth with them to use substances through only "dropping-in" at JVYC. Additionally, after the Omeyocan YES program and the Y2Y program, Gloria was more aware of peer-to-peer modeling as a way to create youth change and promote adolescent health. As such, she chose to work with these young women who were peer leaders. This is a much different model than most traditional after-school models where adults teach youth in a linear manner. Moreover, her approach is significantly different from most alcohol prevention strategies that do not consider the educational context of young people. More traditional strategies also often focus on abstinence rather than accepting where youth are at and identifying present strengths in order to facilitate holistic and contextually embedded development—that is, considering their educational, peer, and after-school contexts. Lastly, Gloria's approach demonstrated that adults would not give up on youth even if they continue to engage in risky behaviors at any level.

6.1.6 Benefits of Youth Leadership

Reflecting on how these changes were made possible, Gloria again emphasizes the role that the financial backing, that came with a new grant that grew out of relationships developed through the STPC, played in the success of their program:

> I really don't think it was until we got our Drug Free Community grant that we had some pretty big money to—we had a lot of ideas of what we wanted to do. We had projects we had seen nation-wide, and that we've seen in other cities that really worked, but we didn't have the resources ourselves to do it, and we didn't have the money. So, this grant came in to play and I think it really just gave us this awesome push that we could really do some awesome stuff with this community, and that's really where we started to see our youth changing. It started with those two girls, it started with these classes, and it just started snowballing into something really big.
>
> And, right now, we're really lucky. We've got a great group of kids, and, you know, if we look at their successes, it's astounding, you know, like, I feel like such a late bloomer! I mean, they have better accomplishments than I've ever had! And I'm jealous and proud at the same time. But, you know, we're just really lucky. We've got some awesome kids and we know that it wasn't something that happened overnight. It's been years in the making, so, we're really excited to be where we are now.

An important message resonates with Gloria: for as much as youth benefit from working with adults in programs such as those run through the JVYC, the adults benefit from the engagement just as much. Gloria spoke at length about giving voice and listening to youth as well as creating opportunities for youth to take on roles of leadership among their peers. The implied and overt subtext of her interview was also clear though—she and the adults at JVYC learned a tremendous amount about youth and how to help youth by engaging the very individuals they set out to assist. Once Gloria and other adults developed that critical consciousness of the youth in their own community, then there was sufficient momentum to not only keep it going but to also build more opportunities for youth. It was their consciousness about the societal context of youth behaviors, combined with a strengths-based approach, that valued, honored, and challenged the youth, inclusive of their cultural background and role as equal contributors to the community.

6.2 Jaime's Story: Laying the Groundwork for Community Transformational Resilience

Jaime Arrieta worked as the youth outreach and prevention specialist at the Southern Arizona AIDS Foundation (SAAF) for 7 years. He played a key role in the South Tucson Prevention Coalition by linking youth with the coalition and providing continual after-school youth spaces for in-depth prevention classes and leadership training for civic engagement. In his time working at SAAF, Jaime created a prevention program called Voz (i.e., translation to the word "Voice" in Spanish) which educated youth about risky behaviors (e.g., substance use, unsafe sexual health practices, self-harm) and worked to develop life skills for community involvement and self-efficacy with youth (e.g., refusal, communication, cultural pride). This after-school program was offered at JVYC and other local areas and helped to develop a youth pipeline for the Y2Y and youth participation in the coalition. One aspect of the Voz program which differentiated it from other prevention efforts was the focus on establishing equitable dialogue among its members—valuing the voice of each individual as being of equal importance to the prevention and educational content presented. This is a fundamental approach to work relying on Freire's (1968) model and participatory action research (McIntyre, 2008). The opportunity to learn and practice these skills in a youth-centric space was an important groundwork for the youth to be prepared to participate as equals in STPC and in future alcohol mapping PAR activities. Although Voz was created as a prevention curriculum for risky behaviors, Jaime understood that in order to truly engage the youth he would need to take a comprehensive approach to participating in youth experiences in the South Tucson community.

6.2.1 *Community Level Voice and Change*

Youth were encouraged to share their experiences as contextualized in their environment and cultural understandings and engaged in dialogue about the influences these contexts had on their behaviors, values, and outlook. Unsurprisingly, many graduates of Jaime's Voz program were the youth who went on to become involved in the future activities of the STPC and Y2Y, such as the alcohol mapping project and the successful protesting of the state granting a liquor license to a local South Tucson Walgreens (see Chap. 9 for a summary). Jaime's involvement with the youth of South Tucson was one component of the larger system of efforts working toward youth health promotion and education, but his hard work stands out as laying the groundwork for the youth-driven community changes that emerged—inspiring youth to believe in the power of their voice.

A key element of the Voz program was the active role the youth played in their learning. Rather than merely relying on presenting facts and information to the youth, the adults involved in Voz facilitated open dialogue about risky behaviors and about how risky behaviors are present in the larger community context. Jaime explained the "*voice in the back of [your] head...that voice is your subconscious. It tells you what's right and what's wrong regardless of how you were raised. In general, you sort of know what's right and what's wrong.*" Developmentally, adolescents can possess cognitive understandings of what is right and what is wrong. Decision-making, however, or deciding whether or not you choose the "right" or the "wrong" option is a skill that adolescents do not master until early adulthood. The Voz program encouraged the youth of South Tucson to be more conscious of their "gut" understandings and how to follow those values through openly dialoguing with informed adults about such sensitive matters. In "*meeting the youth where they were*," Jaime encouraged the importance of participant voice and engagement with the curriculum. The youth were free to ask any questions they were curious about and were given the opportunity to take ownership of their voice. Thus, inspiring voice was twofold for the Voz program and STPC.

Youth participated in a photo-voice participatory action research project through Voz where they took pictures of the aspects of their community that they felt were positive influences and the aspects that they felt were negative influences. Afterward, the youth presented their findings to their youth group and engaged in critical dialogue to raise consciousness (Freire, 1968). Through this exercise, the participants of Voz developed an understanding that their perceptions and experiences mattered and that their opinions were especially important in the context of the communities in which they lived. This type of participatory action research activity laid the groundwork for later youth-led work with STPC where they took their results to the next level of sharing with the broader community of adults and civic leaders. From the Voz activities, youth learned that they could bring about community change through an internalized message that they have the right to take issue with aspects of a community that are detrimental to their health; moreover, they have the insight and ability to help their community change for the better. Some of the negative community attributes that the youth identified were trash, graffiti, alcohol consumption and signage, homelessness, gangs, and drug presence. This work was also a critical precursor for the future work on community alcohol license and signage mapping.

Jaime and Gloria took a clear stance against the faulty deficit-driven view of youth and moved toward a perspective of youth agency and capability through the programs offered and the ways in which they interacted with youth. It was these settings that were created by critically conscious adults that helped to nurture the development of youth leaders who were prepared and confident to participate in the South Tucson Prevention Coalition. Jaime explained how the Voz program challenged the youth to have an active voice in their community:

> It really got the youth to be able to engage in their community and look at their community and [see] what are the problems in our community. We were able to plant some of those seeds on the educational level of like 'Ok this is your community. What are some of the problems you see in it?' I got to interact with these youth and help them create the need… what their need was in their community.

Through the Voz program, Jaime worked to lay the groundwork for youth to believe that they had a voice, were capable of enacting change, and had the right to better themselves and their community. These were key factors in the youth involvement in STPC. Once youth had discovered their voice it was easy to integrate them into working with the adults in the coalition. Some youth were very shy at first, and it took time before they felt comfortable to honestly share their perspectives.

6.2.2 Agency and Respect

Another key component of youth development to which Jaime frequently referred was the concept of agency or efficacy. That is, the belief that one can make decisions for him or herself and influence their self and surroundings. Inspiring the youth who were involved in Voz to believe that they could make a difference in their lives and surroundings was critical to eliciting the final outcome of true community change. It is important to note that these changes did not occur over night. As Jaime explains, "*Community change is very slow. [However] when it happens it kind of has a lot of inertia.*" This statement is very similar to what was noted by Gloria; once there was a breakthrough with adults and youth there are strong momentum that led to bigger changes. When asked about the youth and community reactions to the youth-initiated changes regarding the liquor signage and license denial, Jaime explained that a great deal of respect was given to the STPC and the youth involved. Jaime added that another critical thing he thought the youth took away from being involved in the community and the Voz program was respect—respect for oneself and others and the importance of being an ally. This most basic element is fundamental to working with youth of color, who often face being dehumanized, stereotyped, and disrespected on a regular basis (Garcia-Coll et al., 1996). To facilitate such outcomes, Jaime made it clear that the youth were always treated with respect. He explained:

> I have the grownup insight to pass along to the youth in a language they can understand without discriminating or making them feel less. It's us talking as people not me talking to you. I'll give you the scenario and let's come up with the solution together.

6.2.3 The Role of Dialogue

This concept of supporting a mutual dialogue between leaders and underserved or underrepresented individuals follows a model of exploration and change as established by educational thinker, Paulo Freire (1968). Freire argued against the "banker model" of education where the student was to be "filled" with knowledge or content almost as a transaction of putting money into a vault. Instead, he passionately described a system of co-creation of knowledge between the learner and the learned with both individuals holding each role of the learner and the learned simultaneously. Parsing out the political ramifications of Freire's work, what remains is a core value of humanizing each individual through dialogue—ensuring agency and voice for every person without hierarchy, dominance, or oppression. This is one more critical element of what allowed for such positive changes to occur in the South Tucson community. The youth were treated with respect and dignity and engaged in such a way that they became key participants in their own development.

6.2.4 Seeing Community Change as Collective

In thinking about true community change, it is critical to understand the larger community conceptions of the work being enacted. Jaime explained that outsiders wondered: "That's really cool, how'd you do that? or How does that work?" And he would respond by saying:

> Well, I didn't do it myself. I was just a little small cog in the wheel…and it takes all of those things to make the whole thing function and you just provide whatever you can to make sure that hopefully it works.

Jaime went on to explain the importance of remaining aware of how one's efforts fit into the larger process of change:

> It's kind of like when you're climbing a big hill, all you really do is look down at the ground. You can't look up because you can't see the top of it but when you look back you look [to see] how far I've come. You forget to turn around and look around…and find something that is working. You gotta remember to every now and then look around and keep an eye out for the change because it might happen and you might not see it.

When asked about any advice he had for other communities to learn from STPC regarding youth-direct change, Jaime explained that communities should "*learn about how to organize and get youth buy-in [with] something for the youth to focus on, giving them a project to say 'this is what you have, this is what you get to do with it.'*" In addition, he thought that organizations should "*find out what are the needs of the youth, finding out the needs of the community and…how do you make it work.*" Jaime stressed the importance of the adults who are leading the initiatives getting along and working together toward the larger goals of change.

Through the combined efforts of many individuals, the youth in South Tucson have the opportunity to have a voice and work toward making a change in their community, in part through their participation in STPC. By instilling a sense of agency and capability in the youth through the Voz program, Jaime has clearly worked toward laying the groundwork for youth to believe that they do have a voice and are able to bring about change and create their own realities. Encouraging this agency is no small feat and is truly a beautiful accomplishment. However, as Jaime would point it, bringing about these understandings and goals with the youth was not a one-way interaction from teacher to student. Stressing the importance of dialoguing with youth, colleagues, and the community, Jaime explained that collaboration is crucial for success at every level of the community change process. "*The youth have a voice and it can be heard*."

The work that Gloria and Jaime did with youth in small groups and in providing them opportunities to understand and voice their view of their own community was critical to their ability to step up to leadership within the coalition. When his work was framed in this way and presented back, Jaime was a bit taken aback:

> Robby (interviewer): Just the idea, the core idea, that what the youth have to say—[that] their voices are important—just that idea…it seems like you were really a key person in creating this concept that is so foreign—that we want to hear what you have to say…and that's the groundwork of everything else that came. Jaime: "Thanks, wow, well you sit back and you don't really think about it. It was just something that was fun to do and from my perspective it was empowering the youth to say 'ok these are the problems but how do we attack them'…and coming from a community that didn't have a lot of opportunity or their hands held by their families to do it, a lot of it came from themselves so it was really neat to watch them get inspired by it and do it."

6.3 Conclusion

Just as Jaime made clear during his interview, the most important opportunity that an adult can give a child is a voice. And as both Gloria and Jaime explained, eliciting internalized efficacy over both oneself and context starts with that very voice. By focusing on the roles of community-based organizations (CBOs) in a student's educational experiences, researchers can see a wider scope of ecological factors. For low-income minority families, the social and emotional adjustments of young people influence how they view their own achievements and success (Wong, 2008). The role of adults and the STPC helped to not only build community but also provide opportunities to develop the capacity of the youth by giving them room to examine the structural inequalities. The development of adult critical consciousness about youth and reframing their view of the potential of youth of color was important to the success of STPC. Additionally, the opportunities for continued youth prevention programs that were youth-space oriented were helpful to continue to feed the pipeline of youth who were ready to work with the coalition. They allowed them to examine their identities in the dominant culture and build social capital within their own neighborhood that was more meaningful to them on a cultural and economic basis (Yosso, 2005). By creating the Coalition as a site to create and maintain community norms, values, and trust, youth were given atmospheres to build social capital and examine their membership in their neighborhoods. Youth and adults worked together to create community transformational resilience.

References

Cammarota, J., & Fine, M. (2008). *Revolutionizing education: Youth participatory action research in motion*. New York: Routledge.

Centers for Disease Control and Prevention (CDC). (2008). Youth risk behavior surveillance–United States, 2007. *MMWR Surveillance Summary, 57* (No. SS-4). Atlanta, GA: Author.

Eaton, D. K., Foti, K., Brener, N. D., Crosby, A. E., Flores, G., & Kann, L. (2011). Associations between risk behaviors and suicidal ideation and suicide attempts: Do racial/ethnic variations in associations account for increased risk of suicidal behaviors among Hispanic/Latina 9th-to-12th grade females students? *Archives of Suicide Research, 15*(2), 113–126.

Eaton, D. K., Kann, L., Kinchen, S., Shanklin, S., Ross, J., Hawkins, J., Harris, W. A., Lowry, R., McManus, T., Chyen, D., Lim, C., Brener, N. D., … Wechsler, H. (2008). Youth risk behavior surveillance—United States, 2007. *Morbidity and Mortality Weekly Report. 57,* No. SS-4.

Freire, P. (1968). *Pedagogy of the oppressed*. New York: Seabury.

Garcia Coll, C., Crnic, K., Lamberty, G., Wasik, B. H., Jenkins, R., Vazquez Garcia, H., et al. (1996). An integrative model for the study of developmental competencies in minority children. *Child Development, 67*, 1891–1914.

Ginwright, S., Noguera, P., & Cammarota, J. (Eds.). (2006). *Beyond Resistance!: Youth Activism and Community Change: New democratic possibilities for practice and policy for America's youth*. New York: Routledge.

McIntyre, A. (2008). *Participatory action research*. Thousand Oaks, CA: Sage.

Noguera, P., & Cannella, C. M. (2006). Youth agency, resistance, and civic activism: The public commitment to social justice. In S. Ginwright, P. Noguera, & J. Cammarota (Eds.), *Beyond resistance: Youth activism and community change* (pp. 333–347). New York: Routledge.

Rogalsky J, 2009. "Mythbusters": Dispelling the culture of poverty myth in the urban classroom. *Journal of Geography 108*(4), 198–209.

Romero, A. J., Edwards, L., Bauman, S., & Ritter, M. (2013). *Preventing teen depression and suicide among Latinas*. New York: Springer.

U.S. Census Bureau. (2012). South Tucson census data. http://quickfacts.census.gov/qfd/states/04/0468850.html

U.S. Census Bureau, Department of Commerce. (2013). Current Population Survey (CPS), October 1967–2012. Source: https://nces.ed.gov/programs/digest/d13/tables/dt13_219.70.asp

Wong, N. A. (2008). They see us as resource: The role of a community-based youth center in supporting the academic lives of low-income Chinese American Youth. *Anthropology and Education Quarterly, 39*, 181–204

Yosso, T. J. (2005). Whose culture has capital? A critical race theory discussion of community cultural wealth. *Race, Ethnicity and Education, 8*(1), 69–91.

Zayas, L. H. (2011). *Latinas attempting suicide*. New York: Oxford University Press.

Chapter 7
Youth Perspectives on Youth Power As the Source of Community Development

Joel A. Muraco, Elisa Meza, Oscar Ceseña, Alejandro Gallego, and Michal Urrea

Abstract Within the City of South Tucson, Youth-to-Youth (Y2Y), a positive youth development program, operates within the John Valenzuela Youth Center. A youth-led and adult-guided group, they partnered with South Tucson Prevention Coalition to prevent, reduce, and delay youth substance use including alcohol, tobacco, marijuana, inhalants, and methamphetamines. In the following narratives, the voices of the youth are given a platform in which to tell their truth. Youth leaders Oscar Ceseña, Alejandro Gallego, and Michal Urrea discuss their community, their involvement with the program, and the power of the youth voice. Ultimately, seeking out opportunities to better themselves and their community, they were able to successfully organize and enact positive change to develop community transformational resilience. Collectively, their stories and reflections highlight the power of the positive youth development program when youth are included as equal key stakeholders.

Keywords Youth power • Youth voice • Stakeholders • Community development • Youth leaders

---

J.A. Muraco, Ph.D. (✉)
Human Development and Women's and Gender Studies, University of Wisconsin-Green Bay, 2420 Nicolet Drive MAC C323, Green Bay, WI 54311, USA
e-mail: muracoj@uwgb.edu

E. Meza, M.S.W.
San Francisco Unified School District, San Francisco, CA, USA
e-mail: mezae520@gmail.com

O. Ceseña
Pima Community College, Tucson, AZ, USA
e-mail: cesenao@yahoo.com

A. Gallego • M. Urrea
John Valenzuela Youth Center, Tucson, AZ, USA
e-mail: gallegoclass13@gmail.com; cookie_michal@hotmail.com; michal.urrea@gmail.com

A.J. Romero (ed.), *Youth-Community Partnerships for Adolescent Alcohol Prevention*, DOI 10.1007/978-3-319-26030-3_7

All too often, discussions of how to build better communities do not include building youth involvement and leadership (Ginwright, Noguera, & Cammarota, 2006). The ways youth engage themselves in community spaces outside of school become methodological examples of critical pedagogy based on in the community, *for* the community. The Youth-to-Youth (Y2Y) program (youth-led/adult-guided) was a source of this youth-led critical pedagogy that worked with South Tucson Prevention Coalition (STPC) in order to create community transformational resilience through community-level intervention strategies. These youth-led spaces have the potential to become spaces that develop what scholars refer to as "the social imagination," allowing young people to envision what they would like their community to be like, while acknowledging the current reality (Greene, 2000). Given different "vantage points," (resources and spaces), youth can imagine ongoing achievement individually and collectively as ways of liberating themselves from restraints such as negative stereotypes and prejudice that often disproportionately affect youth of color living in poverty, who may face even more challenges to transforming their community (Freire, 1968). Community spaces can be transformative and thus help youth see that existing inequalities are malleable, and moreover, that youth themselves have the ability to be agentic and enact change.

Within the City of South Tucson, one such positive youth development program is Youth-to-Youth, or Y2Y, which operates within the John Valenzuela Youth Center (JVYC). John Valenzuela was a South Tucson police officer who sought to empower the youth of South Tucson through recreational and educational programs (John A. Valenzuela Youth Center, 2010). Y2Y is a youth empowerment and prevention program (Love, n.d.), designed to be "youth-led and adult-guided" (O. Ceseña, personal communication, November 30, 2010) that operates at the JVYC. The concept of empowerment within the context of positive youth development has been further developed to include ecological determinants of the community they are in as part of a wider strategy to develop their engagement. The understanding of empowerment as described by Banyard and Goodman (2009) is developed through an ecological model to inform how the allocation of resources in a community and the awareness of unequal distribution to youth are a part of its process. The importance of developing empowerment is to define the sociopolitical contexts surrounding the individual, not just the individual themselves. Framing empowerment in a social justice lens supports the need to develop the community as a part of positive youth development.

The assessment of community health is an incredibly crucial component that is missing in traditional school settings. Moreover, most often programs approach community health from a deficit model that only further stigmatizes adolescent behavior. In fact, the Y2Y created many community educational opportunities to provide health education in a manner that was strengths-based and rooted in their own experience living in the community. A critical pedagogy that engages community problems through utilizing novel approaches as way to break away from the status quo rooted in inequalities of their lived situations (Greene, 2000). Once youth develop critical consciousness, they begin to see that social problems, such as youth alcohol use, are multifaceted. However, they also see that solutions have to be multifaceted, and that existing community resources can be marshalled to transform their community. As youth's roles become more connected and interactive within their community, they are more likely to understand how they can improve their environment for themselves, their families, and their peers. In this way, youth can also construct a community transformational resilience by actually changing the infrastructure of their own community, such that it can more readily offer resources and positive development opportunities to many youth while also reducing risks. When youth understand their ecological contexts, their insight can also help identify more specific and relevant solutions to social issues (Flanagan, Cumsille, Gill, & Gallay, 2007). The power in critical pedagogy is to increase youth skills of group decision-making, activity planning, and understanding the broader political contexts they live in (Freire, 1968), which will help them gain critical consciousness and greater empowerment to be agents of change in their community (Cargo, Grams, Ottoson, Ward, & Green, 2003).

Researchers have documented the connection between lower socioeconomic status (SES) and increased alcohol consumption (Van Oers, Bongers, Van de Goor, & Garretsen, 1999) and how after controlling for drinking patterns, lower SES men and women experience more consequences as a direct result of their drinking (Grittner, Kuntsche, Graham, & Bloomfield, 2012). Factors such as social norms regarding alcohol use (Room & Makela, 2000) and availability of alcohol influence prevalence rates and likely are cyclical in their influence. That is: (1) an abundance of alcohol selling establishments are likely to exist in neighborhoods wherein alcohol consumption is a social norm and (2) in neighbors with abundant alcohol selling establishments, the social norm may become one that expects and encourages alcohol consumption. The City of South Tucson was a prime example wherein the social norm from outside, and to some degree from within, was that proximity to alcohol was a positive thing because adults were going to drink.

7.1 Y2Y

JVYC and Y2Y partnered with South Tucson Prevention Coalition (STPC) to prevent, reduce, and delay youth substance use including alcohol, tobacco, marijuana, inhalants, and methamphetamines (City of South Tucson, 2010). Begun in 2002, the Y2Y are a group of youth that attend different schools throughout the City of South Tucson, including charter, public, and alternative schools (J. Alderete, personal communication, January 15, 2015). Initially, members of JVYC attended a Substance Abuse and Mental Health Services Administration conference in Washington, DC where they were first made aware of the Y2Y program. Subsequently, funding became available to take JVYC staff and youth to the Y2Y conference in California

Youth 2 Youth International
Summer 2005 training & conference

Project goals
Brush up skills from the Omeyecan YES graduates
Increase their leadership and empowerment skills.
Offer advanced education on healthily lifestyle choices.
Mentor younger youth (under age 13)
Participate as a member in the South Tucson Prevention Collaboration

To select 10 graduates from the STPC cohorts
The 10 selected will attend the Youth 2 Youth Conference in CA
SAAF will provide workshops & materials on group facilitation
Teens will mentor youth at the 3 safe havens and offer workshops to a minimum of 90 youths

Basic requirements
Must have successfully completed a STPC cohort (Others will be considered, but will require additional Volunteer hours)
Volunteer at any safe haven for a minimum of 25 hours
Recommendation letter from safe haven director or coordinator
Commit to facilitate younger youth workshops during spirit week
Commit to serving on the STPC

Fig. 7.1 Youth-to-youth goals and participation requirements

(see Fig. 7.1). Upon their return, the Y2Y program was implemented. Year to year, the number of youth varies, usually averaging between 8 and 16 youth (J. Alderete, personal communication, January 15, 2015). Many of the youth recruited into the program, such as Oscar Ceseña, have been attending the JVYC for years before they become involved in the Y2Y program.

The Y2Y meet in the evenings to discuss new strategies of raising awareness about substance use issues in their community, often inspired by presentations they have seen and youth retreats they have attended in the past. Through their work, they have organized ways to block corporate chains in the City of South Tucson from obtaining liquor licenses and have written their own scripts to skits performing deeply rooted consequences from driving while under the influence and the importance of confiding in friends and family. The Y2Y gain training skills from attending national youth retreats in other states such as California.

7.2 Beginning Years of Youth 2 Youth: Oscar and Joel

Oscar Ceseña grew up in the City of South Tucson, was a youth in Y2Y, became a Youth Outreach Specialist for Y2Y, and has been a long time member of STPC. Joel (graduate student researcher) was first introduced to Oscar by Dr. Romero at a STPC regular meeting. Joel spent time with Oscar prior to the interview in order to build rapport and to learn more about JVYC mission and resources. Before the interview, Joel also shared the draft of the interview questions and received feedback from Oscar to refine the questions. This exchange was paramount to the success of the interview as it demonstrated what Freire (1968) refers to as "cointentional education" (p. 69). Specifically, this exchange helps to dismantle the preconceived hierarchy that may exist between researcher and participant. Instead, researcher and participant come to be understood as both being subjects whose task it is to recreate knowledge (Freire, 1968). Further, such participation on the part of the community being researched fosters mutual respect of values, strategies, and actions for authentic partnerships (Ahmed & Palermo, 2010). Additionally, from a CBPR framework, it is important for the members of the defined community to have opportunities to participate in the research process (Green et al., 2003).

Joel connected with Oscar several times before their interview, each time working to break down barriers and to get to know each other as people, their lives growing up in Tucson, and issues related to teens. Over the course of 2 weeks Oscar and I spoke, either in person or on the phone, a total of four times. While it was not terribly frequent, it was more often than my training as a researcher had taught me a researcher needs to communicate with a research participant. In my classes, there was next to no discussion about community participation or involvement such that the unspoken understanding was that the researcher only involved the participant as much as was required to ask his or her research questions and debrief the participant after the data had been collected. Either way, four talks led to a mutually respectful relationship to pave the way for a successful interview.

7.2.1 "I Love This Community, Its My Heart"

Oscar Ceseña grew up in the City of South Tucson; he is proud to call it home, stating, "*I love this community… I live in South Tucson, it's, it's my heart.*" It is because the city is his heart that making his community better is so important to him. The youngest of seven children, he witnessed firsthand his brothers and sisters run into trouble, resulting in numerous trips to the juvenile detention center. Oscar says he made a conscious decision early on to be the good kid, and that he "*wasn't going to make my mom cry and make my dad feel disappointed.*" With this resolve, he did well academically and stayed out of trouble. Oscar tells me that because he was doing everything right, his parents left him to his own devices—"*go his own way,*" as Oscar puts it. Compared to his siblings, Oscar took the path less traveled, and he became more involved with the JVYC. Indeed, his commitment to the center is what caught the eye of Gloria Hamelitz-Lopez, the executive director of the JVYC. When the JVYC and STPC partnered and were looking for a youth member, Gloria specifically reached out and asked Oscar to be that member. This increased responsibility served to acknowledge Oscar's good work, which was something he was lacking at home, while also increasing his investment in the work that was being done. Such experiences demonstrate the powerful impact such centers have to transform the lives of youth who may have otherwise followed in the steps of friends and family engaging in detrimental and sometimes illegal behaviors.

It was the praise Oscar received at the JVYC that spurred his interest in community action. Luckily, Oscar found the JVYC early, while in second grade. Oscar says, "*I immediately got a sense of welcome and stuff. So, I started volunteering, after I started growing up a little bit, and doing community service and then, I started an internship, and now I've been working here for almost seven years. So all together I've been coming here for like fourteen years.*" Staff members at the center recognized Oscar as a youth who stood out from the rest and in 2003, when staff members at the JVYV wanted to take a group of youth to the Western States Conference for Y2Y, Oscar was one of seven youth chosen to attend. About the conference and his experience with Y2Y, Oscar says,

> So when we got there it was just really out of our element. We were just like, 'what is this place?' But it was just a bunch of youth running around talking about drug free, doing skits, just a really cool place. So when we got back here we decided to start our own South Tucson Y2Y. So, that's how it started for us. We started developing our own skits also and going out and talking about drug and alcohol free prevention. And now it's been, what is it, seven years since it's been here and we just have a completely new group of kids. Some of them, they started off when they were like thirteen and then they started growing up so they kind of pass the torch to then some of the new kids that are in middle school and stuff. Which is what we wanted. And Youth-2-Youth is, the fundamental guideline is it's youth led and adult guided so I've already done the youth leading and now me and the site director (sic) are the adult guides.

It is his experience both as a youth activist and now Youth Outreach Specialist that distinguishes Oscar from many of his peers. Having had the experience of being an Omeyocan YES graduate, youth member of Y2Y, and now helping to run the youth programs at JVYC, Oscar has incredible insight into the program and its impact on the youth in the community.

7.2.2 Youth Involvement with the Coalition

With Y2Y focusing on drug and alcohol prevention and youth empowerment, STPC found an ally in the Y2Y program when they sought out community youth to add youth voice and perspective to their coalition. Oscar tells the story,

> Yeah. STPC, South Tucson Prevention Coalition, it's they got a grant here in South Tucson to start doing more community outreach for drug, and alcohol, and gang prevention. And so, they needed a youth member so Gloria Hamelitz, the site director here from the center, she asked me to go so I went and we just started doing some stuff with the community that youth, from the perspective of youth. So, that's how we started working with them.

Oscar says that what was really important to the members of STPC was that the youth in the community had an equal voice and that their voice be heard. Oscar comments, "*And so I gave my, I gave my outlook, and they, started listening so it was really important that my voice was being heard and they wanted to know what youth were thinking*." Oscar recognized the importance his words had, stating, "*…at first it was nerve-racking, but just the feeling of them actually listening and wanting to know what I have to say was very fulfilling…*" Through the actions of the STPC members, Oscar felt a sense of empowerment, which was a goal of both STPC and Y2Y.

Essentially, STPC and Y2Y were interested in large-scale social change, which by its very nature requires broad cross-sectional coordination to be successful (Kania & Kramer, 2011). The more organizations and voices at the table, the better the chances of success, with each voice taking and executing its own piece/s. Such an approach helps ensure that each voice, or group of voices organized into a group, can excel in a way that supports and is coordinated with the actions of others (Kania & Kramer, 2011). When asked what concerns he first voiced, as a youth, to STPC, Oscar says,

> Back, back like a couple of years ago South Tucson wa-, it actually now it's still looked down upon, like they say that 'all these bars and alcohol and everything' but actually every year for like the past ten years South Tucson has been, losing a bar. Which is a good thing. But, back then, I was, I still, get mad, but back then I was younger and I use to get really mad that people would say, 'Oh, South Tucson is bad.' And I knew, I mean, living here you see the stuff that happens, but it happens everywhere else, not [just] in South Tucson. But, I really wanted people, my first outlook was that I wanted people to see how good South Tucson could be. So, I wanted to work on that, also, but getting rid of alcohol sales and stuff like that.

Oscar's passion for his community is apparent in his descriptions; moreover, his strong desire to focus on the positive assets in his own community fuels his work. He acknowledges the negative stereotypes and prejudice against his community, and how it was upsetting. Yet, with the help of Omeyocan YES, JVYC, and Y2Y, he was given the skills and support to raise positive awareness about his community and to help transform negative views. When given the tools, youth make the decisions to act on their interpretations of why their environments exist the way they currently are. If given the tools, youth are likely to make informed decisions and to take these opportunities to the next level by sharing their opinions about their neighborhoods. With an opportunity to have input in what should be done in their community, youth of the Y2Y chose to prevent further growth of negative assets and create a way to inform their city council of the injustice being put on their families.

7.2.3 Targeting Community Norms Together

With the help of Y2Y and STPC, the community of South Tucson has since been working on improving the community by taking an active stand against the sale of liquor, the perceptions that drugs and alcohol are normative, and that starting early is okay, among others. One event, the community's biggest events is National Night Out, which Oscar talks about as,

> Well, we had our biggest event (which) is National Night Out, where the whole city, the whole city council right there, they have a big event with a talent show and just a bunch of tables of other agencies, kind of a networking place, we have games going on. So, that is our biggest event and it's really an alcohol or drug awareness day. And so, our kids here at the center, we put on different dances that we choreographed so they would just work really hard. We do costumes and everything. Y2Y does a bunch of skits and they just go out there the parents, and everybody, like the city kind of shuts down for a little bit while everybody is over there.

Through the collaborative efforts of the staff at the JVYC, Y2Y, STPC, the city council, and other local agencies, the community is working to change the perception of their community both to outsiders and insiders.

Oscar talks about how, even though he only sees the youth, he knows that his impact on them is impacting their whole family and thus the community at large.

> The community, like I said before, it's changing, it's changing for the better. Like, people are getting their voices out there and they, the youth, that they come here to the center, they go home and they tell their parents about this stuff and their parents, you know, they don't really, some of the parents aren't, they got work to deal with or kids and everything. So when the kids learn the stuff here and go back home and tell them about it, and then you see their parents and their whole family come out to like National Night Out. It's, (that) they're worried about their city and stuff like that so that's cool that they are. They're getting more aware of the stuff that's happening so they want to change that.

This community shift about alcohol norms was likely instrumental in Y2Y and STPC's endeavors to curb the licensing of new alcohol selling establishments. Specifically, youth participants took the cause directly to their parents, through such events as National Night Out. It is likely that this youth-led event influenced parents more than a data-based or research-based approach from outsiders, such as researchers from the University or health specialists from outside agencies. This engagement is central as parents are a key stakeholder in the change process for adolescent health.

7.2.4 Importance of Collaboration from Youth Perspective

The story *Oscar* tells is illustrative of just how sustainable the impact of Y2Y and STPC has been and will continue to be. Implicit in his description is the notion that this is what is next for Y2Y, that there was not a doubt that Y2Y would continue working toward improving the community. Already, Oscar describes, Y2Y has been working with STPC to deliver presentations to various community members and organizations around the city about the dangers of K2 (synthetic marijuana), adding, "*...And it's not us doing the presentations, it's the Y2Y kids cause I think it will have more of an impact on the other teens*." As part of the process of developing empowerment of youth through community education, the ways in which youth discuss issues in their daily lives are crucial to examine. As a method of validating experience, students learn then that they too can become teachers based on the experiences they hold (Freire, 1998).

The act of learning involves the act of being able to teach each other something new, for Y2Y this was through critical pedagogy. Engaging students to share what they feel is important to them, including what issues they see with their environments, they become teachers in a critical way. Encouraging the development of youth agency becomes part of the larger social context while social context is able to inform teaching practices. The more critical youth become of their surroundings, the more they are able to develop "epistemological curiosity," which is the ability to become more creative as to where and how one learns (Freire, 1968). The condition of only thinking of "education" as occurring within a classroom is disrupted. For migrant communities like ones alongside the Southwest U.S./Mexico border, being able to learn from daily experiences can become transformational for an entire community.

When asked about the success of Y2Y and STPC in the City of South Tucson, Oscar talks about the collaborative effort that is involved and required for everything they do. Oscar gives this example of how collaboration has really helped:

> Well, since, it's not just like one person doing the whole thing. It's a whole, (with) different agencies working together. With STPC when we have our lock-ins(retreats) here at the center, Y2Y since, you know, money doesn't grow on trees, but we can't take them to the Western States Conference anymore in California and we haven't been able to for like four years, Y2Y decided to hold their own mini- one day retreats here at the center. So they have basically everything that's a four day retreat in California crammed into one day here. So, they have workshops, they have skits, they have plays, they have different little groups that they split into, we have quest speakers, and that's where STPC comes in, since we work with so many different people, there they all, we have like networking stuff so we get them to come do workshops here at the center and so that's why I think our events work because we have so many like different people that can help."

Through the collaborative efforts of multiple people from multiple agencies, the community is able to overcome barriers that could easily have ended the progress and momentum of the project. Without funding, Y2Y could have found it difficult to sustain itself over a lengthy period of time; however, with the help of local agencies and STPC, Y2Y has found a creative way to sustain itself and ensure growth—through their own one day mini-conferences that mirror the larger, national conference Y2Y used to attend. Ultimately, for Oscar at least, Y2Y will continue because he is committed to having it continue. Oscar's level of commitment has grown over the years, and arguably, the fact that his voice is equitably heard only aided in that commitment. At the end of our interview, when asked about future life plans and goals, Oscar explicitly talks about his commitment to the center, that no matter where he goes or what he does, "*the center is part of who I am.*"

7.3 Institutionalizing and Expanding Y2Y: Michal, Alejandro, and Elisa

The next generation of Y2Y youth leaders is also included in this chapter, through a 4-week long ethnographic study done at the JVYC; Elisa collected meeting notes, interviews, and focus group discussions to identify the visions youth have for their education and community. After observing and building relationships with these particular youth, she gained critical insight to the value of community-space-based pedagogy as created and led by the youth themselves. Youth that engage in community-based practices understand the societal frame of their realities and also understand that something needs to be done to change the current situation. Being able to establish a relationship between being a student and an influential member of society is important to the development of young people. When youth are engaged in active community participation, their empowerment potential becomes a strategy to improve overall community health and well-being (Cargo et al., 2003).

7.3.1 Building Relationships with Participants

Through subsequent weekly visits to the John Valenzuela Youth Center (JVYC) before Tucson Unified School District's (TUSD) spring break recess, Elisa (undergraduate student researcher) was able to observe programming meetings with the JVYC's youth group, Youth 2 Youth (Y2Y). She learned more about Y2Y's mission and connected with Y2Y members as individuals. The Y2Y consists of students in high school and participants of the JVYC. As part of this approach, Elisa was able to observe who the leading youth were in the group and which particular students would be interested in being interviewed. After months of building a relationship with the JVYC, its staff, and its students, she felt comfortable enough to approach certain students with requests for interviews. Her timeline was elongated based on her prioritization to respect the priorities of the JVYC and the Y2Y. Having respect for the immediate responsibilities of the center allowed Elisa to participate in assisting in other aspects of the JVYC and spend more quality time with the students themselves outside of my active research.

7.3.2 *Observations and Interviews*

With the participants and staff of the JVYC and Y2Y, Elisa conducted semistructured interviews with three youth leaders and staff and was granted opportunities to observe youth-led programming meetings in the evenings after school, which drew approximately 15–20 youth per night. During the meetings, Elisa maintained her role as a listener as youth led their own agendas for planning. Semi-structured interviews were chosen because of the validity of group reflection processing. Through group reflection processing, youth have the ability to hear other ideas and hear the experiences of others, which the youth reference in their interviews. When one youth would respond, other youth would contemplate and respond with their interpretation, thus providing diverse and rounded answers to probing open-ended questions. Probing questions were asked to explore why their retreat was critical for their community and what they gained as a group from organizing a health event for the JVYC participants. The reflection and discussion that resulted from the interview session organically shifted my research to identify other needs in community pedagogical approaches such as community center sustainability and effective outreach strategies

Michal Urrea is a sophomore at Tucson High Magnet School who started coming to the JVYC when she was in the 5th grade. When asked about her involvement in the Y2Y program, she remembers how it was the creative skit performances done by the youth members that drew her attention the most. The skits being performed were created to inform the community of risk factors from underage drinking and being able to avoid situations where alcohol abuse would not be monitored. On how the Y2Y shaped her understanding of environmental factors such as the presence of alcohol in her community, she states:

> When I joined the Y2Y, I started seeing more people's lives and how they started changing and I would see when we started doing skits and stuff it made me realize like, 'Wow, this is a big thing that could really impact someone, you know?' Looking up at like newspapers, you'd see drunk people getting hurt, out driving and stuff, that's what made me say, 'Wow, I don't want to be that. I want to be part of something that prevents people to do it.'

Michal was given an opportunity within the Y2Y space to share her thoughts on current events in her community and come to a conclusion of how to be involved in the prevention of such issues. Being exposed to the ways youth can inform their community of environmental factors that can harm young people was what prompted Michal to also become an active member in the Y2Y.

For *Alejandro Gallego*, a senior attending Tucson High Magnet School, he sees the Y2Y as a place to stay focused, engaged, and committed to his goals. Alejandro has been coming to the JVYC since he was in middle school and continued to remain involved as a volunteer once he transitioned into high school. He chose to stay busy during his gaps between school and going home by participating in the JVYC's night program, which is where Elisa was able to collaborate with him and Michal in developing focus groups to discuss college. His resilience to stay focused has been a factor influenced by his consistent engagement in the Y2Y and also in the Explorers Program, a leadership program with the City of South Tucson Police Department. When asked how these two programs have helped him grow, he states:

> Yeah, it helped me mature a lot, it helped me like, become a leader because that's what everyone tells me, that I'm a good leader. And I think it's because from volunteering and then being in Y2Y and also in Explorers, South Tucson Police Explorers, all those helped me like, become a leader, helped me know and like…it transformed me to become a better person.

Not only had the programs been able to provide him a space to grow as a leader, but building close bonds with the other youth members also impacted his growth. He saw the Y2Y as a place that always had someone reliable to talk to even when it was personal. Alejandro was able to reflect on his own experiences within the community he was from and see himself as a leader within that community.

For *Michal*, being engaged in the JVYC provided her a space where her academic identity could be appreciated without feeling ostracized or seen as different. Because the JVYC is located within her community, that difference becomes what she has in common with the other youth at the center. When asked what it has been like to work with the Y2Y, she states:

> It's been really inspiring and it's been like just seeing my friends like, I wouldn't think of me being a little nerd and just like staying here and being involved in the Y2Y and stuff, but I would also think of it as helping out the community and thinking of going to college and all that stuff. And like I think it's a really good thing, like, I think even as people would look at you and be like making fun of you, I wouldn't think of it that way, but I would think one day they'll think of me as that person that was really involved.

To be conscious of her identity as an active student being seen as something with a negative connotation speaks to the sorts of ecodevelopmental factors schools wouldn't be able to see if Michal's experience wasn't examined more closely. What if she didn't have the JVYC and had to succumb to not being as involved to simply fit in with disengaged students? Her identity thrived at the JVYC which was embedded within her community. Considering how supported she is within her family, it is hard to imagine she would not have found a way to be involved otherwise. But being able to hear her passion and enthusiasm for the Y2Y granting her so many experiences that enabled her activism in her community, this youth center provides an absolutely necessary factor in her positive development.

7.3.3 Y2Y Foundation of *Personalismo*, Trust, and Safety

This semester, the Y2Y decided to replicate a similar retreat structure motivated by the bonds they formed with youth in California. The youth remarked consistently that their inspiration came from the closeness they shared with youth doing similar work in their communities across the country and the confidence they gained knowing there was social justice work being done, youth-led and youth-organized.

During their programming meetings this semester, youth began putting the retreat concept into action and organized to build capacity within the Y2Y and increase overall attendance at the JVYC. Their motivation from being inspired by youth working in other communities complimented their intentions to build their own capacity and numbers is illustrative of sustainable values. Understanding beforehand that in order to organize an effective retreat they must incorporate sustainability into the purpose rounded out their goals to inform their community of issues affecting their families.

The issue the Y2Y decided to focus on for their first youth-led retreat was health and wellness. Through this focus, they would build an environment that was critical of the system feeding their community as well as how to create an atmosphere within the JVYC that will encourage youth to be supportive of each other. In order to create an environment based on trust and confidentiality, the Y2Y created an agenda that began with the development of trust through brainstorming collective rules/guidelines and energizers, to build community and trust. The agenda continued with presentations, multiple options for workshops, a community organization presentation, outdoor relay challenges, family groups for intimate conversations, and finally a closing ceremony with awards and a field trip to a local mini-golf course.

7.3.4 Results and Discussion

After transcribing the focus group discussions and individual interviews, they were analyzed themes that became critical to my interpretation of community pedagogy. Through a system of coding, themes illustrated the following: (1) leadership development, (2) the importance of open climate spaces, (3) critical community pedagogy, and (4) sustainable youth development. Through significant quotations taken from the interviews and focus group discussions, an understanding is developed of the JVYC's implementation of community pedagogy and its impact on education.

7.3.5 Leadership Development

When beginning the open-ended interview and discussion on what the purpose of the JVYC health retreat was for her individually, Michal Urrea was the perfect participant to answer. As a leader in the Y2Y and a junior at Tucson High Magnet School, Michal also participated as a lead organizer and group leader for and during the retreat. For her, it was critical to remember what it used to be like in the past to organize a retreat. She states:

> This year we did it very different than other years because other years, I didn't feel like we were the leaders. I felt like we were just helping other people that were doing the retreat. And now, we were all in charge of it. We were like the young adults that were there, and not just the "kids."

For Michal, the development of leadership was critical to her experience in organizing a retreat. It was important for her to feel influential as a "young adult" and not just as a student in the space. The respect she obtained from the staff at the JVYC while being a member of Y2Y gave her confidence in her leadership abilities. Her excitement to describe the role she had added vibrancy to her statement. The agency she was able to obtain as a leader and feeling directly influential to the education of her peers was a critical observation made during her interview.

7.3.6 The Development of Open Climate Spaces

Before we engaged in discussion pertaining to the content of the health retreat, Michal discussed the importance of having a space to discuss personal issues within the smaller groups formed. As part of the purpose of the retreat, students were given more intimate group spaces designated as "family groups" to discuss deeper issues together. As one of the leaders of a family group, Michal states: "This year, it was more like *opening up.*" The ability to have a space where students feel they can express themselves was a critical part of this retreat, not only for the students but also for the JVYC as a whole. Michal even mentioned what it meant for her to "open up" with the younger students in middle school who attended. When discussing how the space changed for the younger students in center, she states:

> They come here everyday, we talk more. Before, we would kind of talk, but now, we feel it's more open. Now we talk to the little smaller kids…It felt cool to know that they were there. You got to share stories and kinda talk to each other about what's going on.

Not only was it critical to have open climate spaces for more personal discussions, the interaction between the older and younger students proved to be critical to the development of the space. That intergenerational exchange of experiences helped Michal see the younger students in a different way and see her role as a leader in a more critical position as well. By "opening up" to each other, their experiences were interpreted into actionable steps to begin discussing their community environment in more critically conscious ways.

7.3.7 Critical Community Pedagogy

In the process of brainstorming the agenda for the retreat, Michal provided insight to the sorts of presentations the Y2Y wanted to incorporate. The presentations and workshops provided were meant to build a better of understanding of issues that directly affected their community. Besides living healthy lives, eating healthier, and building healthier habits, the Y2Y wanted to address issues that were taboo in their traditional school settings. One of the main presentations of the retreat day was one done by a local community organization called SAAF (Southern Arizona AIDS

Foundation). SAAF facilitators presented a documentary called, "Let's Talk About Sex," which generated a critical response from Michal. Just as the family groups were designed to include intergenerational exchanges, the SAAF presentation on how to discuss sex and global sexual health included younger student participants. Michal states: "*It made the middle schoolers more mature, they weren't laughing. The kids were more open to them [SAAF facilitators], even the ones that rarely talk, I was really impressed with them.*" The change in teaching dynamics, from teachers at school to community organization presenters, generated a critical community pedagogical model that impacted the participation of middle-school-aged youth. They were responsive and engaged with a subject Michal said they would normally not take seriously.

The purpose of having SAAF present was also meant to incorporate discussion on how we talk about health within our own families and communities. The documentary discussed how sex is discussed within these settings across the world. In America, how sex is discussed is extremely different in contrast to other countries. Michal summarized an important point from the film, stating:

> People think of sex being a bad thing. They don't know how to talk about it. But in different countries [not America], they see it like a normal thing. Here [America], if you talk to your mom or dad about it, they get all weird. But I thought it was cool for kids to know.

Michal brings up an intriguing point made about the ways in which critical health discussions are discussed within family settings. In public education, sexual education is meant to fill the gap of knowledge students might not obtain at home. But if there is still a lack of understanding of something as important as sex, not as taboo but as integral to global health, how are youth to know when discussing certain topics is considered inappropriate? Having a presentation done by JVYC, which is an organization that serves the community, is melding together the necessity to bring awareness to issues that affect not only the City of South Tucson, but also communities across the world. A rounded perspective on education that includes perspectives from other communities gave Michal an understanding that her community was not alone in battling systems that continue to repress critical education.

7.3.8 Sustainable Youth Development

As discussed in the prior theme subheadings, incorporating younger students in critical discussions was integral to building a culture at the JVYC. Michal consistently commented on the impact of having younger students in critical dialogue and even mentioned their ability to take critical topics more seriously. As a leader in the family groups, Michal states: "*I felt like really important, like they respected me more than when I'm just like their friend...it felt cool to know they were listening to me and paying attention.*" Whether Michal intended to or not, she created a sustainable model within the critical community learning space. As an older student, she was able to model for the younger students what it meant to also be a teacher for them. She became a model of facilitating critical knowledge, discussion, and group learning processes.

Having another youth like Michal become a facilitator in discussions gave her insight to the dynamics in school that might affect the engagement of younger students. When I had asked Michal to elaborate on why she felt certain topics aren't able to be discussed in classroom settings at school she states:

> In school, I think it's because the teachers are the ones that come up with stuff. And students don't step into do anything. Adults do it. They're gonna do something about it, or tell on us…[in the family groups] we made a bunch of rules like secrecy, 'everything stays here.'

It was extremely critical to acknowledge the point Michal brings up concerning teacher–student dynamics. Being fearful of discussing certain topics in class creates an extremely unsafe environment overall. The only space Michal found to discuss topics like sexual health happened in the JVYC on a day that was not dominated by adult participation. Instead, youth became the leaders in discussions, in choosing the topics being taught, and including all participants of the JVYC no matter what age they were. The students who organized the event broke down multiple traditional learning space characteristics including who was teaching and how they participated. Understanding that the intentions of the organizers were also to bring each other closer created a new learning environment as well. The JVYC became an educational space developing how students think about their community by encouraging them to be the leaders in discussing, planning, and participating.

Keyla Ramirez, an adult JVYC staff member and retreat organizer, provided insight on the development of future goals for the JVYC. Her responses identified the need to build capacity of the center and attendance of new students. From this retreat, they developed a new way of outreach, focusing on maintaining and increasing their numbers. Keyla stated that there is brainstorming currently ongoing in how to create similar retreats for their constituency and in a way that will give youth new experiences such as camping and traveling to other cities. It was important for her to note the difference in the environment at the JVYC after the retreat. More youth were consistently returning to the center, as well as, becoming a lot closer, more engaged in each other's lives, and bringing more positive energy to the space as a whole based on their involvement in the retreat. This is evidence of the central role of personalismo, in other words the organizing means of developing personal relationships in order to mobilize communities for community transformational resilience.

The study Cargo et al. (2003) conducted on Healthy Communities Processes illustrates the impact youth can have on the health of their communities simply by being empowered to think positively towards their family's and community's health. Through a partnership created between adults and youth, youth are enabled to provide feedback to the organizational space, and they are engaged to become active participants in the process of learning (Cargo et al., 2003). This "transactional partnering process" is essential to the improvement of community health and specifically for the development of youth empowerment (Cargo et al., 2003). Students need to feel that their experiences and feelings toward their own health and communities are discussed in spaces where their knowledge isn't construed as inadequate, but rather, the essential component of how we can improve community health. Active control and opportunities for action must be provided for youth ideas to foster innovation and their growth as leaders.

In order to provide opportunities for action, spaces for critical consciousness and civic development must be created, within the community the youth connect to. According to Godfrey and Grayman (2014), "open climates" are what promote critical consciousness among youth. Open climates, specifically in classrooms, refer to spaces in which issues can be openly discussed with respect to all opinions (Godfrey & Grayman, 2014). Critical consciousness then consists of the ability to read social conditions, feelings of efficacy to effect change, and actual participation in these efforts, which Cargo et al. (2003) discuss within the youth empowerment process. However, within the framework of open classroom climates (Godfrey & Grayman, 2014), students not only participate in the development of the space, but in a space specifically facilitated to allow youth to approach controversial issues and utilize their own experiences and opinions to inform the efforts taken to prevent such issues, such as community violence and poverty. Within the "open classroom climate" framework, the focus is less on the partnership between adults facilitating the spaces necessary for youth development, but more on the necessity to build consciousness and empowerment amongst the youth directly to impact change in the community as a pedagogical method (Godfrey & Grayman, 2014). Once critical consciousness has risen, youth can then interpret their own social conditions and take action, which leads to the following qualitative analysis based on the work of youth implementing their critical consciousness within their communities.

7.4 Concluding Comments

In order to build healthier communities, community collaboration is necessary to create programs that address specific local ecological needs. Expanding this collaboration to ensure youth voice increases the scope of experiences and perspectives necessary and important to examine. Finding ways to build youth empowerment is essential to creating positive programming in community spaces, as discussed in the study done by Cargo et al. (2003). Building the capacity, strengths and skills of an entire community is a result of the ability to identify how to apply all of their assets (Banyard & Goodman, 2009). Through open climate spaces (Godfrey & Grayman 2014), youth are able to reflect on their experiences and see their experiences and opinions as essential to improving their communities. Y2Y was successful in youth-led critical pedagogy to raise awareness among peers through youth retreats and to raise awareness in their community through community events. Building positive personal relationships based on personalismo values of trust and safety were key to recruitment and collaboration with adults and with peers. They built on the existing assets of youth identity based on a positive view of their own community. Through after-school programs to develop their empowerment and their voice, they were then ready as leaders to participate with adults in community transformation.

As we continue to strive to find more effective ways of building healthier communities and educating youth, integrating student's community engagement should not be overlooked. Youth involvement in their community has the opportunity to be informative and transformative. When given the chance to become architects of their own ideas, youth agency can become a critical role in healthy community development. Youth like Oscar, Michal, and Alejandro witnessed firsthand the toll alcohol was having on their community. Thus, when the JVYC and Y2Y wanted to tackle alcohol in The City of South Tucson, the youth were predominately supportive. Seeking out opportunities to better themselves and their community, they were able to successfully organize and enact change. Through youth involvement with JVYC and Y2Y, parents also became more involved in bettering the community. The culmination of the collaboration between the community, the JVYC, and Y2Y, came when the City of South Tucson successfully lobbied to keep a national chain from acquiring a liquor license for their South Tucson location.

References

Ahmed, S. M., & Palermo, A. G. S. (2010). Community engagement in research: Frameworks for education and peer review. *American Journal of Public Health, 100*, 1380–1387.

Banyard, V. L., & Goodman, L. (2009). Collaboration for building strong communities: Two examples. In M. E. Kenny, A. M. Horne, P. Orpinas, & L. E. Reese (Eds.), *Realizing social justice: The challenge of preventive interventions* (pp. 271–289). Washington, DC: American Psychological Association.

Cargo, M., Grams, G. D., Ottoson, J. M., Ward, P., & Green, L. W. (2003). Empowerment as fostering positive youth development and citizenship. *Journal of Health and Behavior, 27*, 66–79.

City of South Tucson. (2010). *ST Prevention Coalition*. Retrieved November 24, 2010, from http://www.southtucson.org/user/department.php?choice=department&deptid=15

Flanagan, C. A., Cumsille, P., Gill, S., & Gallay, L. S. (2007). School and community climates and civic commitments: Patterns for ethnic minority and majority students. *Journal of educational psychology, 99*(2), 421.

Freire, P. (1968). *Pedagogy of the oppressed*. New York, NY: Seabury Press.

Freire, P. (1998). Pedagogy of freedom: Ethics, democracy, and civic courage. Rowman & Littlefield.

Ginwright, S., Noguera, P., & Cammarota, J. (2006). *Beyond resistance! Youth activism and community change: New democratic possibilities for practice and policy for America's youth*. New York, NY: Routledge Publishers.

Green, L. W., George, M. A., Daniel, M., Frankish, C. J., Herbert, C. P., Bowie, W. R., & O'Neill, M. (2003). Guidelines for participatory research in health promotion. In M. Minkler & N. Wallerstein, editors. *Community-based participatory research for health*. San Francisco: Josey-Bass, pp. 419–428.

Greene, M. (2000). The ambiguities of freedom. *English Education, 33*, 8–14.

Godfrey, E. B., & Grayman, J. K. (2014). Teaching Citizens: The Role of Open Classroom Climate in Fostering Critical Consciousness Among Youth. *Journal of youth and adolescence, 43*(11), 1801–1817.

Grittner, U., Kuntsche, S., Graham, K., & Bloomfield, K. (2012). Social inequalities and gender differences in the experience of alcohol-related problems. *Alcohol and Alcoholism, 47*, 597–605.

John A. Valenzuela Youth Center. (2010). *About the Program*. Retrieved November 24, 2010, from http://www.pima.gov/nrpr/centers/valenzuela/index.htm

Kania, J., & Kramer, M. (2011). Collective impact. Stanford Social Innovation Review, Winter, 36–41.

Love, R. L. (n.d.). Effective research-based prevention programming for teens: The essence of youth to youth. Retrieved November 24, 2010, from http://www.youthtoyouth.net/about/dl/Essence%20of%20Youth%20to%20Youth.pdf

Room, R., & Makela, K. (2000). Typologies of the cultural position of drinking. *Journal of Studies on Alcohol, 61*, 475–483.

Van Oers, J. A. M., Bongers, I. M. B., Van de Goor, L. A. M., & Garretsen, H. F. L. (1999). Alcohol consumption, alcohol-related problems, problem drinking, and socioeconomic status. *Alcohol and Alcoholism, 34*, 78–88.

Chapter 8
Raising Community Awareness of Alcohol Norms Through Community Events and Media Campaigns: South Tucson Prevention Coalition Phase 2

Andrea Romero, Michele Orduña, Gloria Hamelitz-Lopez, Juan "Johnny" Quevedo, and Maricruz Romero-Ruiz

Abstract The purpose of this chapter is to discuss the relevance of community norms for alcohol use when targeting prevention of adolescent alcohol use. During Phase 2, South Tucson Prevention Coalition (STPC) worked to raise community awareness of alcohol norms through biannual community-wide events and through a bilingual radio media campaign. This chapter also provides more insight into the way in which the coalition members utilized the Community Readiness Model for Change to help identify community norms and to match intervention strategies in order to target current community norms. Shifting community alcohol norms was one step to increase the community readiness for community transformation prevention strategies. Through the chronological presentation and analysis for coalition report summaries and public press releases, we analyze the important function of external funding, training of coalition members, and the way in which activities built on each other to reach a higher level of readiness that lead to community transformational resilience. We also demonstrate the importance of transparent

A. Romero, Ph.D. (✉)
Family Studies and Human Development, The University of Arizona,
650 North Park Avenue, Tucson, Arizona, 85719
e-mail: romeroa@u.arizona.edu

M. Orduña, M.Ed.
House of Neighborly Service, Loveland, CO, USA
e-mail: miorduna@gmail.com

G. Hamelitz-Lopez
John Valenzuela Youth Center, Tucson, AZ, USA
e-mail: gloriahamelitz@hotmail.com

J.J. Quevedo
Pima Community College, Tucson, AZ, USA
e-mail: Tucsonhigh12@yahoo.com

M. Romero-Ruiz, M.S.
United Way of Tucson and Southern Arizona, Tucson, AZ, USA
e-mail: mrruiz1@gmail.com

A.J. Romero (ed.), *Youth-Community Partnerships for Adolescent Alcohol Prevention*, DOI 10.1007/978-3-319-26030-3_8

communication, positive communication, and mission-oriented communication between the coalition, the community, and the local government.

Keywords Community norms • Alcohol norms • Community readiness • Community awareness

It has been argued that there is a need for further integration of community members in the development and implementation of health promotion activities for Latino youth (Castro, 1999). The integration of community is inclusive of the physical environment, community members, and families. During Community Readiness *Stage 6 Implementation* (See Chap. 2), the South Tucson Prevention Coalition (STPC) focused on working together to develop community activities to raise awareness about the risk of alcohol. While the coalition members agreed that they were at a level of readiness to begin planning and implementation, they felt strongly that the local community was at a level of denial or tolerance. Two of the key findings from Chap. 7 were that adolescents identified the negative influence of alcohol accessibility and the pervasive presence of drunk adults in their community. During the first few years of coalition work, STPC's broad community strategy was to raise awareness about the risks of adolescent alcohol use and to change community norms about the wrongness of adolescent alcohol use.

8.1 Alcohol Norms and Community-Level Approaches

A strategic way to prevent adolescent alcohol use is through community-level approaches that target norms of adolescent alcohol use. Alcohol norms are considered to be the degree of acceptability of adolescent alcohol use in the community, another way to consider this is as "how wrong is it for adolescents to drink alcohol." Community-level alcohol norms are important to consider because young people have a strong desire to fit in with normative behavior among their communities. Additionally, by understanding the norms of a community, the prevention strategy can be shaped in a way that is most appropriate for the readiness level and that will be the best match in order to be more effective for prevention. STPC first focused on social norms in their early years by raising awareness on community norms and developing new and positive opportunities for youth and families to gather in alcohol-free environments.

8.1.1 Disapproval, Risk, and Availability

Adolescent alcohol use is strongly influenced by the community norms such as disapproval by family and peers, perception of alcohol risk, and perception of alcohol availability (Burrow-Sanchez, 2006). The degree to which a community feels that it is acceptable or unacceptable for youth to use alcohol is an important factor in adolescent alcohol use. Similar to the norm of acceptability is the perception of degree of risk involved in adolescent alcohol use (Burrow-Sanchez, 2006). These norms reflect the degree of community readiness to work on prevention of adolescent alcohol use (Oetting et al., 1995). When the community perceives minimal risk of adolescent alcohol use and does not strongly disapprove of adolescent alcohol use they are less likely to be ready to engage in prevention or intervention activities. If the community is still tolerating adolescent alcohol use, they are much less likely to be willing to support prevention strategies (Plested et al., 1998; Thurman et al., 2003). Moreover, attitudes that adolescent drinking is okay, or even expected, may in fact undermine prevention strategies (Plested et al., 1998). The adult perception of how wrong it is for youth to drink has the potential to impact decisions about alcohol regulation in their community.

Another key community-level factor for adolescent alcohol use is availability of alcohol, or in other words the ease in which adolescents have access to alcohol. This is associated with accessibility that youth may have within their own home and in their neighborhood. While some stores may not enforce age requirements for purchase, they may also look the other way when adults buy alcohol to give to youth. Another environmental factor is the presence of alcohol advertisements within the youth's environment. There is strong evidence from multiple longitudinal studies which demonstrate that media exposure of alcohol advertising is linked with the likelihood that adolescents will begin drinking alcohol and with heavier drinking among those adolescents who have already started drinking. Community-level strategies have the possibility of impacting many people, including adolescents and adults. There are also drawbacks as it is likely to take more time to build community capacity, collect data, create or change policy, and to change norms. By changing the shared environment through community-level strategies, the results are more likely to be sustainable and to have potential for long-term behavior change for multiple generations of adolescents. According to the Community Readiness Model for Change, once community perspectives are well-understood then community norms can be influenced through raising awareness (Oetting et al., 2001).

Participatory Action Research and Community Readiness Model for Change both emphasize the importance of building on local community and cultural strengths in order to influence alcohol norms. Mexican descent and Native American adolescents have several unique culturally based values and beliefs that influence their social norms related to substance use. To begin with positive ethnic identity is a source of resiliency and strength for minority youth because it protects them against cultural stressors (e.g., discrimination or family cultural conflict) that are linked to more substance use (Cano et al., 2015; Oetting & Beauvais, 1990; Romero, Martínez, & Carvajal, 2007; Schwartz et al., 2015; Romero & Roberts, 2003a, 2003b; Zimmerman, Ramirez, Washienko, Walter, & Dyer, 1998). Additionally, familism, a collectivistic orientation toward family, among minority youth has been linked with fewer risky behaviors, perhaps due to close and supportive emotional connections, as well as daily positive communication and consistent interaction with family members (Romero & Ruíz, 2007; Van Campen & Romero, 2012; Zimmerman et al., 1998). Thus, positive ethnic identity and family context were both important factors that STPC included in their efforts to raise awareness about alcohol norms in the local community. They did this through activities that promoted a positive identification with youth's ethnic background and through outreach to families in all activities.

Overall the cultural context and relevance of social norms are important to consider; this is one reason why community-led activities and youth-led activities can be so powerful, because they have the most authentic understanding of the perspectives of their own community. Community-led activities are more likely to be able to authentically represent both risk and protective elements found in the local community.

8.2 Theory of Change and Logic Model

The mission of South Tucson Prevention Coalition was to prevent and reduce underage drinking. This mission was agreed upon after several meetings and a significant amount of discussion before reaching consensus about how to focus on the mission in a way that the most members felt was the highest priority. This was important because it was always the center point of the coalition that they were able to come back to in order to get refocused. It also helped to facilitate decision-making for intervention strategies on community alcohol norms for adolescents. The mission also helped to focus discussions that were becoming more tangential to the primary mission.

The theory of change for the coalition was to increase the perception of risk/harm of alcohol and to increase the perception of community, parental, and peer disapproval of alcohol use in order to delay the age of onset of youth alcohol initiation and to reduce current youth alcohol use (see Fig. 8.1). The strategies chosen to tackle these goals were community-led events. In order to reach out to the largest number of community members, they hosted the following events block party, Halloween festival, talent show, red ribbon week, and anti-drug coalition poster contest (see Fig. 8.1). The events targeted to youth focused on increased awareness of the consequences of alcohol use in their community and the perception of disapproval of substance use among peers. The events targeted to parents and adult community members focused on the perception of disapproval of substance use by adolescents.

These events evolved over the years, but all were focused on raising community awareness of alcohol norms of disapproval and alcohol availability (see Table 8.1 for list of events). These activities were planned and organized by adults, with a high level of community engagement in the planning and implementation. Adult coalition members and local agencies organized and held events at their sites; however, in the first couple years events were primarily organized by the lead agency. Many of these early events overlapped with existing activities that the Safe Havens would regularly host. Witnessing other agencies and youth participate in these events consistently, responsibly, and collaboratively was critical to develop trusting relationships among individuals as well as among agencies. Each of these events was successful on their own, and they each played a role in developing more presence of

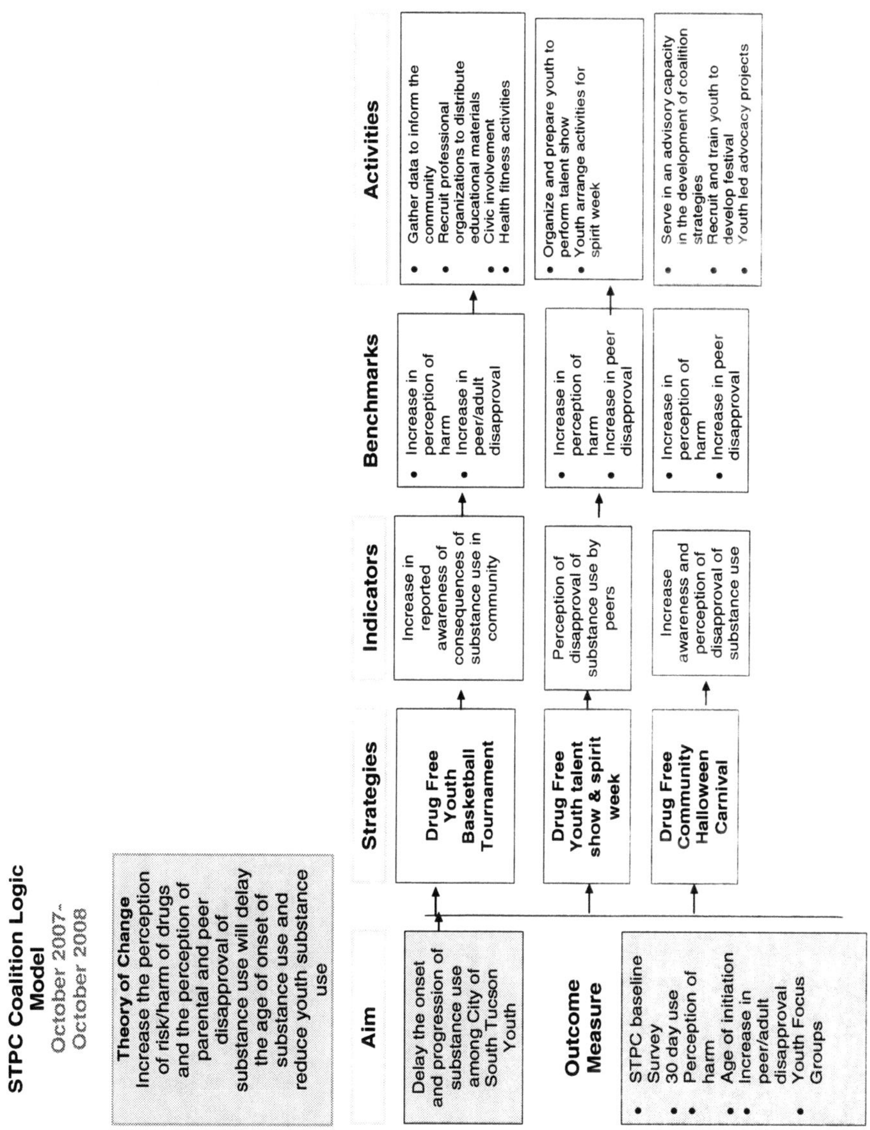

Fig. 8.1 STPC Coalition Logic Model

Table 8.1 South Tucson prevention coalition activities

Date	Event	Who
December 2010	Arizona State Liquor License Board Meeting—Antonio's Bar—withdrawn	City of South Tucson (attorney, city manager, police), UA, JVYC, local business owner
October 2010	Neighborhood Preservation Code Changes	City of South Tucson
August 2010	National Night Out 2010 and Survey	All partners
April 2010	Arizona State Liquor License Board Meeting—Walgreens Liquor License Denied!	Y2Y, JVYC, City Manager, City Attorney, Police, UA, Orduna
March 2010	City Council Meetings (2)—testify to Council and present 600 signatures. Youth Protest.	Y2Y, JVYC, Casa Maria, Eckstrom, STPC, UA
August 2009	National Night Out 2009 and Survey	See list:
July 2009	Movie Nights (2) and Surveys	JVYC, Y2Y, SAAF, UA,
September 2008	Shining Stars Awards	JVYC, Explorers, and others
August 2008	National Night Out 2008	See list
Spring 2008	Report of HNS Needs Assessment	UA, HNS
Spring 2008	Town Hall for Alcohol Mapping Grant	Y2Y, City Council, UA
November 2007	Community Readiness Interviews	Maricruz Ruiz, STPC, key stakeholders
October 2007	Red Ribbon Week	STPC, JVYC, see other list
October 2007	Submit Alcohol Mapping Grant—Funded.	CoST, STPC, JVYC
September 2007	Shining Stars Awards	JVYC, Explorers, and others
2007–2009	SAAF VoZ Prevention Project	SAAF, JVYC, and others
August 2007	National Night Out 2007	See list
Spring 2007	STPC Member Survey	UA, STPC
2007	Public Service Announcements	HNS, JVYC, Y2Y, UA
December 2006	World AIDS Day Press Release/Announcement of Faith-Based Grant Funded ($25,000)	Judge Ron Wilson
2006	Shining Stars Awards	JVYC, Explorers, and others
2006	Anti-Drug Poster Contest	Y2Y, JVYC, Pueblo Optimists Club
March 2006	Town Hall Block Party (342 attended, 65 volunteers)	STPC members and community
May 2006	DUI seminar (30 youth)	CoST Police, JVYC, UA
2005	STPC report to Council	STPC members
2005	HNS Halloween Festival (442 attendees, 50 volunteers)	HNS, STPC
2005	DFC Grant Funded	City of South Tucson, UA
2005	Planning for DFC grant	CoST, Police, HNS, JVYC, SAAF, UA
2004	HNS Halloween Festival (650 attendees)	HNS, STPC
2004	Mission View Talent Show (250 attendees)	Mission View Elementary/JVYC
2004	Y2Y Conference	Y2Y, UA, JVYC
2004	Project YES: Parent Conference	Project YES
2003–2004	Community Capacity Building with Safe Havens to sustain youth prevention programs	JVYC, HNS, Project YES
2002–2005	SAMSHA Grant—Omeyocan YES	UA, City of South Tucson, SAAF, Safe Havens (JVYC, HNS, Project YES)

youth-led activities. Youth-to-Youth (Y2Y) youth members organized fun and brief presentations to gain attention and to share their messages about alcohol norms. They did this through skits at local talent shows, community rallies, community events, and radio public service announcements.

Efforts to create new activities with participation from new partners was challenging at first, until partners learned to trust and work collaboratively. It was this process of community development that led to the creation and execution of truly collaborative coalition activities that were co-led by different agencies and by youth. This was evidenced in the development of the National Night event organized by South Tucson Prevention Coalition, and the success of the co-led event over several years was a significant factor in reaching a large number of community members and raising awareness about adolescent alcohol use prevention.

Through these activities, STPC began to raise awareness among the broader community as well as among local leaders and the local government. In order to target local government, one method was for youth to regularly present their activities and findings at City Council meetings to the local elected leaders, often police and fire department leaders were present at these meetings as well. Ms. Michele Orduña, STPC project coordinator, also provided regular summaries and reports to the city council via written reports and public presentations. Both Y2Y and STPC worked together on these activities to share results and findings in a manner that was supportive and consistent. In the following sections, we provide a chronology of events through summarizing activities and providing historical documents, such as city council reports, press releases, and research reports that provide insight into how the event was conducted, the increasing level of collaboration between the coalition members and participants, the integration of alcohol norm messaging, and the degree of integration with local government leaders.

8.3 STPC Phase 2: Year 1 Activities and Accomplishments

8.3.1 Halloween Festival

A strategy of STPC was to collaborate with existing successful events in the community, as a way to support the existing agencies and also to further integrate and assimilate the alcohol prevention messages in as many venues as possible to reach the broadest population possible. The Halloween Festival took place at the House of Neighborly Service on the Saturday of the Halloween weekend. The festival became a collaborative effort between many different community groups, hosted by the South Tucson Safe Havens, including the House of Neighborly Service (HNS), Tucson Urban League-Project YES, and the John Valenzuela Youth Center (JVYC). Kimberly Sierra-Cajas, HNS Executive Director, comments on the collaboration in her retrospective interview (2010): "*It helped to have more numbers of people helping so we helped each other out. You know for these big events, so it would have been really hard to put it all on by ourselves...We had just tried to plan a Halloween festival on our own, [it had] not been very successful. All three centers went and walked and divided the neighborhood and so, there was a lot of parents they knew very well. JVYC and Project YES knew very well so they would get the word to those parents and then we get the word to the parents of our kids. We really covered a lot of South Tucson that way, but had we tried to that by ourselves it would have been really, really hard. So that you don't have to have all the three times number of staff at one center… and I think our activities were more effective.*"

Since STPC Drug-Free community funding did not support direct services, supplies were donated by local businesses, the South Tucson Police Department, other nearby agencies, and the South Tucson Housing Department. Several groups helped to organize, decorate, set up and operate the Halloween Festival, including students from University of Arizona sororities and fraternities, Presbyterian youth groups, parents from the neighborhood, the South Tucson Police Explorers, the South Tucson Police Department, and staff from the Safe Havens. Indicative of the how these collaborations grew over time is represented in a press release in 2007 (see Fig. 8.2), for Red Ribbon Week for the City of South Tucson that highlights multiple events hosted by different agencies culminating with the second year of the Halloween Festival.

PRESS RELEASE

Red Ribbon Week and National Make a Difference Day 2007 – City of South Tucson

On **Monday, October 22nd**, the City of South Tucson, Mayor Jennifer Eckstrom, City Council Members, and the South Tucson Prevention Coalition (STPC) will host Red Ribbon Week, October 22-31st and on Saturday October 27, will take part in National Make a Difference day.

*Why?** The Red Ribbon Campaign was started when drug traffickers in Mexico City murdered Kiki Camarena, a DEA agent, in 1985. This began the continuing tradition and displaying Red Ribbons as a symbol of intolerance towards the use of drugs. The mission of the Red Ribbon Campaign is to present a unified and visible commitment towards the creation of a DRUG-FREE AMERICA.
Make A Difference Day is the most encompassing national day of helping others -- a celebration of neighbors helping neighbors. Created by USA WEEKEND Magazine, Make A Difference Day is an annual event that takes place on the fourth Saturday of every October.

The City of South Tucson and STPC will be commemorating Red Ribbon Week and Make a Difference Day with the following activities. The activities are free and open to community members. "Working together for a stronger healthier community" (STPC)

*http://www.nfp.org/NFP_RedRibbonGuide07.pdf
http://www.usaweekend.com/diffday/

Date	Event	Venue
October 22, 2007 **6:00 p.m. – 8:30 p.m.**	Movie Night—teenagers enjoy a movie, popcorn, nachos, pizza, drinks and prizes!	Sam Lena Library 1607 S. Sixth Avenue South Tucson, AZ
October 23, 3007 **4:00 p.m. – 5:00 p.m.**	Youth 2 Youth Double Dare—have fun learning, win prizes and goody bags!	Sam Lena Library 1607 S. Sixth Avenue South Tucson, AZ
October 25, 2007 **3:30 p.m. – 4:30 p.m.**	Story time/ Pumpkin decorating—storytelling, poster making, plus pumpkin decorating for youngsters.	Sam Lena Library 1607 S. Sixth Avenue South Tucson, AZ
October 27, 2007 **8:00 a.m. – 12:00 p.m.**	Make a Difference Day—participate in making your community beautiful. Refreshments and lunch provided. Win a t-shirt!	South Tucson Fire Department 1601 S. Sixth Avenue South Tucson, AZ (rear of complex)
October 31, 2007 **2:00 p.m. – 4:00 p.m.**	Halloween—enjoy a spooky afternoon at HNS. Hot dogs and drinks provided, plus	House of Neighborly Service 243 W. 33rd Street South Tucson, AZ

For more information, please contact Michele Orduna, STPC Coordinator at 792-2424 or michelef@u.arizona.edu.

Fig. 8.2 Red Ribbon Week Press Release and Halloween Carnival

The South Tucson Police Explorers Post 317, a member of the STPC Coalition, designed and ran the "haunted house"; police explorers is a national program designed to reach out to middle school aged youth to gain experience and information about careers in law enforcement, where they receive training with police officers. Neighborhood preteens served as tour guides through the "haunted house." Other activities included a cake walk, carnival games, face painting, costume contests, apple bobbing, races, a pie throwing booth, and a scary story telling area. A mini outdoor theater was set up outside where Halloween cartoon movies are projected onto the side of a building. We offered coffee for the parents, punch, cookies, popcorn, and bags of candy. The fee was 50 cents or a can of food for the Thanksgiving food drive. Outreach personnel from the Omeyocan YES or VOZ after-school prevention programs also recruited during the festival for the STPC. The South Tucson School Resource Officer distributes flyers to schools targeting City of South Tucson youth including Ochoa Elementary, Mission View Elementary, and Wakefield Middle School. The community attendance grew from 442 to 500 and up to 650; collaborative Halloween activities between the Safe Havens took place for three consecutive Halloween dates (2005–2007). Here is a brief summary report that was shared with the coalition and the Mayor and Council after the first Halloween Carnival.

City of South Tucson Drug-Free Halloween Carnival
Held October 28, 2005 at House of Neighborly Service
Prepared by Michele Orduña, STPC Project Coordinator

Achievements

- Total attendance at event was 442.
- All City of South Tucson Safe Havens participated.
- 50 volunteers at carnival from 22 different organizations including the neighborhood, St. Andrew's, St. John, Christ, St. Marks, Green Valley, and Presbyterian Campus Ministry, Arizona Blue Chips, Sigma Lambda Beta, Kappa Delta Chi, City of South Tucson, South Tucson Explorer Post 317, Rotary, YAVs, STPC-Drug-Free Communities, Mexican American Studies at the U of A, JVYC, Project Yes, SACASA, SW Center for Economic Integrity, SAAF, Tucson Indian Center, No More Deaths, and Planned Parenthood.
- Many young children and youth dressed in costumes.
- Our Drug-Free balloons were a big hit. We gave away approximately 150 balloons.
- 109 youth signed the pledge entitled "**I pledge the choice for me is to be smoke, drug and alcohol free**"
- Ericka Aguilar, Promotions Manager, from Telemundo did a brief interview with Kimberly Sierra-Cajas, director of HNS, and I (Michele Orduña) about the Halloween event—aired the same night.

Comments obtained from participants from comments cards were positive and demonstrated that the coalition was raising awareness and influencing community norms about alcohol and drug use. This was one of the early methods of data collection for evaluation of the event. For example, in response to the question "***One thing I learned tonight about staying healthy and safe was . . . . .***" participants indicated: "*Say no to drugs*", "*Not to cross the street without looking,*" "*Stay away from drugs,*" "*A lot of help to offer in our community,*" "*Stay out of drugs. They're bad 4 u.,*" "*No smoking,*" "*No drinking,*" "*Stay away from drugs,*" "*Stay in school,*" "*Eat good food!,*" "*No fumar,*" "*I was scared of the haunted house, but I had the best time!,*" "*We loved the good safe time we had.*" These comments demonstrate that not only was the coalition getting across the message about not using alcohol or drugs, they were also promoting positive alternatives, such as alcohol-free events. Positive messages reflected by participants included messages such as stay in school and suggestions about how to be safe by being careful in the streets and eating healthy food. These comments by participants also demonstrate the range of social services and agencies that were included and represented in the activity; the inclusivity of agencies was essential to developing allies and strengthening coalition membership. As an incentive for participants to visit all the booths, they could submit for a raffle prize if they provided a card with stamps from all the participating booths. Additionally, the comments demonstrate that the event was effective at raising awareness about the availability of social services in the local community. Immediate access to social service resources can be critical to the development of youth whose families are living in poverty and may unexpectedly and urgently have needs for food boxes, safe housing, or counseling services.

8.3.2 Quarterly Presentations to Government

Included here is the script for the summary of the year 01 first quarter presented to the City of South Tucson Mayor and Council by the STPC Project Coordinator, Michele Orduña. It was this type of communication that was important to develop a shared agenda and trust with the local government. It is important to note that it clearly describes the grant, the funding, the expectations, and the activities accomplished.

Madame Mayor and Council members, my name is Michele Orduña and I would like to make a report on the Drug Free Communities grant. The local name for the grant is South Tucson Prevention Collaborative: Drug Free Community, or STPC Phase 2. As you may remember, STPC Phase 1 was to deliver and evaluate an educational program for teens (2002–2005). The coalition members were motivated to build on this program by pursuing DFC funding that would allow the community coalition to keep doing new prevention activities and recruit new coalition members. STPC Phase 2 has two main goals (1) prevent/reduce teen substance use in the community and (2) continue to build on community leadership by funding existing coalitions to focus on teen substance use prevention.

In order to reach our goals, the Year 01 objective is to increase coalition membership of STPC Phase 2 (see attached list of organizations that sent letters of support for the grant submission). We meet on the fourth Thursday of each month in the evening at one of the Safe Havens or at the Sam Lena Library at 6 p.m. 23 people attended the meeting in January. We hope to see even more groups represented at our next meeting on February 28th at the John Valenzuela Youth Center at 6 p.m. Our agenda at this meeting is to hear what the community ideas and concerns are about teenage substance use.

In the grant, we have planned to do a community activity one per quarter. The activities are for the benefit of the whole community and not focused on service delivery. The DFC grant does not allow more than 20 % of the budget to be used for direct services. Our first activity of the grant was the City of South Tucson Drug-Free Communities Halloween Carnival held on Oct 23, 2006 at HNS. Attendance was high over 400 people. There was positive feedback about the Carnival. Many people understood the health messages and the drug-free messages. You can find more specific information about the carnival in the packet. We are currently working on the 2nd quarter activity, and you are welcome to attend our STPC Phase 2 meeting tomorrow to give your suggestions.

8.3.3 Block Party

The Block Party was one of the events held in the first year of STPC, and the coalition was still reaching out to new members; in Fig. 8.3 you can see an invitation to participate that was sent from an STPC member. This invitation includes specific information about need for alcohol prevention combined with local statistics as well as specific information about the STPC mission and meeting times. The following are the shared meeting minutes of the STPC members for the planning of the town hall. While, the funding agency encouraged providing "town hall" sessions for presentation of data and discussion, the STPC felt that their community was not ready for this type of strategy. Based on the Community Readiness Model, they felt that while the STPC members were at a more advanced level of planning and implementation, they agreed that the broader community was still at an earlier level of denial or tolerance of adolescent alcohol use. In order to raise community awareness of these issues, they felt that they needed to reach the broadest audience possible, with a specific focus on parents and families. The coalition members felt that the community members who most needed to participate would likely not attend a formal "town hall" for discussion of adolescent alcohol prevention. Juan "Johnny" Quevedo, Y2Y leader, comments, "*The way it all started was to get people to have events and to be involved. (It was a) great way to spread the word about it—to have events. That was the best way to start up, word of mouth to let people know about what is going on and talk about it (adolescent substance use). You have to turn the power around to the ones in need.*"

Dear:

Alcohol use among children and adolescents starts early and increases rapidly with age. A higher percentage of youth aged 12 to 20 use alcohol (29%) than use tobacco (24%) or illicit drugs (14%), making underage drinking a leading public health problem in the United States. To help educate young people and caring adults about the risks associated with underage drinking, the Federal government's Interagency Coordinating Committee for the Prevention of Underage Drinking (ICCPUD) is supporting a series of Town Hall Meeting to take place in communities across America on or around March 28, 2006.

The South Tucson Prevention Collaborative is planning a Resource Fair & Block Party in our area on April 29, 2006 at the John Valenzuela Youth Center, 1550 S. 6th Ave, South Tucson, AZ 85713, from 3-6 pm. This meeting will give us the opportunity to educate parents, teachers, officials, youth, and other community members about the impact of underage drinking and will allow us to develop possible solutions.

As an organization committed to preventing underage drinking, The South Tucson Prevention Collaborative is inviting you to lend your expertise by being a community resource at our Town Hall Resource Fair & Block Party on April 29th. With participation from prominent local organizations, we hope to raise awareness of the risks of underage drinking and to encourage broader use of the many resources that are available to youth, parents, schools, and communities. Media will also be encouraged to cover this Town Hall Meeting.

I will follow up in a few days to inquire about whether you would be willing to participate, or your may contact me at 792-9251. You may now reserve a spot by returning the enclosed response form.

We hope you will join us in educating our community about the importance of preventing underage drinking.

Sincerely,

Maria Jones
STPC Member

Fig. 8.3 Invitation to participate in Block Party

The Coalition debated internally about offering instead a "Block Party" where they felt that youth and families were more likely to attend, and that they could then provide information in a more informal format and fun interactive experiential activities for youth and their families that would help raise awareness. Over time the coalition realized that family participation in community events was key to reaching more people in the community and that involvement of younger children was actually a positive benefit and further extended their prevention efforts to the next generation of adolescents.

At this stage, the STPC was still very wary about collecting new research data or about sharing data with the community; they felt that it would not be received well. They agreed that a "sign-in" table would be acceptable, where participants would be funneled toward in order to gather minimum information about attendance and age (see Chap. 9 for more information). Included here are public meeting minutes describing the plans for the Block Party. At these early stages, the coalition was beginning to integrate the goals and provisions of social services agency collaborators in order to organize the event; however, each event usually had one chairperson who took the lead in ensuring all elements were in place and to ensure communication was shared with all members.

STPC
Block Party & Information Fair
Under Age Drinking Prevention
Updated 4/4/06
Prepared by Gloria Hamelitz, JVYC

Goals:
The Town Hall meetings are part of a national effort to increase the understanding of underage drinking and its consequences, and to encourage individuals, families and communities to address the problem.
Date: Saturday April 29, 2006
Times: 3:00–6:00 pm
Location: John Valenzuela Youth Center 1550 South 6th Avenue
Goal is to reach 300 people

Activities:
The South Tucson Youth to Youth group will be conducting an interactive "maze" available to all ages. The maze will allow people to travel through a simulated driving course and a field sobriety test, while wearing drinking impaired goggles. Specifically youth (ages 10–18) will be targeted. Before they enter, SAAF & Michelle will present each participant with various choices and opportunities to avoid this situation. As a participant navigates their way through, they will be asked questions and given facts regarding the dangers of drinking. The possible two outcomes will result in either ending up in the "Morgue" with their name on a tombstone OR they will end up in a mock jail cell. Their ticket out will require for them to write out their options to drinking.
Upon completing the event, youth participants will receive an incentive for participating.

Games:
There will be four table games that promote drug-free life styles.
A jumping castle and rope course
A cakewalk will be added (we are in need of cakes!!)

Social Services:
Cards will be issued and can be stamped or marked by visitors. Complete cards will be put in a raffle for prizes and incentives to given out at 5:45 pm.
MADD has confirmed

(continued)

TEP's program "Driving Drunk will put your lights out"
Job Corp
Safe Havens & Committee members are encouraged to reserve a table. Thank you HNS & Kerrie for coordinating this!
Gloria will order plastic bags to hold literature
Parents will host a booth
Cope will provide training for the parents before and after the event

Food:
All attendees will be asked to sign in
Upon signing in they will be issued tickets for the food and games.
We are in need of donations of sodas and waters!

Entertainment:
We are looking for all types of talent! Please encourage any talented person or group to fill out Yellow form and return to JVYC.
All the DJ equipment will be provided by SAAF! Any aspiring DJ's need to only bring their music.

Advertisement:
Flyers will be decided at the next committee meeting!
Press Releases will release on April 21st & April 28th to all news and media outlets.
Neighborhood Walk will be on Friday April 21st. Safe havens will split up locations.
Telemundo will be contacted
The daily star will be contacted to place in their calendar

Poster Contest Kick off!
The poster contest will begin at this event. A booth will be available along with rules and requirements. Thank you Paul Diaz for coordinating the prize money of $100! The winner will have their picture on a billboard!

How can you help?
We are in need of Volunteers!!
Please sign up to coordinate a category or volunteer!!
We are also in need of Prizes. A raffle will be held at the end of the evening. We are in need of prizes for families or adults. Any thing will help.
Invite neighbors
Invite any social service organization to have a booth. (Please have them fill out the form or call our office and I can send them a letter)

Decorations
STPC has a helium tank and balloons
Safe Havens will make posters for the event (Alcohol Prevention themed)
Michelle will order a large banner
Any other questions, please feel free to call Gloria at JVYC (792-9251)

8.4 STPC Phase 2: Year 01 Summary Report

Written Quarterly Reports were provided by Michele Orduña, the STPC director, with input from Dr. Romero, the evaluator. Following is one of the public reports shared with all coalition members in meetings and over the email listserv. It is demonstrated in these reports that there is increasing amounts of data integrated into the data collection and evaluations of community events. These reports were also provided in hard copy and presented to the Mayor and Council. The following report describes the Block Party event and Driving Under the Influence (DUI) event. Additionally, it is shown in this report that there are additional trainings of key stakeholder, which expands to more stakeholders over time. Trainings of key stakeholders are a strategic form of intervention to help move to a higher level of community readiness (Plested et al., 2006).

South Tucson Prevention Coalition-Drug-Free Communities (STPC-DFC)
City Council Quarterly Report
Prepared by: Michele Orduña

Coalition Accomplishment
STPC-DFC Resource Fair and Block Party
April 29, 2006 3:00–6:00 p.m.
At JVYC

Over 342 persons attended the April 29th, South Tucson Drug-Free Community Block Party at John Valenzuela Youth Center. Approximately, 143 (42 %) of these individuals were in our target age group between the ages of 9–18 years. Another 85 (25 %) were under the age of 9 years old. The rest of the attendees were adults (over 18 years). One member per group was asked to complete a form with additional information as they entered the event. Based on this information, *68 % of the informants reported that they live in the City of South Tucson. 73 % of those who reported that they do not live in South Tucson reported that they spend a lot of time in the City of South Tucson.* When asked how they heard about the event, respondents indicated: 30 % heard from other family member or friend, 24 % heard from JVYC staff or because they attend JVYC, 18 % flyer, 10 % school, 7 % were driving or walking by, 1 % heard on TV, 1 % HNS, 1 % Luz Social Services. It is estimated that 88 persons completed the DUI maze. Approximately, 65 volunteers were present the day of or spent time assisting planning for the event.

Coalition Accomplishment:
DUI Seminar-Sgt. Marty Harkins-South Tucson Police Dept and AZ
At JVYC at 6:30 p.m.
30 attendees

(continued)

Coalition members and youth at least 12 years old were invited to attend a special presentation given by Sgt. Harkins. Sgt Harkins is a member of the Southern AZ DUI task force and South Tucson Police; he presented slides and deconstructed an archived DUI case. As part of alcohol awareness month, we used this opportunity to reveal real consequences of drinking and driving. After the presentation, many youth discussed among themselves and with JVYC staff how they felt and how drinking and driving could influence their lives. In addition, this was another opportunity to discuss the dangers of alcohol consumption and driving.

Program Duties:
Coalition Monthly meetings
4th Tuesday of every month
Jan 23, Feb 28, Mar 28, Apr 25, May 23, 2006
Complete and submitted 1st biannual report to SAMHSA for DFC on May 15, 2006

Trainings:
Michele Orduña attended a one-day workshop in Reno NV on March 5, 2006. Training topic was the new online reporting system all DFC grantees will need to use.

8.4.1 STPC Phase 2: Year 2 Activities and Accomplishments

The following is the report provided to the City of South Tucson Mayor and Council to describe the goals for year 2 and to summarize progress thus far. It is apparent in these documents that the STPC has developed a regular process for meetings; additionally, it is apparent from the agency participation lists that the coalition has grown tremendously. In particular, they were able to hire an assistant director, Maricruz Romero-Ruiz, who was able to help outreach and further organize events and coalition representation.

The most fundamental accomplishment from Year 01 was that the coalition had converged on a specific mission, rather than broadly addressing all types of substance use; they had identified and agreed that underage drinking was the number one issue in their community. The identification of a specific and narrow topic was key to their future success because it helped them stay very focused. The specific mission also helped to integrate new coalition members so that the coalition could maintain focus while assimilating and expanding membership. This mission was written down at the beginning of each meeting, and it helped to bring members back to topic when there were difficult decisions or disagreements about how to move forward. This was the key mission that everyone agreed on and that everyone felt critically invested in changing. Additionally, this helped to narrow their focus on community norms for adolescent alcohol use and in the future their focus on availability and regulations. Furthermore, this mission was something that could be measured and that was represented in existing local and national datasets.

This period of the coalition is marked by growth in data collection for evaluation (see Chap. 9 for a full description). This period is also marked by new external funding that provided infrastructure and motivation to collaborate on a radio public service announcement campaign that took the coalitions awareness raising campaign to a new level of community reach and also a new level of collaboration.

Also, during this time period there was more training provided to key stakeholders that included county-wide, regional, national-level conferences. More stakeholders were included at this stage, including the STPC project coordinator, assistant coordinator, Gloria Hamelitz, and City of South Tucson staff. The increased integration of the STPC project coordinator and assistant coordinator in county-level prevention groups helped to increase sharing of information through a wider network of prevention professionals. The comparison to other regional and national coalitions also demonstrated how advanced and successful the STPC was becoming in terms of their activities and their collaboration. The stakeholders found that they had more youth involvement than other groups, a wider representation of community sectors, regular successful community-wide events, and a functioning coalition. Overall, they perceived the progress of their community readiness to take on new projects that involved seeking out new external funding sources for new activities, such as the youth-led media campaign. This period is also marked by the beginning of new collaborative community events that were linked with national campaigns, such as National Night Out. This type of expansion and professionalization of activities also demonstrates the changes in community readiness that was being experienced by the coalition during this time period and which is evident in the following community report.

South Tucson Prevention Coalition Report to the City of South Tucson Council
Prepared by Michele Orduña, STPC Project Coordinator
STPC members decided to focus our efforts on ***underage drinking*** in the activities we will plan and hold in the coming months.

Accomplishments

- Monthly STPC meeting held in Oct, Nov, and Dec. 2006 and in Jan, Feb 2007. Monthly meetings are usually held at South Tucson City Hall at 1601 S. Sixth Ave.
- Bi-annual progress report was submitted and accepted by SAMSHA, DFC funding agency. Bi-annual report was approved in Jan. 2007. (see attached)
- House of Neighborly Service was awarded a grant to plan and create several short PSAs for the radio regarding youth HIV and substance use prevention. The youth leaders are finishing writing the scripts, and production will soon follow at Clear Channel. The PSAs are to run from May through August on a several local Clear Channel radio stations.

(continued)

- Michele and Maricruz have been invited and attended several roundtable meetings with Pima County-Tucson Commission on Addiction Prevention and Treatment; one of their current tasks is to take a closer look at and then make recommendations about Special Events Liquor licenses in Pima County. This meeting is usually held monthly.
- Michele and Maricruz also have been attending regular meetings with a new educational program under Planned Parenthood called ***Real Life, Real Talk***. The focus is to bring parents together in entertaining settings and further empower parents/caretakers to talk with youth about not only sex also about the sexuality in our current society, i.e., movies, TV, music, my space, IM, etc. Michele serves on the activities planning committee, and Maricruz serves on the media outreach committee. Several STPC members and community members are planning to attend the facilitator training to bring this opportunity to South Tucson community parents and caregivers; one of our goals is to offer it in English, Spanish or Bi-lingual.
- Michele and Maricruz attended a community prevention form held by the Community Prevention Coalition of Pima County. This was a lunch event where many agencies and various forms of prevention material were brought together to help unify our efforts or at least network each of our efforts.
- Maricruz, Michele, John Irey, Operations Manager at HNS attended the 17th Annual Community Anti-Drug Coalitions of American (CADCA) Conference in Washington, DC the week of Feb 12, 2007. (See Maricruz's report)
- The noncompetitive continuation grant application will be submitted on March 15, 2007. This application is to help ensure STPC is staying on target with our goals. This is a noncompetitive application meaning that we are being looked at on a one-to-one basis.
- Michele and Maricruz have distributed and are currently collecting Drug-Free Communities-South Tucson Prevention Coalition (DFC-STPC) Member Survey. Our goal is to get feedback about activities/events, meeting, and overall goals that STPC has.
- Maricruz continues to work for City Hall 20+ hours a week. She plans monthly meetings and agendas and keeps a liaison between the 12 sectors of DFC, and specifically with the Safe Havens, JVYC, HNS, and Project YES. She also attended various community-wide meetings and committee meetings.
- HNS is in the process of hiring a new Director
- Tucson Urban League/Project YES welcomes new CEO, Kelly Langford

Upcoming Goals/Events

- Bi-annual report will be due in Spring 2007.
- Organize and hold STPC spring community-wide event, a teen basketball tournament in April.
- Attend 2nd annual Statewide Underage Drinking Conference in Phoenix May 1–2, 2007
- National Night Out will be held on Aug. 7, 2007
- STPC is reviewing a new grant application to build our coalition infrastructure over the next 3 years.

8.5 Media Campaign: Radio Public Service Announcements

Media campaigns are successful strategies to raise awareness about community alcohol norms (Flay, 2000; Donahue Hirschhorn, Haskins, & Nightingale, 2008; Kelly, Comello, & Slater, 2006). Moreover, teenagers are savvy and surrounded by media and technology. Disadvantaged economic and underserved communities are active participants in technology and media; moreover, they are especially oriented to popular radio channels in English and Spanish (Paredes Castaneda, 2003). The STPC media campaign was funded through the Faith Partners Contract grant that was awarded to The House of Neighborly Service (HNS), which is a mission of the Presbyterian Church and one of three local Safe Havens in the City of South. HNS was chosen to lead this grant because they are a faith-based agency; additionally, HNS had a strong youth advocacy leader with the executive director, Kimberly Sierra-Cajas. HNS also had the in-kind support staff and the in-kind space for youth to meet and plan their activities; yet, this grant was submitted and implemented in close collaboration with the other South Tucson Safe Havens, including John Valenzuela Youth Center (JVYC) and Tucson Urban League-Project YES (PYES) who each donated four community volunteers at 40 in-kind hours each. STPC's 12 partners donated in-kind, an average of 80 professional hours each, such as partners with expert knowledge about substance use and HIV prevention, including Dr. Romero, assistant professor, at the University of Arizona, Mexican America Studies & Research, Mary Specio-Boyer, MSW, LISAC, Director of Community Health at COPE Behavioral Services, and Jaime Arrieta, program manager for *VOZ*, from Southern Arizona AIDS Foundation. Other key partners that provided human resources include the Safe Havens' outreach personnel: Isaac Durgin from House of Neighborly Service, Jessica Alderete from John Valenzuela Youth Center, and Paul Lyons from Project YES and the STPC director and outreach specialist, Michele Orduña and Maricruz Romero-Ruiz. Other coalition members from the City of South Tucson Police and Fire, local parents, youth, and community members were also additional resources to provide information about substance use prevention and HIV/AIDS awareness. An example of the collaborative spirit of STPC and the integration with the local government for this particular grant is evident in the press release for the announcement of the grant award embedded within World AIDS Day with special speaker Honorable Judge Ronald Wilson making the official statement (see Fig. 8.4).

One strength of STPC has been to build leadership and empowerment among youth in the community. The Youth-to-Youth leadership group (Y2Y) were active members in STPC-DFC with significant training through Southern Arizona AIDS Foundation prevention programs, Omeyocan YES prevention program (see Chap. 4), and VOZ program (see Chap. 6). The additional leadership training of youth program graduates at the Youth to Youth International Leadership camp 2 years in a row also contributed to the youth capacity to take leadership on the media project. The youth leaders had engaged in community outreach for over 2 years by performing skits for younger children and hosting interactive games to inform youth about the dangers of substance use at STPC community events.

South Tucson Prevention Coalition

December 1, 2006

Press Release

Welcome------Michele Orduña

Announcement of award------Kimberly Sierra-Cajas

South Tucson Prevention Coalition, the City of South Tucson and community members support the 18th Annual World AIDS Day on December 1st, 2006. "Stop AIDS: Keep the Promise" is the theme until 2010 when testing and universal access to medication are standard best practices worldwide. Accountability is key among our government, and our local community to fight the preventable life threatening disease HIV/AIDS, which impacts all people.

According to national data from the Center of Disease Control, the Hispanic Community and Women are significantly vulnerable to HIV/AIDS. Hispanic adults, defined as over 13 years old, account for 20% of new AIDS cases in 2004. Minority women account for 27% of new AIDS cases in 2004. HIV/AIDS is the fourth leading cause of death among Hispanic women age 35-44.

STPC and the City of South Tucson are committed to do our part in combating HIV/AIDS. In doing so we are excited to announce a new grant award of $25,000 being made to House of Neighborly Service from the Center of Substance Abuse Prevention and Substance Abuse Mental Health Service Administration. Our goal is to bring additional awareness to youth and community members about the threat of HIV/AIDS. Our mission is to encourage and support youth from our community to develop and create a prevention message about

Fig. 8.4 Announcement of Faith Partners Grant for PSAs

HIV/AIDS and then disseminate that message through radio media in the spring of 2007.

Supporting Speaker-------Hon. Ron Wilson

South Tucson Prevention Coalition

Press Conference – World Aids Day

December 1st, 2006

Judge Ronald A. Wilson

Presiding Judge, South Tucson City Court

Official Statement

Almost every single American knows someone or knows of someone who has been impacted by HIV. Therefore, strong public and private partnerships are needed to ensure sufficient funding for research, prevention and treatment. We must all continue working together to help disseminate accurate information and support the development of age-appropriate programs.

For every "one" person infected by HIV, "thousands" are impacted. This is why public/private partnerships are so important. Thank you, South Tucson Prevention Coalition. You are an example of the partnerships that are needed to mitigate the destruction caused by this devastating disease... And, congratulations, on being a worthy recipient of this $25,000.00 HIV grant.

Fig. 8.4 (continued)

The Y2Y leaders collaborated with a health education specialist from HNS (Yvonne Montoya) and a health education specialist from Southern Arizona AIDS Foundation (SAAF), (Jaime Arrieta) to create a novela to be aired on the radio and represented in comic strips. For both projects, the radio novela and the comic strip youth were compensated for their time and effort by utilizing a stipend. The youth stipend was $7.50 per hour for up to 400 total hours, for both projects. Many of the youth were already working to help financially support their families and/or to help provide for their own needs. The youth stipend was a critical incentive to maintain youth's active involvement in the project over time.

The Public Service Announcements (PSAs) were created to reach youth listeners and pass a message of positive learning about prevention of HIV/AIDS and substance use; however, the use of popular radio channels in English and Spanish ensured that the messages would also reach a broader audience that may include adults. The scripts were created based on the idea of a *novela*, which is similar to what is referred to as a *soap opera* in the United States. Television novelas are very popular in Mexican and Mexican American cultures and are widely accessible also through radio stations (La Pastina, Rego, & Straubhaar, 2003; Slater, 1999; Slater, Kelly, & Edwards, 2000). Television and radio novelas are culturally appropriate modes of interaction with the South Tucson community and one method to reach more youth than using print items alone. Cultural appropriateness was a high priority with the Safe Havens and STPC; staff had completed trainings in the past to increase cultural competency. The novelas used a dramatic, yet comic-like setting, to send messages of basic education about the dangers of substance use and the increased risk of HIV/AIDS. The focus was to increase education and awareness to the greatest number of youth by using radio as a mode of transmission.

The PSAs were created by the youth from the Y2Y (Youth-to-Youth) program in collaboration with adult leaders (Yvonne Montoya and Jessica Alderete) and university undergraduate students (Dominique Calza and Selina Telles). All PSAs were provided in English and Spanish. The PSAs were also recorded by four youth from the Y2Y program (Oscar Cesena, Vanessa Piño, Jesus Mejia, and Gloria Otero). The PSAs aired over the summer of 2007 on the following stations: HOT 98.3 FM, 102.1 FM La Preciosa, and Tejano 1600 AM on Thursday, May 10, 2007. 50 copies of the PSA recordings were distributed to STPC coalition members and to youth. They were also archived by the SPTC coordinators.

As part of this grant, youth also created comic strips that were similar to the PSAs. The creation of the comic strips were done in collaboration between youth and adult leaders, following the Y2Y philosophy of youth-led/adult-guided. Youth decided to create a total of six comic strips that directly reflected the text found in the six radio novelas. Each youth was responsible for designing at least three comic strips, and then they voted to select the final comic strips to use in their project. Youth created a poster presentation of the six official comic strips for use in STPC community events. Five of the youth presented the comic strips at STPC's first National Night Out on August 2007. Attendees (adults, children, and adolescents) frequented the table to view the comic strips and ask questions about the project. Additionally, the event's disc jockey frequently played a copy of the PSA's/radio novelas between announcement and songs throughout the evening.

8.6 National Night Out

National Night Out is a national campaign to promote crime prevention through community-hosted block parties to bring police and community members together. The leaders of STPC upon learning about National Night Out felt that this was a great opportunity to create a new community event that truly could be jointly hosted by STPC partners. National Night Out seemed ideal because it is billed as an annual community-building campaign and one that specifically emphasized creating a positive activity for police and community members to join forces to improve the safety of the community. The police often witness the most extreme consequences of underage drinking, or they are contacted by family when they face a problem with underage drinking. However, education and outreach is often not a consciously scheduled part of their activities. However, National Night Out was a great event to integrate police in a positive manner on an annual basis. Moreover, National Night Out was a good opportunity for police to share the information that they receive from other agencies.

The National Night Out event in South Tucson was held annually on the first week of August, which is one of the hottest times of year in Arizona with temps regularly reaching over 100°. Yet, it proved to be a great opportunity for youth to engage in positive fun activities and also to stand up to crime in their neighborhoods. Youth often provided fun and brief presentations to raise awareness about the risks of alcohol and drug use. This event was truly co-hosted by multiple agencies and members of STPC (see Fig. 8.5 for First Year Letter of Request). John Valenzuela Youth Center often took the lead in organizing youth, who participated in dance presentations, skits, and fun activities for children. Juan "Johnny" Quevedo, Y2Y youth leader, STPC Coalition member, recalls in his retrospective interview:

> National Night Out is the annual event at the end of the summer program. We all came together and pulled out a show—out of no money—you feel the pressure and adrenaline rush, and doing a show—we are going to have people Our goal was to have the community come together. We wanted the family, parents, friends, we wanted everyone to be there. It was our chance, once a year, to inform, it was an opportunity to inform people of all ages about what was going on in our city. Everyone was there. We can all be together in one huge parking lot in front of city office. (A lot of)people asking to have tables, because they knew that many people would come by, and right on 6th avenue, (which is) always a busy street and (we) definitely got attention. This was a chance for Youth 2 Youth to let people know what was going on. It made me care.

At the event, the police and the junior police group, the Explorers, would often offer hot dogs or other food. Many social service agencies participated by hosting a booth with fun activities, giveaways, and health information. Gospel Rescue

July 14, 2006

Ruben Villa
Acting City Manager
1601 S. Sixth Ave
Tucson, AZ 85713

Dear City Manager,

South Tucson Prevention Coalition (STPC) in conjunction with the South Tucson Explorers, the Youth to Youth Leadership group, and the South Tucson Police are planning to partake in the 23rd National Night Out (NNO) on August 1, 2006. National Night Out is designed to support crime and drug prevention, including local anticrime programs, strengthen local communities and police-community partnerships and send a message to criminal that the community is organized and fighting back. This will be the first year our local community will be participating in the NNO campaign.

The planning committee has would like to ask the City of South Tucson for use of the front courtyard, in front of City Hall, from 5:00-8:00 p.m., on August 1, 2006. The front courtyard has been identified as a prime space for the community to come and show their support of NNO. The planning is on-going however, a few of the activities included for NNO is a youth talent show, drug prevention table top games, and we will have Mc Gruff the Crime Dog, as well we will announce the winner to our STPC summer youth poster contest. The South Tucson Explores will be selling food and the Youth to Youth Leadership Group are planning to do a skit for the audience.

On behalf of the Coalition and the planning committee, we invite the City Mayor and Council members to join us on NNO. We look forward to our further collaboration, and strengthening of our local community. If there are any questions or concerns please feel free to contact me.

Thank you,

Michele D. Orduña M.Ed.
Project Coordinator
South Tucson Prevention Coalition-Drug Free Communities
1601 S. Sixth Ave
Tucson, AZ 85713
O:520.792.2424 F:520.628.9619
michelef@u.arizona.ed

Fig. 8.5 Letter of request for First National Night Out

Mission would often bring their truck to offer food and clothing. The fire department would regularly bring a fire truck to the front of the activity and organize a piñata activity for the children at the end of the evening.

The event was always hosted in the front plaza of the City of South Tucson government buildings. The event was typically attended by 400–600 people, every year from 2006 to 2010. STPC had good media coverage at this event almost every year. For several years, they were featured in interviews with local television news programs. In one newspaper article (Kalaitzidis, 2007), the event is described as "*drug prevention was the central theme of the National Night Out event at the South Tucson City Hall*" with quotes from youth Jesus Mejia, 15 years old, 10th grader, and Y2Y member, "*People played 'double dare'. If they could answer a question about drugs right, they got a point. The winning teams got prizes.*" There were also quotes from adult allies, such as Jessica Alderete, youth program coordinator at John Valenzuela Youth Center "*About 500 people attended the South Tucson event. It was a success, bringing the community together.*" These are excellent examples of the integration of community and the visibility of a South Tucson in a positive light.

8.7 Conclusion

Community alcohol norms play an important role in shaping the expectations, availability, accessibility, and regulation of adolescent alcohol use. South Tucson Prevention Coalition was guided by the Community Readiness Model for Change and identified the need to first raise awareness among the community about the risks associated with adolescent alcohol use. During the first few years of the coalition activities, they focused on collaborative efforts to offer community-wide events that were safe drug-free family-oriented activities where they could offer information and activities to reinforce community messages about the wrongness of adolescent alcohol use. Over time, the coalition grew in membership and in level of readiness in part through additional training of stakeholders and through the support of external funding. The highlight of the community awareness of alcohol norms initiative was the youth-led media campaign for bilingual radio public service announcements. This was the highlight because it demonstrated that the coalition was able to obtain new funding together, to work together collaboratively to support a youth-led project that was highly successful and highly visible. It was through these small steps of incremental change that the STPC was prepared to expand and institutionalize their changes in the next step of their work to target the prevention of liquor licenses.

References

Burrow-Sanchez, J. J. (2006). Understanding adolescent substance abuse: Prevalence, risk factors, and clinical implications. *Journal of Counseling and Development, 84*, 283–290.

Cano, M. A., Schwartz, S. J., Castillo, L. G., Romero, A. J., Huang, S., Lorenzo-Blanco, E. I., … Szapocznik, J. (2015). Depressive symptoms and externalizing behaviors among Hispanic immigrant adolescents: Examining longitudinal effects of cultural stress. *Journal of Adolescence, 42*, 31–39.

Donahue Hirschhorn, E., Haskins, R., & Nightingale, M. (2008). Using the media to promote adolescent well-being. *The future of children*. Princeton-Brookings.

Flay, B. R. (2000). Approaches to substance use prevention utilizing school curriculum plus social environment change. *Addictive Behaviors, 25*(6), 861–885.

Kalaitzidis, K. (2007). No crime, no drugs allowed. Tucson Citizen, August 8th, 2007. http://tucsoncitizen.com/morgue/2007/08/08/59566-no-crime-no-drugs-allowed/

Kelly, K. J., Comello, M. L. G., & Slater, M. D. (2006). Development of an aspirational campaign to prevent youth substance use: "Be under your own influence". *Applications, 12*(2), 14.

La Pastina, A. N. T. O. N. I. O., Rego, C. M., & Straubhaar, J. D. (2003). The centrality of telenovelas in Latin America's everyday life: Past tendencies, current knowledge, and future research. *Global Media Journal, 2*(2), 1–15.

Oetting, G. R., & Beauvais, F. (1990). Orthogonal cultural identification theory: The cultural identification of minority adolescents. *International Journal of the Addictions, 25*(5-A-6-A), 655–685.

Oetting, E. R., Donnermeyer, J. F., Plested, B. A., Edwards, R. W., Kelly, K., & Beauvais, F. (1995). Assessing community readiness for prevention. *International Journal of the Addictions, 30*, 659–683.

Oetting, E. R., Jumper-Thurman, P., Plested, B., & Edwards, R. W. (2001). Community readiness and health services. *Substance Use and Misuse, 36*(6&7), 825–843.

Paredes Castaneda, M. (2003). The transformation of Spanish-language radio in the U.S. *Journal of Radio Studies, 10*(1), 5–15.

Plested, B. A., Jumper Thurman, P., Edwards, R. W., & Oetting, E. R. (1998). Community readiness: A tool for effective community-based prevention. *The Prevention Researcher, 5*(2), 5–7.

Plested, B. A., Edwards, R. W., & Jumper-Thurman, P. (2006). *Community readiness: A handbook for successful change*. Fort Collins, CO: Tri-Ethnic Center for Prevention Research.

Romero, A. J., Martínez, D., & Carvajal, S. C. (2007). Bicultural stress and adolescent risk behaviors in a community sample of Latinos and non-Latino European Americans. *Ethnicity and Health, 12*(5), 443–463.

Romero, A. J., & Roberts, R. E. (2003a). Stress within a bicultural context for adolescents of Mexican descent. *Cultural Diversity and Ethnic Minority Psychology, 9*(2), 171–184.

Romero, A. J., & Roberts, R. E. (2003b). The impact of multiple dimensions of ethnic identity on discrimination and adolescents' self-esteem. *Journal of Applied Social Psychology, 33*(11), 2288–2305.

Romero, A. J., & Ruíz, M. G. (2007). Does familism lead to increased parental monitoring?: Protective factors for coping with risky behaviors. *Journal of Child and Family Studies, 16*, 143–154.

Romero, A. J., Edwards, L., Fryberg, S., Orduna, M., & Calza, D. (Under review). Adolescent discrimination resilience model: Protective effects of ethnic identity development. *Developmental Psychology*.

Samaniego, R. Y., & Gonzales, N. A. (1999). Multiple mediators of the effects of acculturation status on delinquency for Mexican American adolescents. *American Journal of Community Psychology, 27*(2), 189–210.

Schwartz, S. J., Unger, J. B., Baezconde-Garbanati, L., Zamboanga, B. L., Lorenzo-Blanco, E., De Rosiers, S., … Szapocznik, J. (2015). Trajectories of cultural stressors and effects on mental health and substance use among recently arrived Hispanic adolescents. *Journal of Adolescent Health, 56*(4):433–439.

Slater, M. D. (1999). Integrating application of media effects, persuasion, and behavior change theories to communication campaigns: A stages-of-change framework. *Health Communication, 11*(4), 335–354.

Slater, M. D., Kelly, K. J., & Edwards, R. W. (2000). Integrating social marketing, community readiness, and media advocacy in community-based prevention efforts. *Social Marketing Quarterly, 6*(3), 125–137.

Thurman, P. J., Plested, B. A., Edwards, R. W., Foley, R., & Burnside, M. (2003). Community readiness: The journey to community healing. *Journal of Psychoactive Drugs, 35*(1), 27–31.

Van Campen, K. S., & Romero, A. J. (2012). How are self-efficacy and family involvement associated with less sexual risk-taking among ethnic minority adolescents? *Family Relations, 61*(4), 548–558.

Zimmerman, M. A., Ramirez, J., Washienko, K. M., Walter, B., & Dyer, S. (1998). Enculturation hypothesis: Exploring direct and protective effects among Native American youth. In H. I. McCubbin, E. A. Thompson, A. I. Thompson, J. E. Fromer, H. I. McCubbin, E. A. Thompson, ... J. E. Fromer (Eds.), *Resiliency in Native American and immigrant families* (pp. 199–220). Thousand Oaks, CA: Sage Publications.

Chapter 9
Community–University Collaboration to Examine and Disseminate Local Research on Underage Drinking

Andrea Romero, Payal Anand, and Ana Fonseca

Abstract The purpose of this chapter is to discuss the university and community collaboration efforts to collect new data on community alcohol norms. This chapter describes the challenges that exist for university collaborations in low income and ethnic minority communities. This chapter describes the use of participatory dialogue to build relationships and trust between university researchers and community members. The critical discussion about the flaws of regional, state and national data was an important process that raised awareness of community members about the need for local data collection. This process led to the community-led and community-created surveys. Participatory dialogue was utilized again to collaboratively analyze and interpret local survey findings for community alcohol norms and perception of alcohol accessibility for adolescents.

Keywords Community-led research • Participatory dialogue • Community-led surveys • Reflection • Data interpretation • Research dissemination

All Participatory Action Research (PAR) emphasizes a collaborative approach to research that builds on community strengths through equal participation in all research components (Minkler & Wallerstein, 2008). However, the ideal of equal participation is often difficult to achieve. Finding the balance between community goals and research rigor is challenging; thus, scholars describe multiple levels of community involvement with PAR (O'Fallon & Dearry, 2002; Turnbull, Friesen, & Ramirez, 1998). Effective collaboration can be challenging because community members and researchers often have different, or even conflicting, agendas (Israel et al., 2005). Even when research projects are completed, there are challenges to shared interpretation of findings and dissemination of findings that effectively reach community audiences as well as research audiences (Plested, Edwards, & Jumper-Thurman, 2006). Moreover, linking research findings to community action in meaningful and

---

A. Romero, Ph.D. (✉) • P. Anand, M.P.H. • A. Fonseca, M.A.
Family Studies and Human Development, The University of Arizona,
650 North Park Avenue, Tucson, AZ 85719, USA
e-mail: romeroa@u.arizona.edu; payala1@email.arizona.edu; anafonseca@email.arizona.edu

A.J. Romero (ed.), *Youth-Community Partnerships for Adolescent Alcohol Prevention*, DOI 10.1007/978-3-319-26030-3_9

understandable ways is often elusive. In the current chapter, we discuss how changes in community readiness led to South Tucson Prevention Coalition's (STPC) community and university collaboration to produce research findings that were actionable.

A multiyear perspective demonstrates the iterative spiral of activities that lead to community-led research and dissemination of findings that helped to not only raise community awareness on adolescent alcohol use but also led to community action to prevent liquor licenses (Cousins & Earl, 1992; McIntyre, 2008). The goal of the STPC community-led research was not so much to evaluate the STPC activities, but rather to use it as a means of collective reflection on the group's progress. The dialogue for reflection on survey results led to a united front about how to prevent adolescent alcohol use in the local community. The coalition members were more willing to accept research findings when it was their own data, as compared to data that was collected by state or national entities. As such, this process further contributed to a unifying vision for action among community agencies, community members, and university researchers. Community-led research contributed to STPC's successful joint decision-making about next steps for community prevention strategies. In this chapter, we discuss the process of research integration and the unique and collaborative roles of community members and university researchers.

In fact, community readiness was key because over time community awareness increased about the issues of underage drinking. Additionally, as the community came together around the issue of adolescent alcohol use, community awareness also contributed to their capacity and willingness to use research to advance their prevention efforts. In part, we describe how changes in community readiness lead to an openness to discuss existing data and to begin to open the door to integrating research into existing activities. Additionally, the community-readiness perspective of taking small incremental steps towards change was instrumental in moving towards community-led research. In this chapter, we describe how research resistance changed to acceptance within the coalition and evolved to community–university collaborations. Some of the lessons learned include (1) mutual benefits for community members and researchers, (2) mutual use of data for community agendas and comparison to national data, (3) equal participatory dialogue to identify research questions and for interpretation of data, and (4) trust between community members and university researchers.

9.1 Participatory Action Research Process

PAR principles provided a structured process that was amenable to the community. In fact, it was through the use of PAR principles that community members began to embrace equality and trusting relationships with university researchers. We describe how the iterative spiral of PAR activities contributed to this process of community-led research, which included dialogue, implementation, reflection, and refining of data collection procedures (McIntyre, 2008). The PAR process was critical to the deepening of respect for research and the integration of research findings into group discussion and group decision-making. PAR can increase ecological validity of the study with practical outcomes while retaining conceptual and theoretical integrity because of the balance between technical rigor and community-driven issue identification. By ensuring methodological appropriateness that promotes recruitment and retention, researchers can be assured that internal and external validity will both be strengthened.

In fact, tracking coalitions over time and evaluating their effectiveness is difficult because they often take on a life of their own with ebbs and flow in growth, action, and success or failure. Most evaluations of coalitions are post hoc and rely primarily on qualitative data based on interviews, documentation, and meeting minutes (Grekul, 2011). However, a benefit of using PAR is that there is often a focus on process and identification of factors that contribute to success. This process is based on open dialogue and reflection after joint activities are completed (Freire, 1968; Godfrey & Grayman, 2014). The focus of reflection is on identifying lessons learned that help build a strong foundation for the development of the next activities. This type of process further nurtures relationship building and trust among members.

9.1.1 Challenges to Equal Participation of Community and Researchers

The development of the PAR process and equal participation takes time, particularly among low-income communities and ethnic minority communities with a history of being taken advantage of by researchers (McIntyre, 2008; Minkler & Wallerstein, 2008). Before Dr. Romero began to collaborate with community members, they had legitimate concerns about research because of previous negative experiences that portrayed their community in a one-dimensional stereotypical manner by researchers. The community had rarely been included in the development or interpretation of research. Often low income and ethnic minority communities are resistant to working with outsiders, especially university researchers (Harper & Salina, 2000; McIntyre, 2008). Too often researchers conduct what is termed "helicopter research," where community members are not included in the aforesaid dialogue (Ferreria & Gendron, 2011). In these cases, research is not conceived as giving back to the community. Moreover, in some unfortunate cases, researchers promise some kind of output to the community, but do not provide the outcome promised. It is these types of clashes or unfulfilled promises that can lead to community distrust of researchers (Harper & Salina, 2000). Thus, it is not surprising that community-based projects are often not inclusive of researchers as equal participants in the process and may in fact be resistant to research and university researchers. Yet, there is great potential in university and community partnerships that can lead to gains for both groups (Harper & Salina, 2000).

However, PAR is one way to achieve a research method that may be more ethical, valid, and reliable with underrepresented populations, as compared to traditional research methodologies (McIntyre, 2008; Minkler & Wallerstein, 2008). In some PAR projects, it is the community that is in the driver seat, such that they decide who is researched, what is researched, where it is researched, when it is researched, why it is researched, how it is researched, and what ultimately happens once the research is complete. This approach only leaves university researchers with limited outside consultant roles (Plested et al., 2006) in which it is assumed that there is no overlap in agendas. It also assumes that there is no potential for mutual benefit of community and researchers. Conceiving of a university researcher's role as external to PAR leaves little room for the equal voice of researchers in the discussion of topics or data procedures; additionally, it leaves little incentive for researchers to be involved in participatory research models.

However, we will argue that the equal participation of researchers should be considered because they have the potential to play a critical role in the development and utilization of research. Researchers can bring unique skills and resources to contribute to community-based research projects that can help the success of PAR. In particular, their expertise in data collection and the organization and interpretation of results can help community utilization of research. There are many reasons why community members may not be able to complete research projects or that their projects may not lead to action-oriented results. One of the reasons is that community members may not be able to remain continuously involved in projects over the extended time that may be required to complete research and/or disseminate findings that leads to action (Harper & Salina, 2000). In fact, the turnover of community participants is one reason why continued commitment to projects may be limited. Another aspect of the critical role of university researchers is that they may be able to see certain strengths and weaknesses from a third-person lens that may be difficult for community members to consciously identify. These are some of the reasons as to why both the community and the university researcher elements should be considered in PAR projects.

9.2 STPC Readiness and Research

Often the first step in community readiness is to obtain community feedback about adolescent alcohol use in the community and their interpretation of national data (Plested, Jumper Thurman, Edwards, & Oetting, 1998). A participatory dialogue method, based on problem-posing, was used by STPC to review existing research, including national, state, and regional data (see Chap. 3 for more details). This was an effective technique for community members to engage in critical thinking about the existing data. In the open climate, they could express whether they felt that the existing data was representative of what they witnessed in their own community. Moreover, this process further emphasized the need for local data collection in order to really understand what was happening in their community. This approach helped community members and researchers to come to critical consciousness about how they wanted to phrase their own questions to understand the unique setting of their own community.

9.2.1 Participatory Dialogue

Identifying local issues to work with is an important process. Individuals within a community may feel that there are other "better" issues to work with, and this is where it becomes important to prioritize the community's needs. Often researchers may have already identified what they perceive to be the most critical health issue afflicting a community; yet, the community may perceive a different health issue as more important. Participatory dialogue can be a useful tool to employ to discuss through problem-posing combined with reflection and action-oriented outcomes to achieve consensus for the coalition goals. Essential to effective PAR methods is engaged dialogue around problem posing, in a manner such that all members are equal participants and co-learners, including researchers and community members (Freire, 1968). This can be a challenging process to leave all ages, socioeconomic status, egos, and titles at the door and to welcome and facilitate comments from ALL participants in an equal manner, and equally to listen in a respectful manner to all comments. It is likely that community members and researchers at first will not always agree on how to define the topic. However, as a result of dialogue and consensus, the result is significantly more likely to be conducted within a real problem context, with more immediate solutions for action.

A problem-posing strategy for discussion is likely to limit didactic presentations of statistics by focusing the discussion through posing questions to participants so that they can work together to uncover the root causes of the issue within their own community. Central to effective problem-posing dialogue is asking participants to consider socioeconomic, political, cultural, and historical aspects of the problem during their discussion, which is more likely to lead to understanding the problem within a larger context. This is also a way in which to develop group critical thinking processes to work through identification of the common issues and to create strategies for community level change.

9.2.2 Critique of Existing Regional Data

Phase 1 of STPC provided rigorous and nationally situated longitudinal survey data collection with youth through the Omeyocan YES project (see Chap. 4). These Phase 1 results from the STPC baseline data were used to help guide discussions during the first year of STPC coalition meeting discussions about the mission. The baseline data from STPC indicated that 72 % of the youth had used alcohol in their lifetime, 45 % of the youth had used alcohol in the past 30 days, and 26 % were drunk in the past 30 days (see Table 9.1). Compared to national and state level data at that time, it appears that the local survey is representative (30 day use: 52 % Arizona 2003, 47 % Arizona 2005; 45 % U.S. 2003, 43 % U.S. 2005; drunk in past 30 days: 35 % Arizona 2003, 31 % Arizona 2005, 28 % U.S. 2003, 26 % U.S. 2005), if not slightly lower than

Table 9.1 Regional data on alcohol norms

	2003–2005 STPC: Phase 1 $N=125$	2006 Arizona Youth Survey Tucson High School (10th Grade)
Lifetime alcohol use	72 %	80 %
Past 30 days alcohol use	45 %	42 %
30 days drunk	26 %	n/a
Age of first alcohol use	13.4 years	13.2 years
Friends think it is wrong or very wrong to use alcohol	37 %	60 %
Parents think it is wrong or very wrong to use alcohol	n/a	85 %

state averages (Johnston et al., 2014). Thus, it was clear that alcohol was the most often used substance, and this was one factor that helped focus the coalition's decision to focus on underage drinking rather than substances in general.

However, in the first few years of STPC Phase 2, Drug-Free Community, there were too many barriers to collect new survey data. There was a perception that community members were asked to do too many surveys. Additionally, there was not sufficient funding from the Drug-Free Community mechanism to fund a large-scale longitudinal data collection; thus, data collection was not feasible for university researchers. Thus, it was agreed to utilize the preexisting Arizona Youth Survey data that could be parsed out by specific local areas. This survey already collected data on youth alcohol use, other substance, alcohol norms of parents, alcohol norms of peers, and perception of riskiness. These were the key factors identified in the STPC theory of change and the focus of the logic model (see Chap. 2).

The Arizona Youth Survey, a state-wide survey conducted at specific high schools, was collected every other year. So the first year of relevant data for STPC was the 2006 survey, and the closest high school that completed the survey was Tucson High School. However, the City of South Tucson was zoned for youth to attend two different high schools, and Tucson High School was only one of those schools. Additionally, Tucson High School represented youth from several other surrounding neighborhoods and even from across the city given the open-enrollment policies. In general, demographics for the Tucson High School were much more diverse than the City of South Tucson for race, ethnicity, and socioeconomic status. Thus, the STPC community felt that the data was only marginally relevant. However, data from the 2006 survey were utilized for STPC coalition discussion (see Table 9.1). The results suggested slightly higher rates of lifetime alcohol use compared to the STPC Phase 1 data, but lower rates of alcohol use in the past 30 days. The Arizona Youth Survey also suggested much higher rates of friend disapproval of alcohol use compared to the STPC Phase 1 data (see Table 9.1). It is important to note that 85 % of the parents felt that alcohol use was wrong or very wrong, which once again points out the critical role that parents and family members can play when considering adolescent alcohol use.

In the first year (2006), Dr. Romero and the STPC project coordinator developed a coalition member survey that was several pages. However, they found that coalition members were not motivated to complete and return the survey. In 2007, the coalition received formal training about the use of the community readiness interview. After this, a small subset of coalition members agreed to collect interview data and to analyze results to determine community readiness levels (see Chap. 2 for details). There were a handful of interviews that were conducted guided by the community readiness dimensions; however, it was challenging to obtain surveys from all members (Plested et al., 2006). Moreover, the compiling of the results and analysis of findings provided to be challenging. The activity was useful as a means of reflection, and anecdotes were shared and contributed to the participatory dialogue. These were some of the steps that led to different approaches of the role of community and researchers in developing research strategies where each played a significant role that catered to their own expertise.

9.2.3 Incremental Steps Toward Data Integration

Collecting data specifically on norms can be useful to understand how the community feels about how wrong it might be for adolescents to use alcohol. In the beginning, there was a level of concern about the collection of data at the community-wide events. In fact, at the initial community STPC events (e.g., Halloween Festival, Block Party, see descriptions in Chap. 8), the data collection was limited to counting of the number of participants. At another early event, there was a sign-in desk, where participants could answer a couple questions on a small slip of paper (see Fig. 9.1). Even though the community was coming together around a common issue and working effectively to offer community-level events to raise awareness, there was still not an embracing of the utility of data collection or its purpose.

Do you live in the City of South Tucson?
_______Yes
_______No (Do you spend a lot of time in the City of South Tucson? _____Yes_____No

How many people came with you today? __________
How many of them are between 9-18 years old?______________
How many are under 9 years old?__________

How did you hear about our event? ______________________________________

Fig. 9.1 Original Block Party Survey

9.3 Community Developed Surveys

Once the community had reached a higher level of readiness, one of implementation, they were more open and prepared to consider evaluation strategies (Oetting, Jumper-Thurman, Plested, & Edwards, 2001). When STPC first began community events in 2005–2006, they were developed from preexisting events (see Chap. 8). There was resistance to add surveys or data collection to existing events. Truly, at this time the focus was on building collaboration between agencies not on data collection readiness. However, at the first STPC-hosted Block Party (see Chap. 8), the coalition agreed for Dr. Romero to collect demographic information. The coalition reviewed the survey (see Fig. 9.1). The data from this survey was included in reports to the coalition and to the City Council as a means to demonstrate the attendance. It also helped to demonstrate to the City Council that the majority of attendees were from the City of South Tucson.

However, there was significant progress in the coalition functioning and level of readiness by 2009; STPC was at a stage of community readiness where they were beginning to focus on confirmation and expansion of prevention activities (see Chap. 2). At this point, the coalition members were all highly aware of adolescent alcohol use as an issue of concern, and they had moved through preplanning activities and effectively initiated new joint prevention projects with success. In order to better assess the local community needs, STPC took the lead in organizing community surveys (paper–pencil) for youth and adults to be collected at the National Night Out event (see Fig. 9.2). The starting point for this survey was based on the alcohol norm questions that were utilized in the national/regional surveys that STPC has already reviewed. Survey questions were selected by input from community members and recommendations from Dr. Romero during regular STPC meetings. The coalition reviewed not only the wording of the question but also the wording of the responses. The survey was created in both English and Spanish (translations were conducted by STPC members), and both versions were reviewed and edited by coalition members.

Coalition members added new survey questions, such as questions specifically about perceptions of community norms, as opposed to peer norms. However, they agreed that the emphasis should be on "getting drunk" similar to binge drinking (4 or 5 drinks), rather than any drinking at all. Again, at this stage even the coalition did not want to include experimental drinking, rather they focused on binge drinking. They added their own re-worded version of disapproval with responses that included "That it is ok," "That it is NOT ok," and "I don't know." This change was made in order to make it easier for the community to understand and respond to the question. However, it was also agreed to keep a second question with the standard national wording, in order to compare to national data at Dr. Romero's recommendation. In addition, the coalition and the community repeatedly discussed the importance of parents and family when considering prevention of adolescent alcohol use. For this reason, the coalition also chose to create an adult survey (see Fig. 9.2), with questions specifically worded for adults about the same alcohol norms that were asked of the youth. In the previous review of national and regional data, there is only access to youth survey results, and there are no national or regional surveys of adult or parent populations.

The first survey met with such success (see discussion of findings below) that the following year the coalition expanded and revised the survey for another data collection point during the National Night Out Event in August 2010 (see Fig. 9.3). Once again a similar process of dialogue contributed to the development of both

STPC National Night Out Youth Survey

1. Teen Survey - National Night Out, August 4th, 2009

Please answer these questions to help South Tucson Prevention Coalition learn more about how to help teens in your community.

1. Do you live in the City of South Tucson?

A. Yes B. No

2. How old are you?

3. What grade will you start this year in school?

4. Are you a . . .

A. Boy B. Girl

5. What would your parents/guardians think if you were very drunk from alcohol (beer, wine, or hard liquor)?

A. That it is o.k. B. That it is NOT o.k. C. I don't know what my parents would think

6. What does your community think about teens being drunk from alcohol (beer, wine, or hard liquor)?

A. That it is o.k. B. That it is NOT o.k. C. I don't know

7. How wrong do your parents/guardians feel it would be for you to drink beer, wine, or hard liquor (for example, vodka, whiskey, or gin) regularly?

A. Very wrong C. A little bit wrong
B. Wrong D. Not at all wrong

8. How easy would it be for you to get alcohol in the City of South Tucson?

A. Very Easy B. Easy C. Not Easy

THANK YOU FOR YOUR HELP! HAVE A GREAT TIME AT NATIONAL NIGHT OUT!

2. Encuesta de Adolescentes: NNO 4 de agosto

Page 1

Fig. 9.2 2009 National Night Out Community developed surveys for youth and adults

STPC National Night Out

1. Adult Survey: National Night Out, August 4th, 2009

Please answer these questions to help South Tucson Prevention Coalition learn more about how to help the community.

1. Do you live in the City of South Tucson?

A. Yes
B. No

2. Are you the parent or guardian of a teenager between the ages of 13-18 years old?

A. Yes
B. No

3. What would you think if your teenager was drunk from alcohol (beer, wine, or hard liquor)?

A. That it is o.k.
B. That it is NOT o.k.
C. I don't know

4. What does your community think about teens being drunk from alcohol (beer, wine, or hard liquor)?

A. That it is o.k.
B. That it is NOT o.k.
C. I don't know

5. How wrong would it be for your teen to drink beer, wine, or hard liquor (for example, vodka, whiskey, or gin) regularly?

A. Very wrong
C. A little bit wrong
B. Wrong
D. Not at all wrong

6. How easy would it be for someone under 21 years old to get alcohol in South Tucson?

A. Very easy
B. Easy
C. Not easy

THANK YOU FOR YOUR HELP! HAVE A GREAT TIME AT NATIONAL NIGHT OUT!

2. Ecuesta de Adultos

Spanish version adult survey

Por favor responda las siguientes preguntas y asi podría asistir a South Tucson Prevention Coalition aprender mas sobre como ayudar a los jóvenes de la comunidad.

1. Vive usted en la ciudad de Sur Tucson?

Si
No

Page 1

Fig. 9.2 (continued)

youth and adult versions of the community survey, and all were administered in English and Spanish. However, this time the coalition was significantly more comfortable with this process, and the questions went beyond the basic alcohol norm questions of the last survey. This time the coalition added questions about education, perception of improving the community, and cultural events.

Additionally, during that year Arizona had approved a new bill, SB1070, that would increase police enforcement of undocumented immigration, otherwise known as the "show me your papers" bill. There was significant concern in the local community about the impact of this bill on youth and families, given that 30 % of the community was foreign born. However, the South Tucson Police had been a strong coalition member since the beginning of the Drug Free

Please answer these questions to help South Tucson Prevention Coalition learn more about how to help the community.

1. Do you live in the City of South Tucson? (boundaries are: West:10th Ave; North: 26th 1/2 Ave, South: 44th St., East: 2nd Ave)

A. Live in South Tucson B. Do not live in South Tucson

2. How old are you?

3. What school do you go to? (please indicate if you will not go to school this fall)

4. How important are art and cultural events in your community?

A. Very important B. Somewhat important C. A little important D. Not at all important

5. How wrong would your parents feel it is for you to drink beer, wine, or hard liquor (for example, vodka, whiskey, or gin) regularly?

A. Very wrong B. Wrong C. A little bit wrong D. Not at all wrong

6. How important is it that you graduate from the university?

A. Very important B. Important C. A little important D. Not at all important

7. How likely is it that other kids from your neighborhood will graduate from high school?

A. Very likely B. Somewhat likely C. A little bit likely D. Not at all likely

8. How easy would it be for you to get alcohol in South Tucson?

A. Very easy B. Easy C. Not easy D. I do not know

9. Has SB 1070 changed the way that you and your family live your daily life?(not going to church, not going to school, not going to doctor/hospital, or not using resources from federal, state or local agencies)

A. A lot B. A little bit C. Not much D. Not at all

10. Would you like to know more information about SB 1070 and your rights?

A. Yes B. No

11. How confident are you that City of South Tucson Police will enforce SB 1070 fairly?

very confident somewhat confident not very confident not at all confident

12. How safe is your neighborhood?

A. Very Safe B. Somewhat safe C. Not very safe D. Not safe at all

Fig. 9.3 2010 National Night Out Community developed surveys for youth and adults

STPC National Night Out Adult Survey 2010

Please answer these questions to help South Tucson Prevention Coalition learn more about how to help the community.

1. Do you live in the City of South Tucson? (boundaries are: West:10th Ave; North: 26th 1/2 Ave, South: 44th St., East: 2nd Ave)

A. Live in South Tucson B. Do not live in South Tucson

2. How important are art and cultural events in your community?

A. Very important B. Somewhat important C. A little important D. Not at all important

3. Are you the parent or guardian of a teenager between the ages of 13-18 years old?

A. Yes B. No

4. How wrong would it be for your teen to drink beer, wine, or hard liquor (for example, vodka, whiskey, or gin) regularly?

A. Very wrong B. Wrong C. A little bit wrong D. Not at all wrong

5. How important is it that your child graduate from the university?

A. Very important B. Important C. A little important D. Not at all important

6. How likely is it that children from your neighborhood will graduate from high school?

A. Very likely B. Somewhat likely C. A little bit likely D. Not at all likely

7. How easy would it be for someone under 21 years old to get alcohol in South Tucson?

A. Very easy B. Easy C. Not easy D. I do not know

8. Has SB 1070 changed the way that you and your family live your daily life? (such as not going to church, not going to school, not going to doctor/hospital, or not using resources from federal, state or local agencies)

A. A lot B. A little bit C. Not much D. Not at all

9. Would you like to know more information about SB 1070 and your rights?

A. Yes B. No

10. How confident are you that City of South Tucson Police will enforce SB 1070 fairly?

A. Very confident B. Somewhat confident C. Not very confident D. Not at all confident

Fig. 9.3 (continued)

Community grant. In fact, many of the STPC activities in the past years, particularly with the National Night Out event, had worked to improve relations between police and local community. Thus, the coalition felt strongly that questions about the perception of SB1070 and the local enforcement of this policy by police needed to be included in the survey. During discussions, Dr. Romero expressed hesitancy about including these questions and concern that community members may not want to complete the survey because the questions might be seen as too invasive. However, the coalition discussed these concerns and agreed that the questions, as they are phrased, needed to be included because of the importance of the topic. The changing and heated political environment at the time may have not only potentially impacted adolescent alcohol use, but importantly it may have impacted STPC's ability to outreach into the community. It may have also impacted community member's ability or willingness to attend large community events. It was for these primary reasons that the coalition chose to include the questions. These questions mirrored the changes and expansion of the coalition to consider the relation between adolescent alcohol use and the broad context of unique community factors, both positive and negative.

9.4 Analysis and Interpretation of Data with Community

Data was collected during the National Night Out events in August where approximately 500 people attended each event. Approximately, 20 % of the attendees completed the surveys. Participants completed surveys voluntarily and anonymously. There were no incentives to complete the surveys. Dr. Romero, coalition members, and youth volunteers worked together to collect surveys from attendees. Dr. Romero and a research assistant entered the data into an on-line survey database and then prepared charts for the questions to share with the coalition at the next meeting. An aspect of the mutual benefit of this process for Dr. Romero and the research assistants was that it was utilized for students to complete criteria for undergraduate honor's thesis projects or independent study projects.

The results are compiled in Table 9.2 for comparison to national datasets on alcohol norms. Here we provide a brief summary of the results from both surveys. The data between 2009 and 2010 cannot be directly compared because the questions were asked differently, and the samples are not confirmed to be the

Table 9.2 Community-Led National Night Out alcohol norms

	2009		2010	
	Youth	Adults	Youth	Adults
Parental disapproval				
Very wrong or wrong	96 %	97 %	92 %	100 %
A little bit wrong	4 %	1.3 %	6 %	0 %
Not at all wrong	0 %	1.3 %	2 %	0 %
Alcohol availability				
Very easy or easy	42 %	79 %	56 %	75 %
Not easy	58 %	16 %	17 %	9 %
I don't know	0 %	5 %	27 %	16 %

same because the surveys were anonymous, so they could not be matched between years. In 2009, 101 surveys were collected [76 adults and 25 youth (average age 13.6 years)] at the annual STPC sponsored event to gather data on the accessibility of alcohol. The majority of participants reported living in the City of South Tucson (54 % adults; 84 % youth). In 2010, data was collected with 143 individuals [91 adults and 52 youth (Youth average age 15.15 years of age)], where the majority of participants reported residing in the City of South Tucson (46.7 % adults; 53.8 % youth). In 2010, slightly more than double the amount of youth in 2009 completed the survey, while this may suggest more acceptance of the survey, and also more effective data collection efforts, it does make it difficult to compare between 2009 and 2010. However, a similar number of adult surveys were collected both years.

In both years, the vast majority of youth and adults felt that it was "very wrong" or "wrong" for adolescents to get drunk (2009: 96 %, 97 %; 2010: 92 %, 100 %). The slight changes among youth may be attributed to the difference in sample size. It was encouraging to see that adults moved from 97 % to 100 % across these years. The disapproval rates from local data obtained from the Arizona Youth survey at a local high school in 2006 were also lower at a rate of 85 % of youth who felt that parents would feel it was wrong or very wrong to use alcohol. The disapproval rates in 2009 and 2010 are significantly higher compared to regional findings for Pima County where 85 % of youth in 2008 and 85 % in 2010 reported that parents felt adolescent alcohol use was very wrong or wrong (Arizona Criminal Justice Commission, 2015). These rates are also significantly higher than national rates between 2006 and 2010, where they hover between 70 and 80 % for 10th graders (Johnston et al., 2014). Overall, the coalition felt that they had been successful in raising awareness about alcohol disapproval norms in their community.

The rates for alcohol availability were not consistent between adults and youth, which may explain the difference in perspectives between youth and adults about alcohol availability in the local community. However, more adults felt it was "very easy" or "easy for youth to obtain alcohol (79 % in 2009 and 75 % in 2010). Whereas, 42 % (2009) and 56 % (2010) of youth felt it was "very easy" or "easy" to obtain alcohol in South Tucson. The change over time that is demonstrated here is that there is a decrease in the number of youth and adults who feel it is "not easy" to obtain alcohol in South Tucson from 2009 to 2010, and many more indicate that they "don't know." It is difficult to interpret these results, but it may suggest that STPC was raising some awareness about adolescent access to alcohol, because whereas in 2009 many more youth and adults felt sure that it was not easy to get access to alcohol, these numbers decreased quite a bit in 2010. Interestingly, Pima County findings from 2008, 2010, 2012, and 2014 report that the most popular source of obtaining alcohol reported by youth is *by someone under 21 years of age*, *someone else who bought it*, and *someone not family over 21* (Arizona Criminal Justice Commission, 2015). However, these rates are higher compared to national data that suggests that 10th graders who feel that alcohol accessibility is "fairly easy" or "very easy" is between 80 and 90 % during the years 2006–2010 (Johnston et al., 2014). The findings on alcohol availability clearly pointed the coalition to prioritize on their next prevention strategy to limit liquor licenses in the community as a means to limit alcohol availability.

9.5 Dissemination of Results

9.5.1 How Results Were Prepared

Dissemination of results was very important to community-led research (see Appendices 1 and 2). The whole point of collecting local data was to share it with the local community as a means to raise awareness about alcohol norms. It was important that the results were understandable and available to the largest segments of the population possible. The coalition members discussed the results of the survey; they asked in-depth questions that guided Dr. Romero and her assistant to prepare the community report. Coalition members were interested in questions related to gender, age, and comparisons to national data. Dr. Romero and an undergraduate honor's student compiled the data into a community report that was shared with key stakeholders who provided feedback and edits. Dr. Romero worked closely with undergraduate or graduate research assistants to prepare community reports that had a mixture of graphs and written explanations to share the most critical findings to the largest audience. The reports were disseminated in hard copy at coalition meetings and at City Council meetings. There were also disseminated on-line to coalition members. Dr. Romero presented them to the coalition members during a regularly scheduled coalition meeting.

9.5.2 Content of Reports and the Importance of Context

The community reports are comprised of the following elements: (1) STPC mission, (2) background of who prepared the reports, (3) when/where the report was presented, (4) demographics of the survey, including how many lived in the City of South Tucson, (5) results of alcohol norm questions, including comparison to national data, (6) opportunity for discussion or suggestions about how to get involved, and (7) Thank you and acknowledgement of STPC and City Council Members (see Appendices 1 and 2). These reports were compiled by Dr. Romero with the help of a research assistant in order to input the data and to produce graphs using a user-friendly on-line survey tool. However, the content of the reports and the style of presentation were very much determined by the community coalition members. These reports are presented in full in Appendices 1 and 2 not only to provide templates for other communities but also to represent in full the extent of community-led data collection and manipulation of the data. It was very important to coalition members that the results were reported within a context of national data. It was also critically important to include the names of all coalition participants and to thank all key stakeholders in their community audience.

9.5.3 Interface with Local Government

There were regular presentations to the City Council that slowly integrated more data over time. First, the Youth-to-Youth (Y2Y) group began to take the lead in preparing these presentations with use of pictures and anecdotal descriptions of the impact of alcohol on their community. This was an effective way to increase awareness about adolescent alcohol use among the city council members, who were much more open listening directly to adolescents who lived in South Tucson. Regular reports were distributed to the city council by the STPC project coordinator; these reports included a description of the events and a summary of any data collected. Often these were one page memos provided prior to the council meeting or very brief 1 paragraph descriptions or summaries of the events that had occurred (see Chap. 8 for more information). This proactive approach to informing and involving local government members was an effective strategy to raise awareness of factors that contributed to adolescent alcohol use in the local community.

9.5.4 Action-Oriented Goals

The primary findings of the community-led research over this time period was that (1) both youth and adults perceived that adolescent alcohol use was wrong and (2) alcohol was perceived to be more available to adolescents in the City of South Tucson compared to state and national data. Thus, these findings combined with the alcohol saturation findings from the youth-led alcohol mapping project clearly led STPC to focus on alcohol availability as a point of action. The results provide insight to help unite community members to act to prevent adolescent alcohol use. Through using action research in STPC, we were able to generate practical knowledge within a real societal context that helped to unify the coalition and focus their mission (Bryndon-Miller, Greenwood, & Maguire, 2003). Moreover, the data helped STPC members clearly decide the next action steps for their coalition to prevent adolescent alcohol use.

9.6 Conclusion

This chapter demonstrates how one community utilized community readiness approaches of incremental change to raise awareness of adolescent alcohol use and PAR techniques to develop their interest and acceptance of incorporating data collection. It was not until the level of community readiness had advanced among coalition members that they were aware of adolescent alcohol issues in their community, and they were working together as a functioning collaborative when they were ready to take on their own community-led research. At the beginning of the project, the community members were still silo-ed in their own agencies and their own age groups. They had high distrust of outsiders, especially university researchers. Moreover, the community was not united and working together for adolescent alcohol use. Community readiness strategies suggest that sharing of national and regional data can be used at early phases to increase awareness. This was done with coalition members, who were already identified key stakeholders for adolescent alcohol prevention. However, it was the process of using PAR that helped the coalition deconstruct and critique the national and regional data. This process was motivating to develop trust with university researchers and also to motivate community members to take on their own data collection procedures.

The first year of community-led research was so successful that the coalition further embraced this strategy in the final year of their work, to further expand the survey questions and to utilize the research findings to motivate their actions to limit alcohol licenses in their own community. The increased awareness of the local context of underage drinking helped this community to pinpoint their local action strategies for prevention. In this chapter, we provide a multiyear perspective that considers how multiple studies piece together as part of a larger puzzle that is influenced by community influence during and between projects. This can only be done over time through developing equitable and trusting relationships. However, high quality research is also more likely to lead to action-oriented solutions that can be leveraged in order to share in public spaces, such as with local government. There are many research strengths to utilizing PAR; for example, it can increase ecological validity of the study with practical outcomes while retaining conceptual and theoretical integrity (Minkler & Wallerstein, 2008). By ensuring methodological appropriateness that promotes recruitment and retention, the researchers can be assured that internal and external validity will both be strengthened. Moreover, the achievements of successful collaboration, breaking down silos, and developing community-led research led to the next steps of youth-led research that focused more specifically on alcohol sales within the City of South Tucson.

9.7 Appendix 1: South Tucson Prevention Coalition Community Report 2009

9.7.1 South Tucson Prevention Coalition Community Report Fall 2009

9.7.1.1 Report of Youth and Parent Surveys Collected at National Night Out 2009

Andrea Romero, and Jessica Blaire
University of Arizona, Tucson, AZ, USA

STPC DFC Mission

STPC members focus our efforts on ***underage drinking***.

National Night Out is a crime prevention activity and is held annually in the first week of August. It is a good opportunity for youth to engage in positive fun activities and also to stand up to crime in their neighborhoods. 10 groups participate in the National Night Out, including: John Valenzuela Youth Center, Safos Dance Theater, Dancing in the Streets, Southern Arizona AIDS Foundation, Gospel Rescue Mission, Youth Explorers Post Y2Y, South Tucson Police, South Tucson Fire Department, and the City of South Tucson.

The following is a report prepared by Jessica Blaire, University of Arizona, Honors Student, for completion of her honors track in Mexican American Studies course 280: Chicano/a Psychology under the supervision of Dr. Andrea Romero. She entered the data, analyzed the findings, and prepared the following report.

This report was presented to key coalition members on Wednesday, December 16, 2009 at the John Valenzuela Youth Center.

Who Completed the Survey?

25 youth and 76 adults completed this survey at the STPC National Night Out (NNO). Approximately, one-half of the NNO attendees completed the survey.

- What age were the youth who participated? How many boys and girls participated?
  - All youth were between the ages of 11 and 18 years old.
- How many boys and girls participated?
  - The survey was completed by 10 boys and 15 girls.
- Where do they live?
  - 84 % of the youth said that they live in the city of South Tucson.
  - 64.5 % of the adults said that they live in the city of South Tucson.
- Who were the adults?
  - 50.7 % of the adults said that they were the parent or guardian of a teenager between the ages of 13 and 18 years old.

Teen Perspective on Teen Alcohol Usage
The youth that participated in the STPC survey were overall very aware of their community's views on underage alcohol usage. The majority of teens did not think that their parents would approve of any type of alcohol usage.

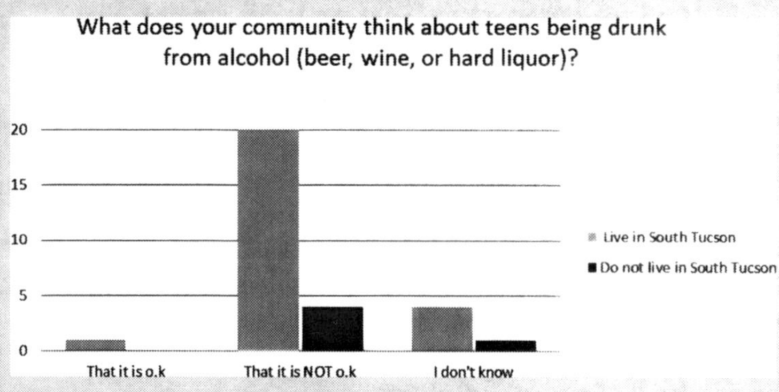

- When asked what their parents or guardians think about alcohol…
  - 80 % of teens said that their parents would <u>not</u> think it was o.k. if they were very drunk from alcohol.
  - 88 % of teens said that their parents would feel it is very wrong for their teens to drink alcohol regularly.
- 79.2 % of teens said that their community would think it was very wrong for them to be drunk from alcohol.

The majority of youth feel that their parents and their community would not be ok with them using alcohol.

- National Reports indicate that most (89.7 %) adolescents reported that their parents would strongly disapprove of their having one or two drinks of an alcoholic beverage nearly every day, which was similar to the rates in 2007 (89.6 %) and 2002 (89.0 %).
- Youths aged 12–17 who believed their parents would strongly disapprove of their using substances were less likely to use that substance than were youths who believed their parents would somewhat disapprove or neither approve nor disapprove. (http://oas.samhsa.gov/NSDUH/2k8NSDUH/2k8results.cfm#Ch6)

Adult Perspective on Teen Alcohol Usage

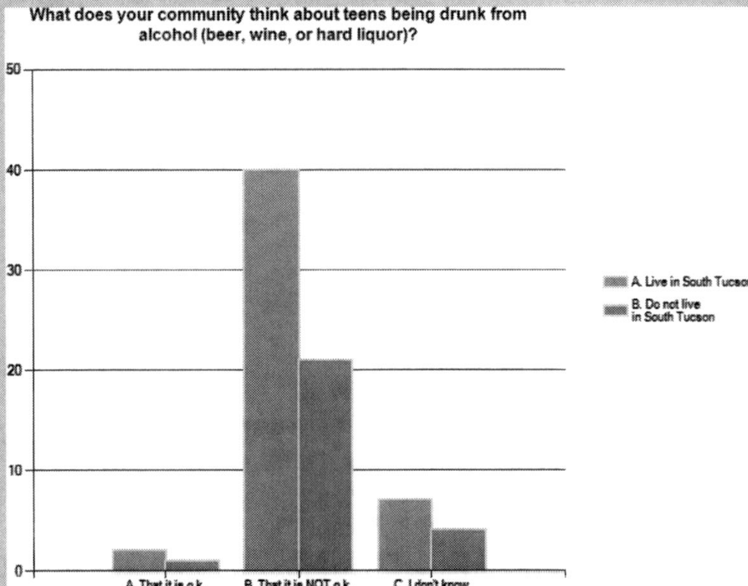

- When asked what they thought about their teenagers using alcohol…
  - 87.8 % of adults said that they would not think it was o.k. for their teenager to be drunk from alcohol.
  - 88.2 % of adults said that it would be very wrong for their teenage to drink alcohol regularly.
- 81.3 % of adults said that their community would not think it is o.k. for teens to be drunk from alcohol.

The majority of adults said that they would not be ok with their kids using alcohol and that their community would not be ok with kids using alcohol.

Accessibility of Alcohol in the Community

- 41.7 % of teens feel that it is very easy—easy to get alcohol in the city of South Tucson
- 78.9 % of adults feel that it is very easy—easy for someone under the age of 21 to get alcohol in the city of South Tucson

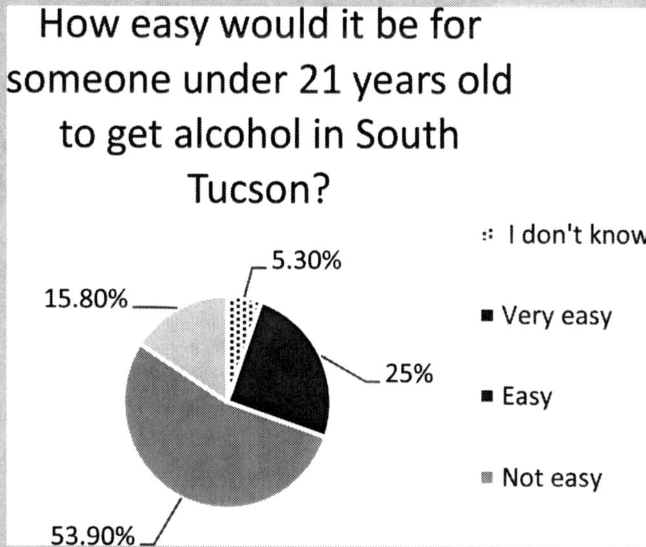

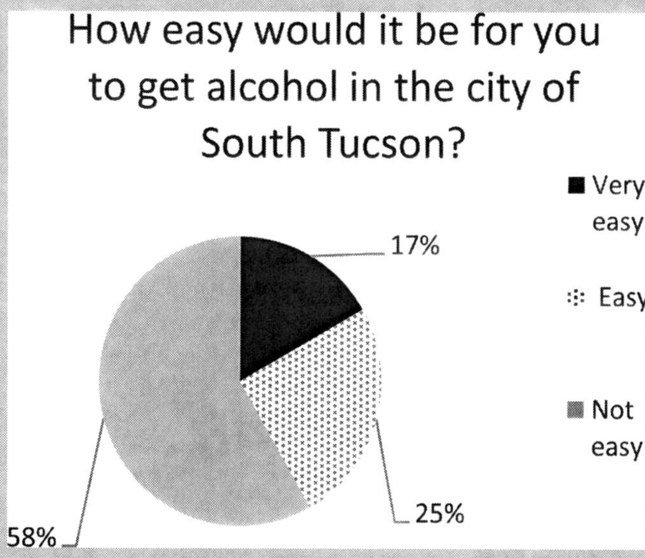

The majority of adults feel that it is easy for youth under the age of 21 to get alcohol in their city. Almost half of the youth feel that it is easy for them to get alcohol in the city of South Tucson.

How Can Parents and the Community Get Involve?

- Talk to your teens
  - Parents can talk to their teens about what they know about drugs and alcohol and what they have learned about their effects.
- Encourage teens to participate in 4 Elements: Hip Hop Prevention Program
  - 4 Elements has a summer retreat program for teens that helps them develop in positive ways to prevent teen risky behaviors.
- Submit Youth Nominees for the Shining Stars Awards
- Parents and teens participate in or attend National Night Out
- Learn more about the Social Host Ordinance and let your Council members know that you support it.
- Join South Tucson Prevention Coalition to help prevent teen alcohol and drug use in South Tucson.
- Form Community Watch Groups
- Send youth to John Valenzuela Youth Center activities, House of Neighborly Service, Aztlan Boxing, etc.

THANK YOU
SOUTH TUCSON CITY COUNCIL
AND
SOUTH TUCSON PREVENTION COALITION MEMBERS

9.8 Appendix 2: South Tucson Prevention Coalition Community Report 2010

South Tucson Prevention Coalition
STPC
A Drug-Free Community
Working together for a stronger healthier community

9.8.1 *South Tucson Prevention Coalition Drug Free Community Fall 2010 Report*

9.8.1.1 Report of Youth and Parent Surveys Collected at The City of South Tucson's National Night out 2010

Andrea Romero and Henry Gonzalez
University of Arizona, Tucson, AZ, USA

South Tucson Prevention Coalition (STPC) Drug Free Community (DFC) Mission

STPC members focus our efforts on ***underage drinking***.

National Night Out is a community activity that works to support families and the community to prevent teen risky behaviors, such as underage drinking, drug use, crime, and school dropout. The event is held annually the first week of August. It is a good opportunity for youth to engage in fun and positive activities, as well as to stand up to issues in their neighborhoods. **21** groups participated in the 2010 National Night Out, including:

Bike Ambassador Program, Organizing for America, Border Action Network, Brown Berets, Tucson-Pima County Bicycle Advisor Comm., Ochoa Elementary School, Our Family Services, Su Voz Vale, Luz Southside Coalition, We Reject Racism, First Things First, Community Prevention Coalition (CPC), Aztlan Youth Program, Gospel Rescue Mission, Primavera, Kool Smiles Dental, Retirement Plan Advisors, C.A.S.T (Clean and Sober Theater), Sin Puertas PPP, EL Paso SW Greenway Bike Path, Kingian Non-Violence.

English and Spanish one page surveys for teens and a separate survey for adults were administered to National Night Out attendees on August 3, 2010 during the evening between 5 and 8 p.m. Dr. Romero, Veronica Moreno, and Denise Valencia asked adults and teens to complete a survey so that they may obtain a form that would enter them in a raffle to win one of many prizes (mostly family board games). Most individuals came to the front check-in table to complete the survey; however, survey administrators also walked around the event and asked individuals to complete the survey. All completed surveys were placed into a labeled box on the front check-in table. Individuals only completed one survey.

The following is a report prepared by Henry Gonzalez under the supervision of Dr. Andrea Romero. He entered the data, analyzed the findings, and prepared the following report.

Who Completed the Survey?
52 youth and **91** *adults* completed surveys at the 2010 STPC National Night Out (NNO). Approximately, **one-half** of the NNO attendees completed the survey.

52 **Youth (Total):** ***29*** **South Tucson Residents and** ***23*** **non-South Tucson Residents the following descriptions are only for the 29 South Tucson residents:**

- What age were the youth who participated?
  - All youth were between the ages of 8 and 19 years old.
- What school do they go to?
  - 18.5 % Tucson High School
  - 29.6 % Safford Middle School
  - 3.7 % Pueblo High School
  - 48.1 % Other (Omos, Roskruge, Pima Community College, Arizona Virtual Academy, DACR Academy, PASS Alternative, Ombudsman, Tortolita, Rincon, Catalina, Ochoa, PPEP Tec H.S., Utterback)
- What language did they complete the survey in?
  - 3 youth completed the survey in Spanish
  - 25 youth completed the survey in English

91 **Adults (Total):** ***43*** **south Tucson Residents and** ***48*** **Non-South Tucson Residents the following descriptions are only for the 43 South Tucson residents:**

- Who were the adults?
  - 66.7 % of the adults said that they were the parent or guardian of a teenager between the ages of 13 and 18 years old.
  - 13 adults completed the survey in Spanish
  - 30 adults completed the survey in English

Results for South Tucson Teens
Teens Perspective on Teen Alcohol Usage

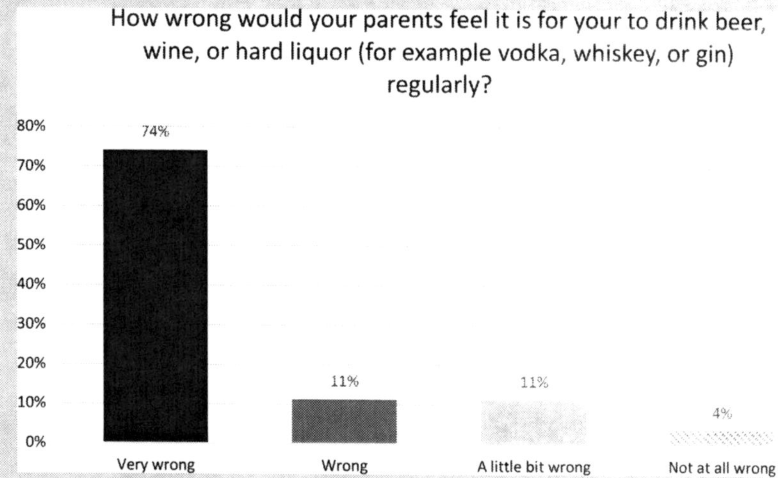

The majority of teens (74 %) felt that their parents would feel it was "Very Wrong" for them to drink regularly.

- 91.3 % of the youth who were NOT from the City of South Tucson reported that their parents would feel it was "**very wrong**" from them to drink regularly.
- National Reports indicate that most (*89.7 %*) adolescents reported that their parents would *strongly disapprove* of them having one or two drinks of an alcoholic beverage nearly every day, which was similar to the rates in 2007 (89.6 %) and 2002 (89.0 %).
- National reports indicate that *youth aged 12–17 who believed their parents would strongly disapprove of their using substances were less likely to use illicit substances* compared to youth who believed their parents would somewhat disapprove or neither approve nor disapprove. (http://oas.samhsa.gov/NSDUH/2k8NSDUH/2k8results.cfm#Ch6)

Results for South Tucson Adults
Adult Perspective on Teen Alcohol Usage

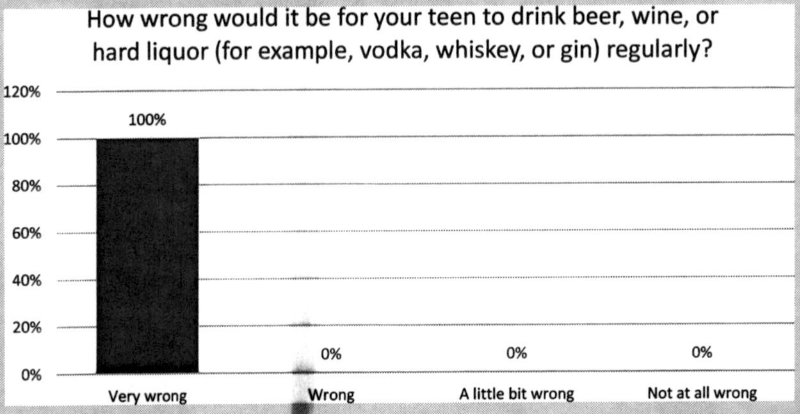

- When asked what they thought about their teenagers using alcohol regularly…
  - 100 % of adults said that it would be "very wrong" for their teenage to drink alcohol regularly.
  - 100 % of the adults NOT from the City of South Tucson felt it would be "very wrong" for their teens to drink regularly.

  Question: Why is there a discrepancy between what adults report and teens?
  How can we change this?
  How can parents get this message across to their teens?

Results for South Tucson Residents
Accessibility of Alcohol in the Community

- 39.3 % of teens feel that it is <u>very easy</u> to get alcohol in the city of South Tucson. On the other hand, *35.7 % said it was <u>not easy or that they did not know</u>*.
- 50.0 % of adults feel that it is <u>very easy</u> for someone under the age of 21 to get alcohol in the city of South Tucson.

Adults

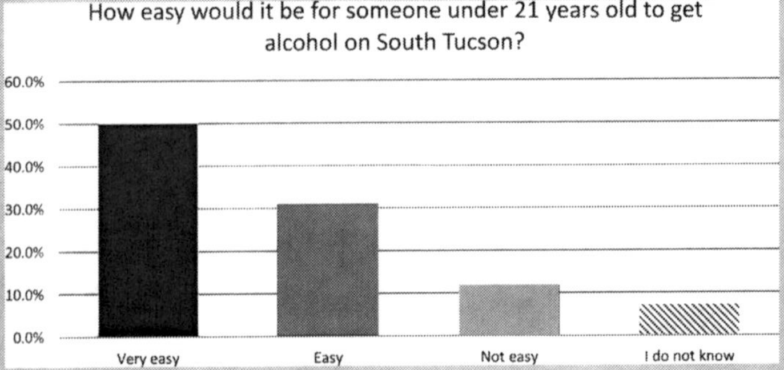

Teens

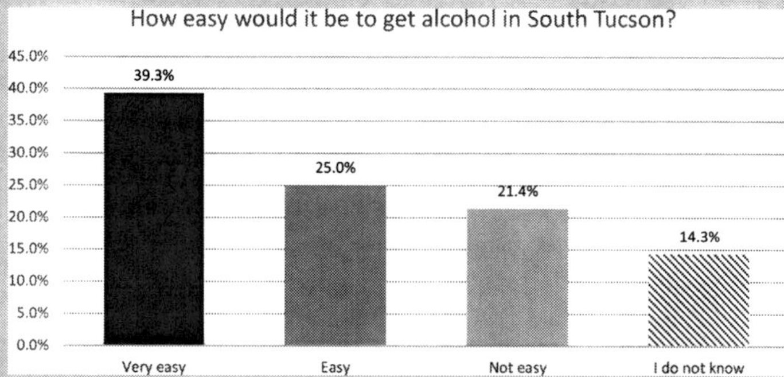

- 50 % of adults NOT from City of South Tucson felt it was "very easy"
- 26.1 % of youth NOT from City of South Tucson felt it was "very easy"; 56 % said they did not know or that it was "not easy"

Question: How can adults help make it less easy for teens to get alcohol?

Results for South Tucson Residents

Neighborhood Safety

Adults

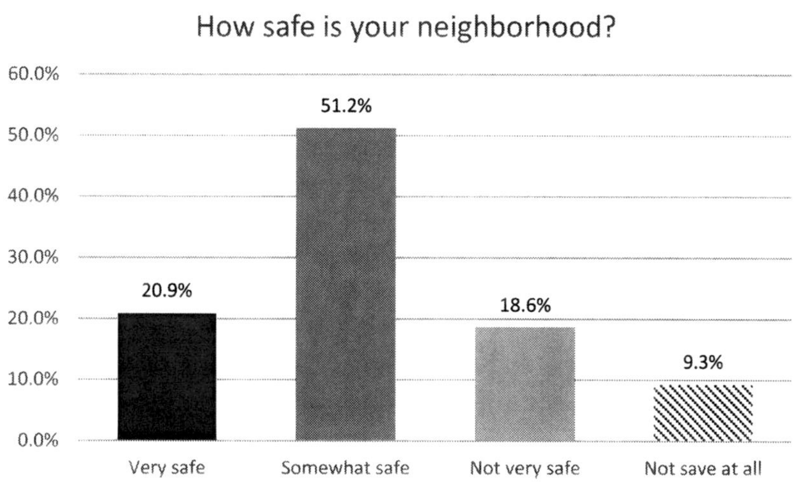

Teens

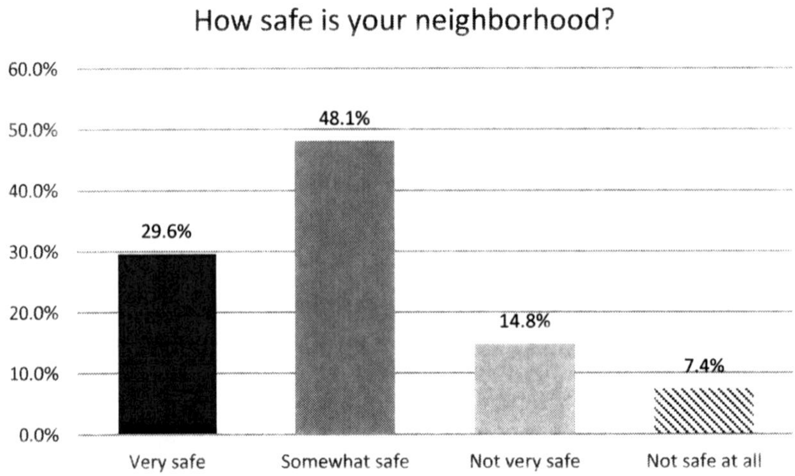

Results for South Tucson Residents

Can you make South Tucson a healthier and safer place?

Adults

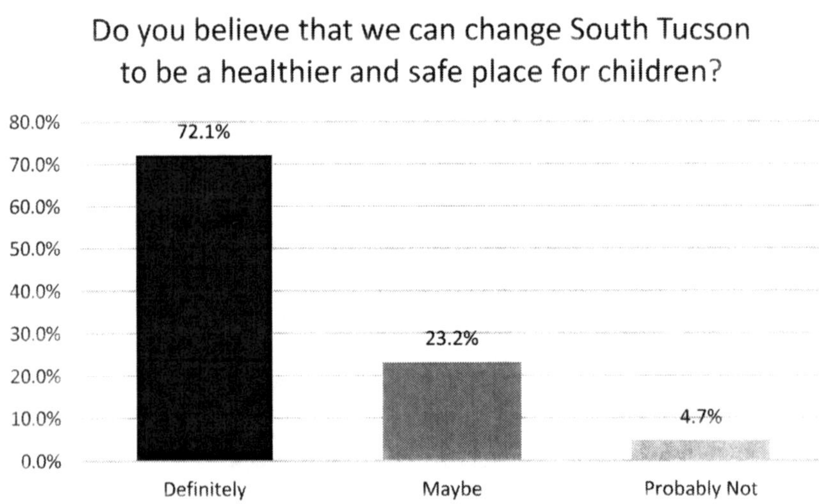

Teens

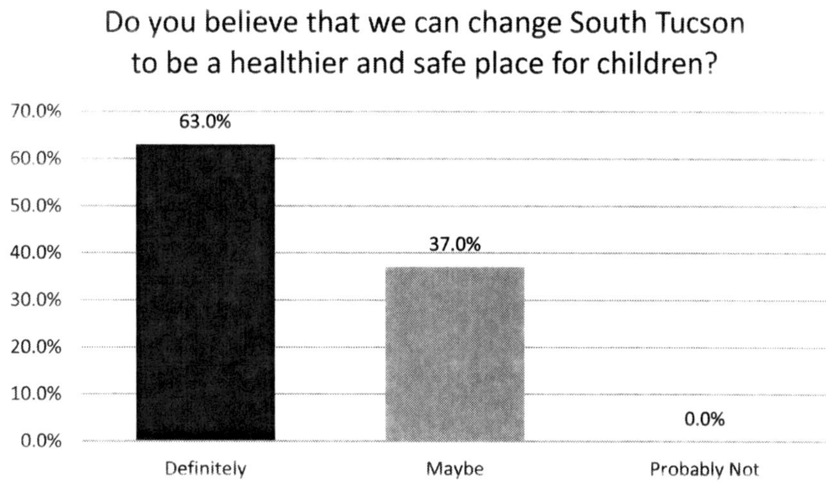

Results for South Tucson Residents

Are South Tucson children college bound?

Adults

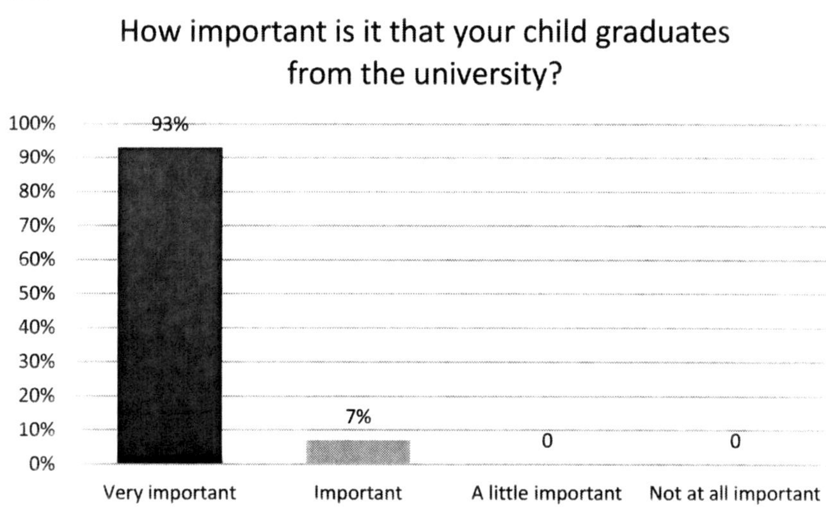

Teens

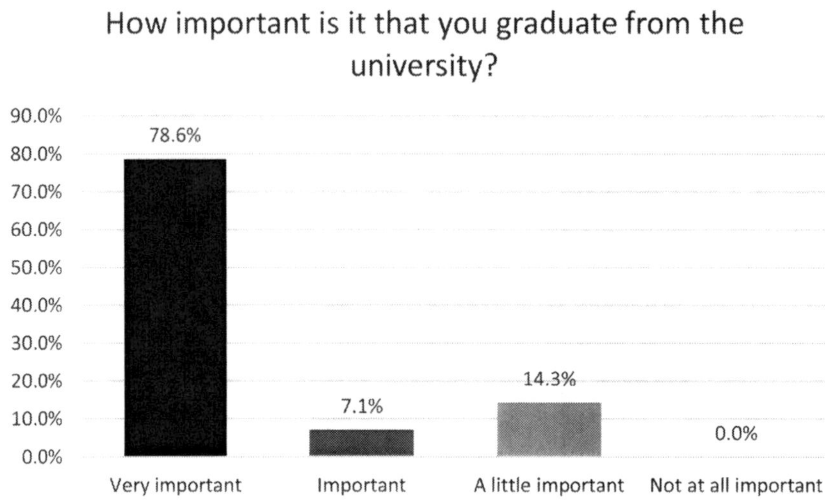

Results for South Tucson Residents

Education Norms

Adults

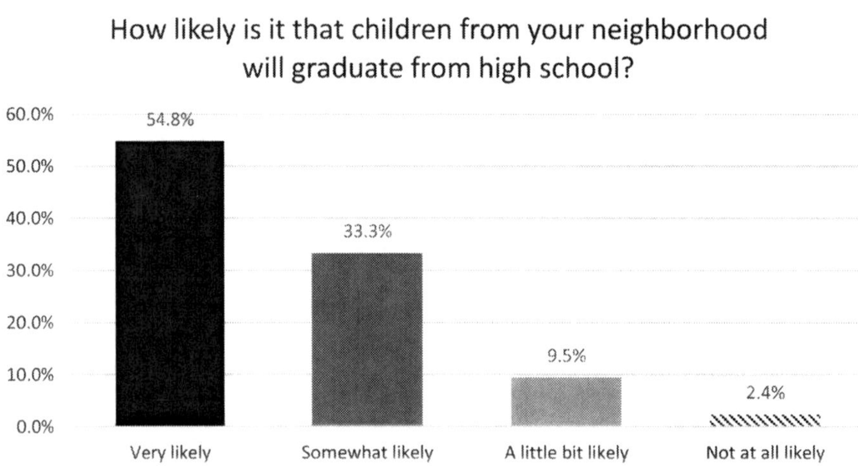

Teens

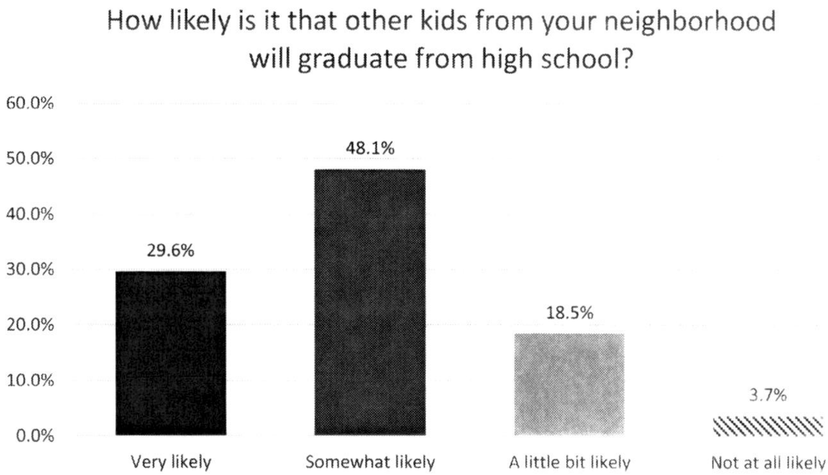

Results for South Tucson Residents

Arts and Cultural Events

Adults

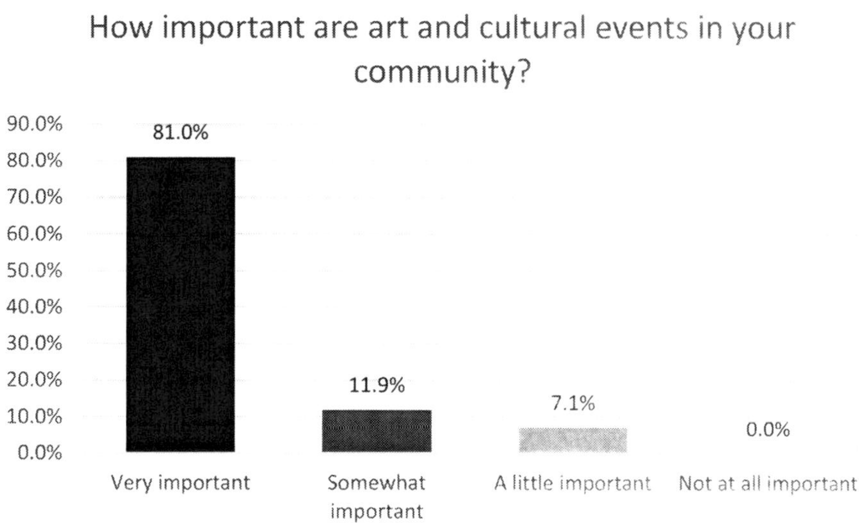

Teens

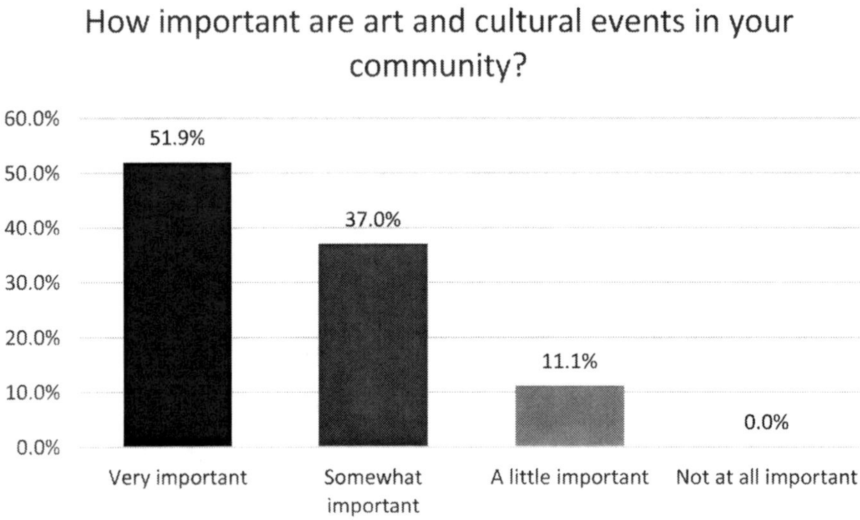

Results Comparing South Tucson Residents and Nonresidents

- Nonresidents were less likely to be parents of teens (65.2 %) and the majority (87.2 %) completed the survey in English.

The Effects of SB1070 on Family and Daily Life

- 45.2 % of Adults and 48 % of youth who live in the City of South Tucson reported that SB 1070 had already changed their daily life "A lot."
- Whereas, 31.9 % of adults and 30.4 % of youth who do NOT live in the City of South Tucson reported that SB 1070 has "not at all" changed their daily life.

Adults

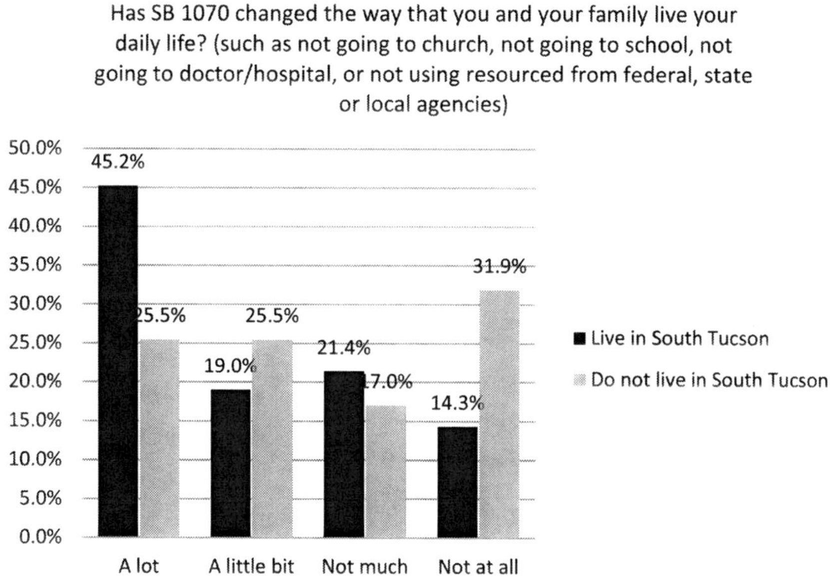

Teenagers

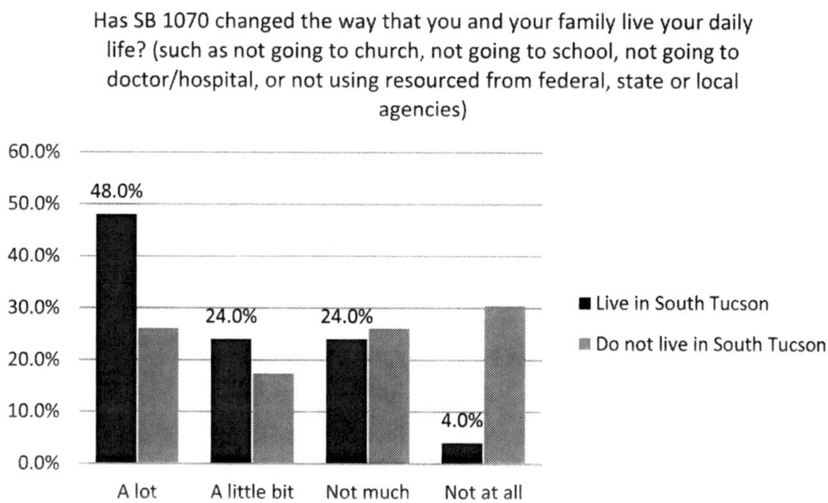

Request for More Information About SB 1070

- The majority (average 75 %) of adults and youth both in the City of South Tucson and outside the City reported that they would like to know more about SB 1070 and their rights.

Adults

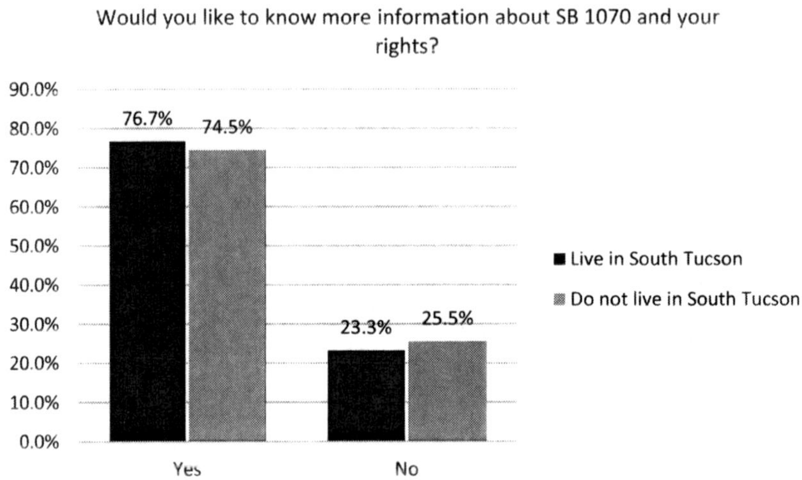

Teenagers

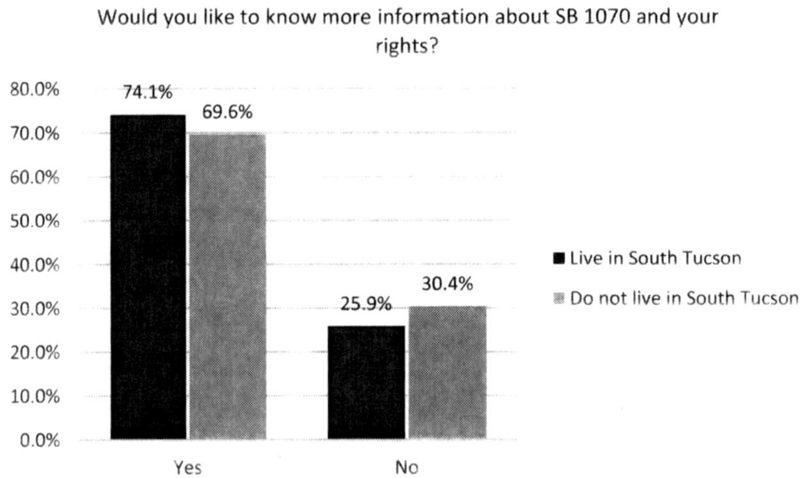

South Tucson Police, SB1070 and Fair Enforcement

- On average, adults and teens are confident that that City of South Tucson police will fairly enforce SB 1070.
- However, 17 % of teens who do NOT live in South Tucson felt "not at all confident" that South Tucson police would fairly enforce SB 1070.

Adults

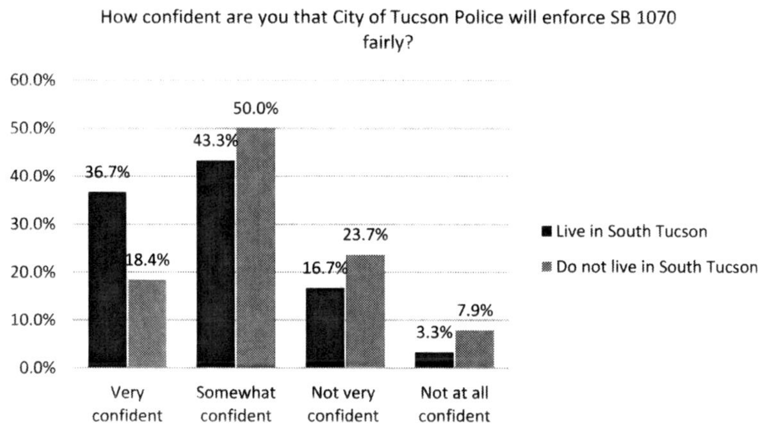

Teenagers

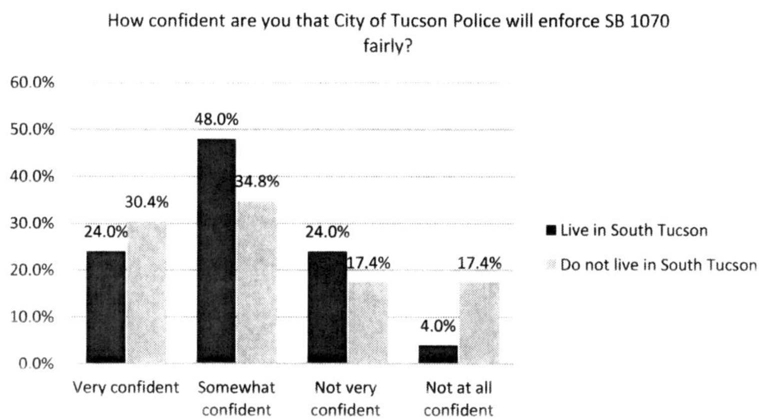

Discussion: How can Parents and the Community Get Involved?

THANK YOU
SOUTH TUCSON PREVENTION COALITION MEMBERS

References

Arizona Criminal Justice Commission. (2015). Arizona Youth Survey. http://www.azcjc.gov/ACJC.Web/sac/AYS.aspx

Bryndon-Miller, M., Greenwood, D., & Maguire, P. (2003). Why action research? *Action Research, 1*(1), 9–28.

Cousins, J. B., & Earl, L. M. (1992). The case for participatory evaluation. *Educational evaluation and policy analysis, 14*(4), 397–418.

Ferreria, M. P., & Gendron, F. (2011). Community-based participatory research with traditional and indigenous communities of the Americas: Historical context and future directions. *International Journal of Critical Pedagogy, 3*(3), 153–168.

Freire, P. (1968). *Pedagogy of the oppressed*. New York, NY: Seabury Press.

Godfrey, E. B., & Grayman, J. K. (2014). Teaching citizens: The role of open classroom climate in fostering critical consciousness among youth. *Journal of Youth and Adolescence, 43*, 1801–1817.

Grekul, J. (2011). Building collective efficacy and sustainability into a community collaborative: Community Solution to Gang Violence. *Journal of Gang Violence, 18*(2), 23–45.

Harper, G. W., & Salina, D. D. (2000). Building collaborative partnerships to improve community-based HIV prevention research: The university-CBO collaborative partnership (UCCP) model. *Journal of Prevention and Intervention in the Community, 19*(1), 1–20.

Israel, B., Eng, E., Schulz, A., & Parker, E. (2005). Introduction to methods in CBPR for health. In B. Israel, E. Eng, A. Schulz, & E. Parker (Eds.), *Methods in community-based participatory research for health* (pp. 3–26). San Francisco: Jossey-Boss.

Johnston, L. D., Miech, R. A., O'Malley, P. M., Bachman, J. G., & Schulenberg, J. E. (December 16, 2014). *Use of alcohol, cigarettes, and number of illicit drugs declines among U.S. teens*. Ann Arbor, MI: University of Michigan News Service. Retrieved 06/30/2015 from http://www.monitoringthefuture.org

McIntyre, A. (2008). *Participatory action research*. Thousand Oaks, CA: Sage Publications.

Minkler, M., & Wallerstein, N. (2008). Introduction to community-based participatory research. In M. Minkler & N. Wallerstein (Eds.), *Community-based participatory research for health: From process to outcomes* (pp. 5–19). San Francisco, CA: Jossey-Bass.

O'Fallon, L. R., & Dearry, A. (2002). Community-based participatory research as a tool to advance environmental health sciences. *Environmental Health Perspectives, 110*(2), 155–159.

Oetting, E. R., Jumper-Thurman, P., Plested, B., & Edwards, R. W. (2001). Community readiness and health services. *Substance Use and Misuse, 36*(6 &7), 825–843.
Plested, B. A., Edwards, R. W., & Jumper-Thurman, P. (2006). *Community readiness: A handbook for successful change*. Fort Collins, CO: Tri-Ethnic Center for Prevention Research.
Plested, B. A., Jumper Thurman, P., Edwards, R. W., & Oetting, E. R. (1998). Community readiness: A tool for effective community-based prevention. *The Prevention Researcher, 5*(2), 5–7.
Turnbull, A. P., Friesen, B. J., & Ramirez, C. (1998). Participatory action research as a model for conducting family research. *Research and Practice for Persons with Severe Disabilities, 23*(3), 178–188.

Chapter 10
Preventing New Liquor Licenses Through Youth–Community Participatory Action Research

Andrea Romero, Elisa Meza, Josefina Ahumada, Oscar Ceseña, Michele Orduña, Juan "Johnny" Quevedo, and Michal Urrea

Abstract This chapter examines how youth-led participatory action research to map the locations of liquor licenses in their city led to youth and adult collaboration to prevent new liquor licenses. Alcohol accessibility is a significant factor associated with adolescent alcohol use. Youth living in lower income neighborhoods often have higher than typical exposure to alcohol accessibility. In many ways, this chapter demonstrates how the South Tucson Prevention Coalition (STPC) worked together to create community transformational resilience because they were able to transform their environment in order to limit risk factors for adolescent alcohol use in a manner that would impact all youth in the city for many years. Their example demonstrates how a community can transform their environment to enhance opportunities for youth positive development and to limit exposure to risk factors.

A. Romero, Ph.D. (✉)
Family Studies and Human Development, The University of Arizona,
650 North Park Avenue, Tucson, AZ 85719, USA
e-mail: romeroa@u.arizona.edu

E. Meza, M.S.W.
San Francisco Unified School District, San Francisco, CA, USA
e-mail: mezae520@gmail.com

J. Ahumada, M.S.W.
School of Social Work, Arizona State University, Mesa, AZ, USA
e-mail: josefina.ahumada@asu.edu

O. Ceseña • J.J. Quevedo
Pima Community College, Tucson, AZ, USA
e-mail: cesenao@yahoo.com; Tucsonhigh12@yahoo.com

M. Orduña, M.Ed.
House of Neighborly Service, Tucson, AZ, USA
e-mail: miorduna@gmail.com

M. Urrea
John Valenzuela Youth Center, Tucson, AZ, USA
e-mail: cookie_michal@hotmail.com; michal.urrea@gmail.com

A.J. Romero (ed.), *Youth-Community Partnerships for Adolescent Alcohol Prevention*, DOI 10.1007/978-3-319-26030-3_10

Keywords Liquor licenses • Alcohol accessibility • Alcohol availability • Youth leadership • Alcohol mapping • Youth-led participatory action research

Youth are often left out of sociopolitical spheres and thus, they are also left out of decision-making about how to improve their communities (Flanagan, 2003). However, engaging youth in transforming systems of inequity in their community may lead to honest youth insight into how to generate community health assets while also limiting risky factors for students (Walsh, DePaul, & Park-Taylor, 2009). Giving students the tools to understanding the context of their health behaviors can build their own capacity within their communities and provide their families with their own positive developmental resources. In fact, minority youth can become more empowered when they understand how their community is shaped by racial inequities associated with education, health care, and a hostile receiving context for immigrants. Engaging youth in their own environments through meaningful roles is likely to expand their understanding of the influence of environment on their lives. Moreover, it is an innovative way to develop community transformational resilience, where youth can lead transformations in their community to increase more protective factors and reduce risky factors.

In this chapter, we will discuss a youth–community partnership for a participatory action research project to limit alcohol availability in one city. This collaborative study examines how to utilize research and collective action to create a healthier community with youth-promoting resources that also limits access and availability of risky health behaviors. We present here the experiences of the youth and adult allies who participated in a liquor license-mapping project that was used to connect Positive Youth Development (PYD) and asset-building community models for alcohol use prevention. As youth became advocates for social justice and health, they also became resourceful assets to their community as a whole. This chapter demonstrates how context can shape the life of minority adolescents, and also how agency and education can be leveraged to create change in those contexts that contribute to youth and community resiliency. However, it was all the work prior to this activity that led to increased community awareness of alcohol norms and alcohol availability. It was the increased capacity of the community members to work together effectively and the fact that community leaders were listening to youth. This activity was also critical to community acceptance and embracing of research because it was led by youth and community members in partnership with university students and researchers. In this chapter, we will tell the story of how participatory action research principles for collective research, collective action, and most importantly the humanizing of minority youth lead to the success of preventing new liquor licenses in one city, which also lead to changes in city policy to promote protective factors and limit risky factors.

10.1 Limiting Alcohol Availability as a Community Strategy

Specific environmental strategies often focus on alcohol regulations and alcohol availability through targeting enforcement of existing laws (e.g., minimum age purchase), server/seller training, reducing use of false identification. It was the process of youth-led participatory action research and coalition collective action that lead to consensus about a need in South Tucson to control alcohol outlet density because of the specific geographic boundaries and the higher than usual count of existing alcohol outlets. The coalition agreed that limiting new alcohol retail licenses would be a proactive and strategic method to further limit the growth of alcohol availability in their community.

Availability refers to the time, energy, and money that must be expended to obtain a commodity (e.g., alcohol, marijuana, and cigarette); in other words, the more resources required to obtain something, the lower the availability. The research on availability could not be clearer; when the availability of drugs, alcohol, and tobacco is limited, the use of alcohol, tobacco, and other drugs goes down (Burrow-Sanchez, 2006). STPC focused on availability of alcohol in the following few years with youth alcohol-mapping projects and sharing of data. This is the time during which the coalition engaged the most seriously in participatory action research. **Regulation** includes laws, rules, and policies that specify acceptable and unacceptable behaviors and that specify sanctions for violations. Regulations can specify who may use alcohol, tobacco, or other drugs (e.g., minimum age restrictions, sale of certain drugs by prescription only), where alcohol, tobacco, and other drugs may be used (e.g., designated smoking areas, restrictions on drinking in public places, workplace drug policies), who may sell alcohol, tobacco, and other drugs (e.g., licenses for alcohol and tobacco retailers, controlled substance numbers for doctors), and where, when, and how alcohol, tobacco, and other drugs may be sold (e.g., restrictions on sales of alcohol at community events or at gas stations, restriction on giveaways and discounts, restricted hours of sale, and ban on cigarette vending machines).

During the final few years, the coalition was prepared and ready to focus on issues of regulation and to work most directly with the local government. This was achieved after several years of raising awareness of adolescent alcohol issues, adolescent prevention programs to develop critical consciousness and leadership capacity, and coalition development work. The STPC chose to focus on limiting alcohol outlet density in the community by targeting new requests for liquor licenses; this was partially based on the results of their community-led surveys (see Chap. 9) but also based on the youth-led research for alcohol mapping.

An extremely important ecological factor when working with youth directly in the City of South Tucson is their contextual environment. A city that seems divided within the larger city of Tucson creates a border illustrated by obvious differences with sociogeographic markers (i.e., billboards prominently advertised in Spanish, more pedestrians, street vendors, etc.). Civic education in understanding these ecological differences as compared to their peers located on the north side of Tucson can become a developmental asset to their community by the ways youth view the potential of seeing their community grow. The City of South Tucson is a city within the greater city of Tucson where context dissimilarities are obvious and observable. Unequal resource allocation and provisions of support need to be considered as risk factors for youth alcohol outcomes (Dupree, Spencer, & Fegley, 2007). Yet, central to success of STPC is that youth were included as equal partners in the coalition to develop prevention strategies; this decision was based on previous research and theories such as the Community Readiness Model for Change and Participatory Action Research.

10.2 The Importance of Youth Leadership: Humanization of Youth of Color

Males (1996) argues that the USA is one of the most anti-youth societies, because there are few human rights extended to youth, yet there are a significant number of restrictions (e.g., curfews) and consequences (policing policies) specific to youth behavior. Even though youth in general have positive outcomes and many problematic issues are decreasing, such as substance use, school dropouts, and teen pregnancies (Males, 1996), they are still often portrayed in a negative and stereotyped light as if they are disaffected, uninvolved, and unsuccessful. Furthermore, views of ethnic minority youth are often even harsher than the views of youth in general, and they are portrayed as not fully human or deserving of rights or voice (Cammarota & Fine, 2008). For example, Latino youth are most often portrayed in society in a negative light. Stereotypes are negative generalized assumptions of an entire group; stereotypes of Latinos and Native Americans include assumptions that they are heavy drinkers, gang-affiliated, and with little education (Flores Niemann, 2001). These views of youth of color can be stigmatizing and can be even more pervasive for individuals who live in neighborhoods with high poverty.

Youth living in the City of South Tucson discuss being negatively stereotyped by those in the outside community; they describe being portrayed as being involved in gangs, crime, school dropouts, poor, and immigrants (see Chap. 7). These are just a few of the reasons why YPAR and CBPR are important methodological strategies to working with marginalized, yet resilient, communities, because it offers one way to rehumanize them within a group setting through offering respectful ways of interaction and the dignity of sharing their voice and their action as a group. Thus, working with youth in South Tucson had a clear mission to begin with respectful treatment of youth to provide settings with dignity and safety.

Central to Youth Participatory Action Research (YPAR) is that the youth are situated as constructors of their own reality, as researchers and as leaders (Torre & Fine, 2006). In fact, researchers across many studies have found that ethnic minority adolescents are eager to provide sharp critique of the system they see around them and to challenge the current strategies; however, the majority of this research has been focused on educational outcomes or civic engagement (Cammarota & Fine, 2008; Ginwright, Noguera, & Cammarota, 2006; Rodríguez & Brown, 2009). Furthermore, many of the published studies focus on the work with youth and youth allies, and do not discuss the outreach and work done to engage community leaders and other adults who may not be youth allies (Ginwright et al., 2006). While, many of these studies discuss the importance of civic engagement and development of youth as citizens, few have been able to link youth work with actual policy changes (Cahill, Rios-Moore, & Threatts, 2008; Ginwright, 2008). While YPAR is highly relevant and useful for educational settings, we also argue that this approach to youth organizing and policy making is applicable to health promotion and alcohol prevention even though there are few published YPAR projects specifically for substance use prevention (Allen, Mohatt, Beehler, & Rowe, 2014; Berg, Coman, & Schensul, 2009).

There are several key elements of Youth Participatory Action Research that have been described by Ginwright and Cammarota (2007) and Rodríguez and Brown (2009) that include (1) youth have human rights; (2) youth have agency to transform the status quo of their environment; (3) youth work needs to be inquiry based in a manner that considers youth experiences within their economic, political, and social contexts; (4) youth positive development is a ***collective response*** to current marginalization of all youth; and (5) equal youth participation is necessary for all stages of knowledge production. We follow these key principals in much of our work with youth. Each of these principles really focuses on how adults view youth, and each is a reminder about the humanity and autonomy of youth. These principles are emphasized because so often youth are dehumanized and infantilized because they are not adults yet and do not have adult individual rights (Ginwright & Cammarota, 2007). By considering the broader context of youth health and focusing on collective responses to create change, YPAR hones in on the means by which to create societal level changes to improve youth health.

10.2.1 Youth as Civic Leaders

Martín-Baró et al. (1994) argued that the action and reflection cycle that is inherent in the PAR process is essential to youth development as civic activists. Ginwright (2008) argues that a central goal of YPAR is to develop youth as active participants in the democratic process; however, this takes on a new and unique meaning when working with youth and families in South Tucson, given that many parents are immigrants and almost one-third of youth are immigrants (U.S. Census Burearu, 2010). This reality puts into question the use of the term citizen and the meaning of the democratic process as something much more complex than voting alone. Thus, our inclusive view of civic and sociopolitical engagement lays out multiple ways in which individuals of all backgrounds can still have voice and impact on the political structures within their communities (Watts & Flanagan, 2007). We rely on the definition of citizen put forth by Cahill and colleagues (2008), which states that citizenship is "being recognized as a decision maker and an agent of change." Yet, the focus should not only be on their future participation of youth in the voting process but also what they can do as adolescents by emphasizing the presence of their voice and their perspective in order to shape policies and legislation, particularly those with direct relevance for their lives.

Effective engagement with civic activities has been linked to positive youth development, via self-esteem and political self-efficacy (Morgan & Streb, 2001). However, it is not only community service that matters, it is the community service component when linked with critical consciousness that can truly lead to collection action and activism to change the existing community structure (Sherrod, 2007). In sum, there is evidence that youth who are involved in community issues are more likely to report feelings of social responsibility, social connectedness to their community, higher self-esteem, and a better understanding of social issues (Ginwright et al., 2006; Yates & Youniss, 1996). A key component of individual empowerment has been defined as sociopolitical control which includes self-efficacy, motivation, competence, and perceived control within a sociopolitical sphere. This specifically includes aspects of leadership competence and policy control (Peterson, Peterson, Agre, Christens, & Morton, 2011; Zimmerman & Zahniser, 1991). Christens and Peterson (2012) demonstrate the critical role of perceived sociopolitical control as a mediating variable between ecological supports and positive development. Peterson et al. (2011) found that youth with more perceived sociopolitical control were also more likely to be engaged in their communities and less likely to report alcohol use.

A fundamental aspect of STPC's success with youth was that there were continuous opportunities for youth to participate in after-school prevention programs (Omeyocan YES and VOZ), and the programs were always based on cultural assets with a critical pedagogy to understand health within a larger societal context. Watts and Flanagan (2007) suggest that youth first develop a critical worldview of their environment, and then youth are significantly more likely to be involved in sociopolitical behaviors, that include civic voice, activism, organizing, as well as voting. As such, sociopolitical development is critical to linking youth of color with the civic processes of their community as an essential part of their healthy development into adulthood. Opportunities for this type of sociopolitical development and civic engagement in general may be particularly important for immigrant adolescents or adolescents with immigrant parents who may find unique challenges to access socialization into the US civic processes. Schools are often traditional sources of democratic socialization; yet researchers found that there are few opportunities for open climates in the public schools that allow for discussion of controversial political issues, including immigration (Godfrey & Grayman, 2014). It is also crucial to note that civic education classes in public schools seems to have become less of a national priority due to the health of the nation as a whole (Torney-Purta, Barber, & Wilkenfeld, 2007). These are reasons why low income and immigrant communities may need to offer additional opportunities for open discussion with adults and inclusion of adolescents into adult civic activities. In fact, adolescent's immigrant context and ethnic minority status are likely to inform their contributions to their community in a manner that is based on their own experiences of inequity and social justice (Sanchez-Jankowski, 2002).

10.2.2 Youth and Adult Community Partnerships

In order for youth to effectively be engaged in civic activities, there is an intergenerational component that must be integrated, and this may mean moving outside the sphere of working with adult allies. The presence of opportunity structures to teach youth and to support opportunities for action is essential to the process of youth sociopolitical development (Watts & Flanagan, 2007; Watts & Guessous, 2006). Youth cannot move alone; they are more likely to have success if they can work in partnership with adults (Ginwright & Cammarota, 2007). Moreover, in order to ensure the continued democratic participation of any community, it is important to consider how youth are being socialized to participate in the democratic process, not only through voting but also through volunteering, using their voice and gaining knowledge about the political process (Ginwright & Cammarota, 2007; Watts & Flanagan, 2007).

Some empirical studies have demonstrated that opportunities for youth experiences and for social interaction rooted in civic changes are the strongest predictors of youth agency and political awareness (Yates & Youniss, 1996). Yet, at times when sociopolitical contexts are changing rapidly, some adults choose to further exclude youth; however, some argue that this is exactly the critical time to increase participation of youth in their community civic activities (Christens & Peterson, 2012; Ginwright & James, 2002). Youth involvement is likely to increase the inclusivity and diversity of democracies. Moreover, some argue that conscious exclusion of youth in civic process is a form of age discrimination or age segregation (Christens & Peterson, 2012). Often because of stigma against youth, and especially youth of color, they are most often excluded from decision making about services aimed at teens (Watts & Guessous, 2006). However, several scholars also remind us that the most effective blends within programs find a way to balance youth-led opportunities with adult-guided structure and support (Flanagan, 2003). Zeldin, Christens, and Powers (2013) argue that the most effective programs have the following definitive elements: meaningfulness, authenticity, opportunity to impact others, collaborative action, and partnerships with adults. Towards the middle and through the end of the STPC project, it was clear that all of these elements were in place and functioning together. It was these factors that contributed to the success of youth-led research and then collective action of youth and community partners to affect decisions about liquor licenses.

The Y2Y attended retreats out of state, in California, for the International Youth-to-Youth Conference. At those retreats, the youth were able to connect with others throughout the nation, expanding their networks and building a wider analysis of the sorts of issues other youth face in their communities. This made the alcohol availability issues within the City of South Tucson seem like reoccurring themes throughout the nation, which reminded the youth that they were a part of something a lot larger than what they initially realized. Juan "Johnny" Quevedo, Y2Y leader, comments about the importance of the international conferences to build the youth leadership skills and confidence.

> Attending the annual Y2Y international conference, we gained information from other people, our peers. The discussions that we would have were much more different. (Other youth groups) would describe their "battles" against drugs and alcohol, and we were there to give advice. Everyone else had issues, like offering drinks and drugs, and I would say much more than they would ever imagine, like, talking about us doing the liquor count, their community wasn't as involved as we were (even though we were a small city).

The conferences also provide new opportunities for South Tucson youth to be leaders at a national level, and both Oscar and Juan became leaders at the national conference. As minority youth on a national stage, they also found ways to embrace and share their experiences about their ethnicity and language. While, it was one thing to talk about cultural and language assets in the bicultural community of South Tucson. It was also transformative for Juan to share his personal story about immigration and learning English on that national stage. He describes it as:

> The best time was at the annual conference in California. We were so excited to let others know about what we did. I was a speaker. I talk about my life story at the conference. There were 700–800 people. I was asked to speak because my life story was fascinating to others, coming to a new country, not knowing the language, feeling lost, stupid, I felt really really behind. The center and the fun things that I would do, to help elementary school age children—it helped mold me into something great. The fact that they invited me to speak, I talked about where I was from, and how confusing my life was, being a teenager, being Mexican, being gay, and coming out to my adopted family—and being Arizona. It was a lot, but I managed to do a lot more.

10.2.3 Alcohol Retailer-Mapping Proximity to Youth

The Alcohol Retailer-Mapping Proximity to Youth (ARMPY) project was funded by the Arizona Governor's Office for Children, Youth, and Families. Given the previous success of the youth-led prevention public service announcements (described in Chap. 9), a very similar method of implementation was used again, with youth leaders who were chosen to carry out the alcohol retail mapping. They were recruited from the Y2Y and the South Tucson Explorers group. Adult allies also worked with youth, including Jessica Alderete (JVYC Youth Specialist), Dr. Andrea Romero, City of South Tucson Planners, and Michele Orduña (STPC Coordinator). Youth engaged in several hours of group participation in planning and organizing.

Their goal was to collect data about liquor license density and proximity to youth activities. They did this through collecting data in order to map the locations of the liquor licenses in the City of South Tucson. They also specifically identified whether the liquor licenses were on-sale (e.g., consumed on the site where they were sold, such as in a restaurant) or off-sale (e.g., consumed off the location where they were sold, such as in a grocery store or market) and the youth attractions (locations where children and youth gather, such as schools or youth centers). Juan "Johnny" Quevedo, Y2Y youth leader, describes some of what the youth found as part of the process, "*There were so many good things, library, fire station, convenience stores, Walgreens, restaurants, local stores, famous restaurants, I was surprised that there were a lot of places to visit, store, museum, one pet clinic (we didn't know about), barber shops, things you always pass by and you miss. I liked the fact that we, the teenagers, got that done, with the help of STPC. It is appreciated much more when it is hands on and not just listening to an adult talk to us. We learned that we had several businesses in the city that are beneficial to the community. We also learned how to work with one another.*"

In the City of South Tucson, youth found 22 liquor license businesses, 15 of which were on-sale retailers and 7 were off-sale (see Fig. 10.1). They also found that there were 52 youth attractions within .25 mile radius of the liquor retailers. Youth attractions were defined as any place that youth can go under the age of 21, such as schools, day cares, parks, churches, community centers, auto shops, restaurants, and grocery stores. Youth also took pictures that demonstrated the proximity of liquor sales to locations where children and youth spent a lot of time (see Fig. 10.2).

10.2.4 Youth-Identified Benefits of ARMPY

Youth participants identified the benefits they experienced as a result of the ARMPY, which include (1) Leadership, (2) Knowledge, (3) Teamwork, and (4) Responsibility. The aspects of leadership were for both youth and adults. While youth learned leadership skills, they also contributed leadership to the coalition by helping to make the community better. Youth learned leadership through the mapping project because they saw how they were making the community better through putting their best foot forward. By their work doing research to gather knowledge and to share their findings, they helped lead to future innovative ideas for prevention strategies in the community.

Even though all the youth were from South Tucson, they also felt that they gained knowledge through their participation because it helped them to understand how many liquor retailers were in the community. They acknowledged that their research on the liquor retailers helped them distinguish between important nuances, such as on-sale and off-sale vendors. This distinction was important to understand how drinking in restaurants and bars differed from buying alcohol and taking it home. Yet, this distinction also shed light on the neighborhood phenomenon of individuals who bought alcohol and drank in the streets. These individuals were often passed out or drunk in the streets or near the location selling alcohol. It also increased youth and adult awareness about how easily alcohol was available in all the local grocery stores and convenience stores. Youth noted how near alcohol was placed to healthy

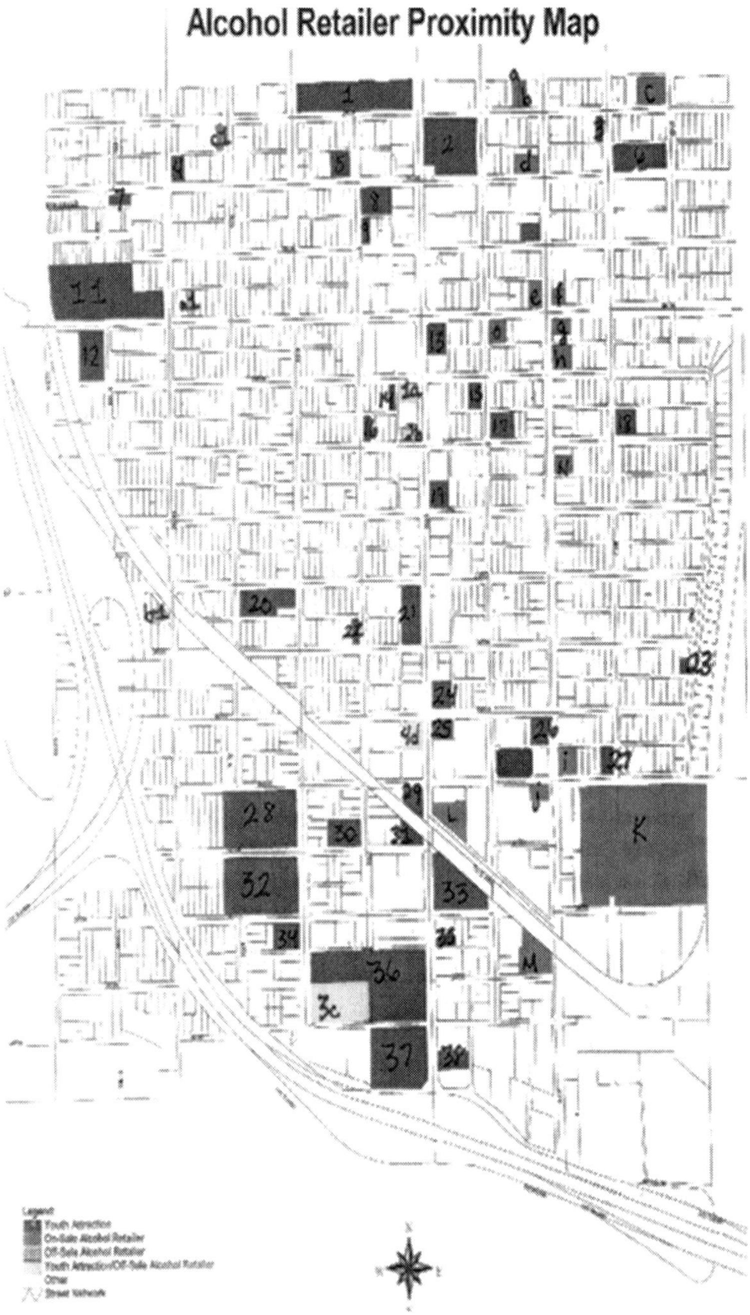

Fig. 10.1 Alcohol retailer proximity map, youth attractions are numbered and that on-sale alcohol retailers are lettered. Off-sale alcohol retailers have numbers and letters

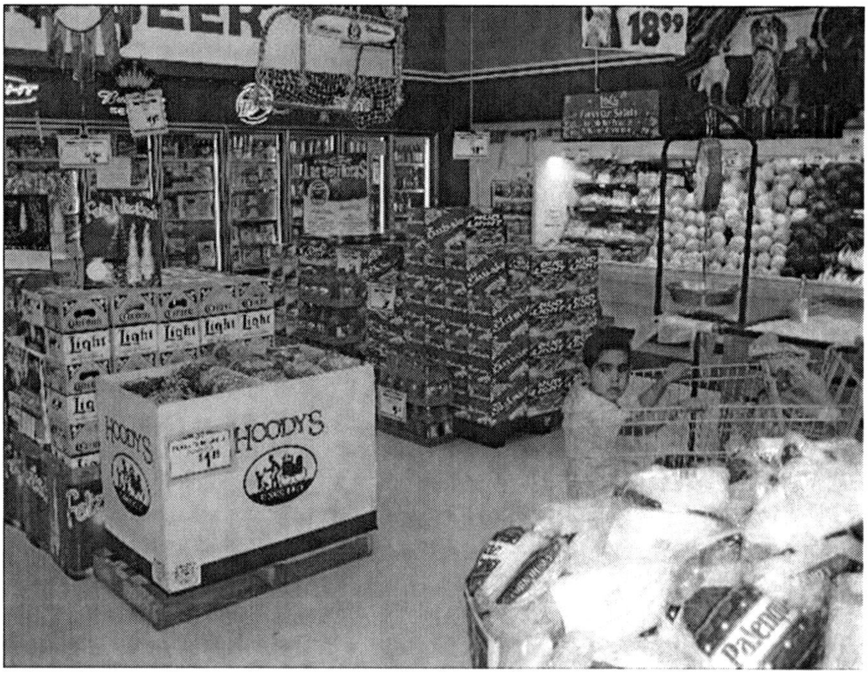

Fig. 10.2 Youth pictures of alcohol retail proximity to youth. These pictures depict the proximity of beer sales to healthy food and areas where children are present

foods, such as fruits and vegetables. They stated "*There are too many liquor places close to youth attractions and it's affecting our youth because it seems so easy for them to acquire liquor.*" This comment gets to the heart of the community alcohol norms on availability. The tangible visual results of this project helped youth to share their knowledge and to make a strong rationale to limit the number of liquor licenses (see Fig. 10.1 for map).

Through this process, youth also identified teamwork as a benefit. They learned to work together through the process, as they gathered information. The project was too big for only one or two people. As a result, the teens learned to rely on each other to gather information in different sectors of the community. The resulting map pulled together all their efforts into one cohesive tangible result. They also felt that sharing the results with STPC and other adults through town halls helped them understand that prevention was a community level issue. They realized that to create change in the community, it would require more teamwork beyond just youth members. Lastly, they felt that one of the benefits was responsibility. The youth reported feeling that they learned responsibility because they were accountable to adults and other youth to be on time and having to report their findings to the team after data collection activities. They felt that this was a positive benefit of the activities.

10.2.5 Youth-Identified Community Benefits of ARMPY

Youth participants also identified community benefits that they felt resulted from the ARMPY, which include (1) raising awareness and (2) ideas for future projects. To begin with, the youth felt that awareness about on-sale versus off-sale liquor licenses was important for the community to be aware of. Additionally, they felt that the awareness about the proximity of alcohol selling to location where youth spent a significant amount of time was important for adults to be aware of. Often adults overlook youth activities and locations that youth frequent because it is not very conscious; it can be almost invisible to adult perception. One of the results of the map was to demonstrate to adults exactly where youth spent time in the city. This helped raise adult's awareness about youth activities. Yet, the map also raised awareness about how close in proximity adult activities, such as drinking, were in relation to youth activities. It also raised awareness about how adult activities could impact youth and children who witnessed their actions in the community. Another key benefit for the community was to increase ideas for future prevention strategies, both youth-led and adult-led. The youth were very inspired and motivated by their findings, and it led them to come up with more ideas about youth-led projects that could identify environmental factors to reduce underage drinking.

The information from the ARMPY project was presented by youth and adult allies during the Fiesta de La Comunidad on April 26th, during a STPC town hall on May 13th, and to the Mayor and City Council in the same month. Youth proposed that the solution to the issue of too much liquor sales in near proximity to youth attractions was to reduce alcohol advertising outside of buildings in off-sale locations, like local markets (see Fig. 10.2). Not long after these presentations, the City Council chose to pass an ordinance to stop advertising alcohol outside of off-sale locations.

The second solution proposed by youth was to reduce liquor licenses or prevent new ones. This proposed solution was reached after much reflection on the data collected by youth. Youth at the JVYC were committed to bringing attention to the variations within the City of South Tucson by participating in community-mapping projects to highlight the excess presence of alcohol consumption throughout their community. Youth became critically conscious of the negative impact of so many liquor licenses within one city. However, initiating this solution to prevent new liquor licenses was still a process, and it required collaboration of youth and adults. The first opportunity that presented itself was in the middle of the national economic recession in 2010; Walgreens, a large corporate pharmacy and market, entered 135 applications to sell alcohol across Arizona. Michele Orduña, STPC Project Coordinator, recalls first being contacted by Gloria Hamelitz-Lopez, JVYC Executive Director, to ask if STPC would support a youth protest against Walgreens's liquor license application in South Tucson.

> Gloria called me, in the 3rd year of the grant, and said 'Michele, have you read the paper? There is all this stuff about how all Walgreens in the state want to apply for liquor licenses.' At first, I said 'I don't understand what this has to do with us at all.' She said 'The teens

> want to protest the liquor license.' I remember thinking 'They want to do what? Gloria, I don't even know what that entails, I don't even know what that means?, but if they want to . . She (Gloria) was asking 'they (youth) want to know if the coalition will help them' I replied 'sure, I don't know what that means, but yes, why not.' With that, at the next meeting we brought it up and the coalition as a whole wanted to do it, and we then embarked on a 9-month journey about protesting this liquor license. It is a lengthy process to begin with, once you apply for a liquor license, you need community input, a community recommendation, it goes up to the board, then a two-week waiting process. So we agreed to stand beside the youth as they made this protest, and this argument against this liquor license.

As part of this youth-led and adult-guided model, there were several meetings with youth and adults to critically think through how to protest the liquor license application. One of the most critical decisions that they made together was how to craft the campaign message. The youth and adults agreed that making a social argument, such as to deny the liquor license because of underage drinking, overconsumption, theft, nuisance, or stealing, would fall flat because the decision is primarily a business decision, rooted in the quality of the business, and how it would add to local and state economy. So, they reached consensus that the campaign message would be "We don't want one more liquor license in South Tucson." This message was derived from their previous alcohol-mapping research, from which they knew that Circle K already had a liquor license and was only 88 feet away from Walgreens. Moreover, they felt that they could argue that South Tucson was oversaturated with liquor licenses, and there was no need for an additional one. Michele describes some of the reasons why this campaign message was important and effective:

> We just don't want another one (liquor license), it is close to schools, it is in our community, it is on a major intersection, it is right in the center of South Tucson. It was made clear early on, and this was important to everyone in the fight against the liquor license, that we don't have an issue with Walgreens, because everybody loved the Walgreens, you can find everything there, and it was the only pharmacy in South Tucson. We just didn't want to do it as a whole blanket that Walgreens was bad because they wanted the liquor license, or that they were no good now, it was 'We just don't want the liquor license, we don't want one more.'

Youth collected over 600 signatures on a petition to protest the liquor license in a city with approximately 1500 people. Michele describes the next steps of a public march and rally to protest the liquor license in front of Walgreens (see Fig. 10.3) "*Youth went on public sidewalks in front of Walgreens one day and held signs and protested that they didn't want a liquor license, and it was a cold and windy day that day. They did press releases that day and they got some media coverage. We started a petition and asked everybody to sign that petition.*"

Youth also attended the City Council sessions, along with over 100 other locals who filled up the room. There was extensive discussion, and a second City Council meeting had to be scheduled to continue the discussion. During the call to the audience, many people including youth stated that they were against the approval of this liquor license. Youth presented the petition signatures to the City Council; there were another 200 signatures collected by a former city council member. Michele states "*Mayor and council were very open, they were, I think, a little taken by surprise at the presentation the youth gave, how much thought, effort, and energy went*

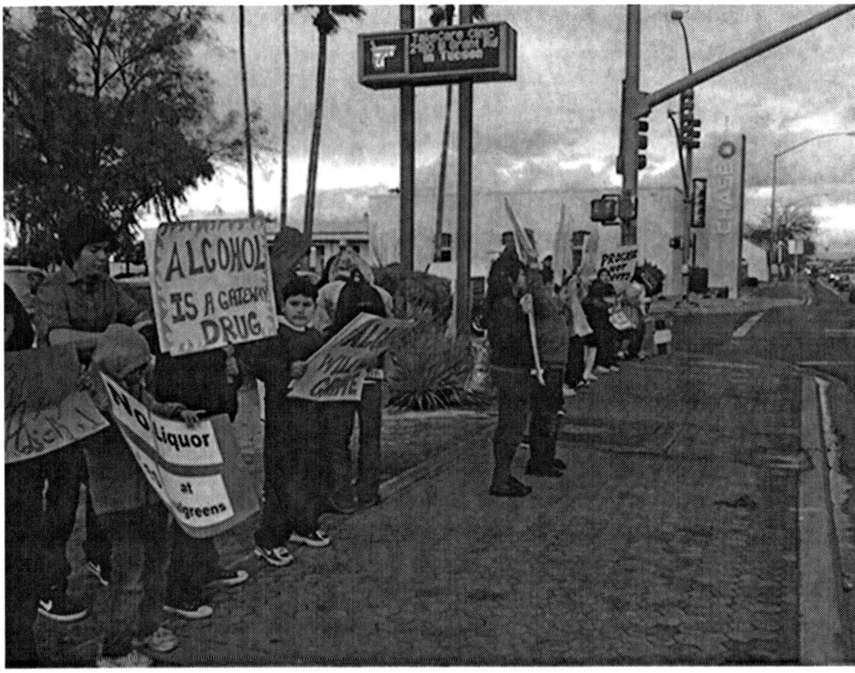

Fig. 10.3 Youth protest against the liquor license

into it, and how much they were willing to go up in front of mayor and council and speak and tell that story. Mayor and council validated their argument and offered to not recommend to the liquor board." That was all that the City needed to do, was to not recommend the application for the liquor license; however, this denial only moved the final decision to the state liquor license board.

Michele describes the next stage of the process that moved to the state liquor license board meeting in Phoenix, the state capitol. The state liquor license board meets monthly and is comprised of a 7-member bi-partisan committee that has set term limits. The board often strongly represents the business community at the state level.

> Once (the license application) gets to the board review, there are not many people come to provide an argument, you are allowed to send up all this information and all these arguments on paper. The reason that I say this is that the room is small where the committee meets. It is usually, maybe two people from the neighborhood associations, never a group of people. When we went, we decided, well, this is a community-based effort, we are going to take teens, we are going to take fire, police, JVYC staff, UA staff, so it was going to be a cross-section of people who live there and some that don't work there too. It was a weekday and we had to caravan up to Phoenix, they had a schedule, but we didn't know there was a lot of waiting, there were a lot of other applications being reviewed that day. So, we go, and it is real intense, you can cut the tension with a knife, and there is almost no one in the room.

Youth mobilized so that they and other STPC members could attend the state board meeting; this was in the state capital (1½ h away) on a school day. This required quite a bit of organizing, obtaining permission to leave school, and obtaining transportation.

The representation from the City of South Tucson was strong at the state board meeting, with representation from at least nine youth and many adults including the City Manager, City attorney, a representative from the City police, STPC director (Michele Orduña), John Valenzuela Youth Center Director (Gloria Hamelitz), and Dr. Romero (see Figs. 10.4 and 10.5). So, in this very formal business-like and government setting, there sat the liquor license board and about 15–20 townspeople from the City of South Tucson. Michele describes what happens next.

> We are excited, we are ready, we are prepared. We waited hours. The room is really quiet, and you are not supposed to react to thing. They figured out we are not going anywhere, we are from Tucson, so we are not going anywhere. So they make some changes to the agenda. They were not used to that many people coming up to protest a license, and we find out that not everyone can speak, only 4–5 people can speak. We had to figure that out quickly. The

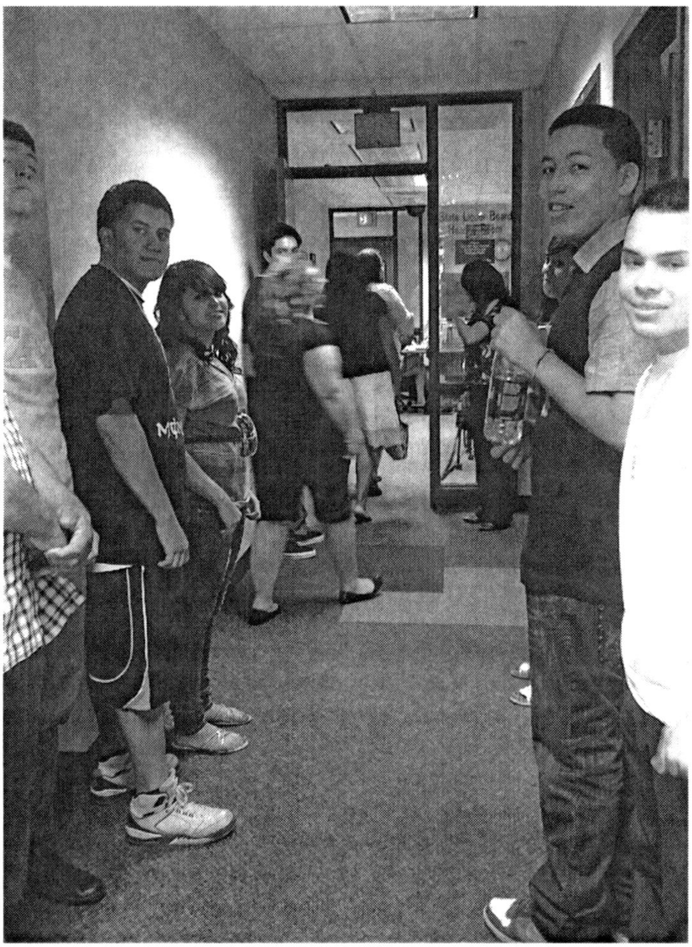

Fig. 10.4 Preparing to go into the state liquor license board meeting in Arizona State Capital, Phoenix

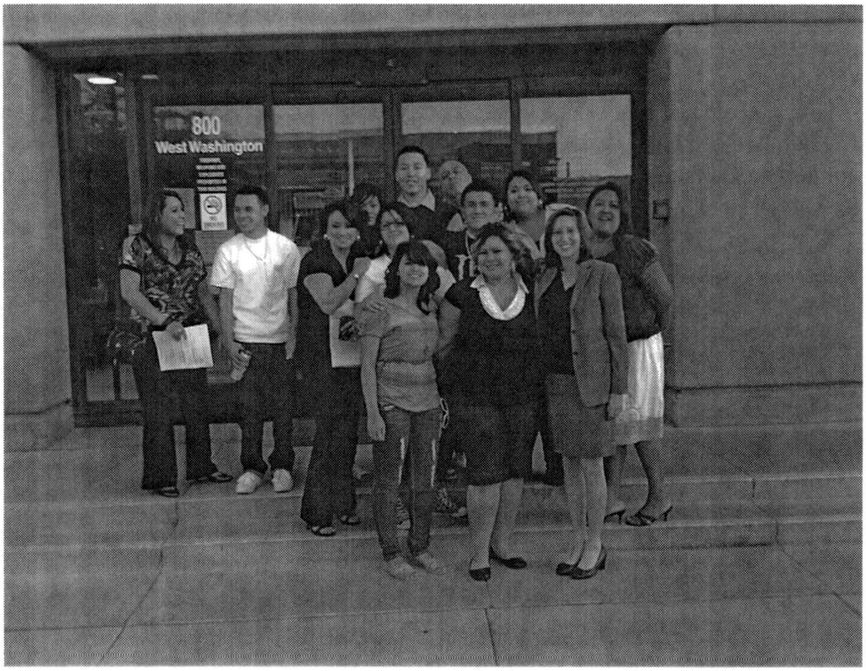

Fig. 10.5 Celebrating after the state liquor license board decision to deny the liquor license

> city manager and the city attorney went—because you have to be represented through the city attorney, because you have to be represented by the local government, which is the City of South Tucson. If we didn't have him (the city attorney) there we wouldn't have been allowed to speak. So we decided who was going (to speak) and in what order. It was one of the most intimidating things I've ever done in my life, kind of like this whole journey was. You didn't know how finite these rules are or these regulations or this policy or how things are conducted, so it is kind of scary the first time. So, we give our argument. A couple teenagers testified, the police chief (or staff), I testified, and Dr. Romero. The argument was the same—'We don't want another one (liquor license)'.

All city reps, Ms. Orduña, Ms. Hamelitz-Lopez, two youth, and Dr. Romero provided sworn testimony and responded to questions from the Walgreens representative lawyer during this session. Afterwards, there was at least 20–30 min of discussion by the board. Michele describes some of the public discussion by the board members.

> A board member said, this is a really tough decision, and it shouldn't be, because Walgreens is an upstanding reputable business. I've never known any Walgreens to have any issue with a liquor license, they've never been on probation, they've never been pulled, they are a good company. This is a business decision, because this is sales to the state. Why would we deny money coming into the state, and why would the city deny that because that trickles down? But then I am looking at the people who are here and make this argument, and it is a different argument then we usually get. So they couldn't easily justify one more liquor license. Other board members felt challenged about what decision to make. In that moment, you are like, I don't know if it is going to work or not, and there is no recourse. **They came back and officially denied the liquor license. We stood our ground.**

In the end, the board voted unanimously to deny the liquor license to Walgreens in the City of South Tucson location; in fact, it was only 1 of 2 applications denied to Walgreens in Arizona that year. There was an op-ed written by the STPC Project Director, Michele Orduña, published in the main local newspaper that describes the prevention of the liquor license (see Fig. 10.6).

June 11, 2010 12:00 am • Michele Orduña Special To The Arizona Daily Star

0

This spring the Walgreens in the city of South Tucson was one of 30 Walgreens stores applying for new liquor licenses.

South Tucson officials, teens, parents and children became concerned when the South Tucson Walgreens, at 1900 S. Sixth Ave., was identified among the others, because of the efforts of South Tucson's mayor, council and administrators to reduce liquor licenses in our community.

Just a few decades ago we had over 40 liquor licenses in our 1.2-square-mile city at bars and liquor stores. Today, there are about half that number of licensed alcohol vendors, and most of those are restaurants.

Teens from the South Tucson John Valenzuela Youth Center (JVYC) were among the first to protest the new liquor license. JVYC's mission is to continue the vision of South Tucson police Officer John A. Valenzuela by promoting the positive development of youth with recreational and educational programs that espouse healthy living.

JVYC leaders had often shared their concerns about underage drinking and its connection to the many liquor outlets in our tiny city. In 2006, they participated in an alcohol-mapping grant funded by the Arizona Governor's Office of Children, Youth and Families. The youth walked and charted the proximity of youth attractions to liquor outlets.

That mapping exercise inspired JVYC to make the community healthier and more drug-free.

Fig. 10.6 South Tucson pulls out all the stops to prevent a new local liquor license

In May, Walgreens went before the Arizona State Liquor Board to make its case for another liquor license in South Tucson to sell beer and wine.

Back in March, the city of South Tucson's mayor and council held two public hearings to get input from community members before making their official licensing recommendations to the liquor board. JVYC youth helped organize a public protest in front of the South Tucson Walgreens store, with children and teens holding posters stating, "No more liquor licenses."

Next, the teens collected over 600 signatures to enter as official opposition at the City Council meeting. Ildefonso Green, a resident and former city of South Tucson council member, collected another 200 petition signatures.

Based on those efforts, Mayor Jennifer Eckstrom and the council voted unanimously for a "disapproval" recommendation against the South Tucson Walgreens.

During the Arizona Liquor Board hearing in Phoenix on May 6 sworn testimony was given from the South Tucson city attorney, the city manager, the deputy police chief, two local teens, a University of Arizona professor, and the director of the John Valenzuela Youth Center. Based on the testimony of those community members, the board denied the South Tucson Walgreens liquor application.

One member of the liquor board later said that he had never seen "as many community members attend a license board hearing." South Tucson residents, youth and organizations like the Pima County Community Prevention Coalition, went to Phoenix to fight the South Tucson Walgreens liquor license application.

Fig 10.6 (continued)

It was a huge victory for a tiny city, inspired by the leadership of our JVYC youth. It could have gone differently; after all, the great majority of businesses that request them are granted liquor licenses.

But that day we had decided that there would not be even one more liquor license in South Tucson.

That effort by our teens and other community members was a wonderful reaffirmation of how diligent, civic duty by youth and adults has its rewards.

Michele Orduña is director of the South Tucson Prevention Coalition. E-mail her at MiOrduña@gmail.com.

Fig 10.6 (continued)

10.3 Youth Reflections on the Liquor License Prevention Success

Oscar discusses the evolution of the efforts of Y2Y and STPC that ultimately led to the successful protesting of Walgreens. He links the work of the alcohol-mapping project to the decision and the work to protest the liquor license:

> …but other than that we've done, alcohol-mapping grants where myself and a couple of Y2Y members, we went out and we actually walked the entire city counting how many liquor establishments there were next to youth attractions and there's, right now there's like 22 liquor establishments and which is better than, like a couple years ago when it was like 52. So, you can see how over the years it's gone down a lot. But it was really cool, because we mapped the entire city, we broke it down into four quadrants and for a month we walked down, um, the entire quadrant, all of us. And then we gave all the data to, the people on the STPC board. And what was cool about that is that it got nationally recognized, where they actually did a whole presentation about it in Tennessee. So myself and one of the other Y2Y members, that was part of that, we got to go over there and see it. So that's pretty cool. And then, more recently they wanted to do a liquor license at the Walgreens here so we really protested that. We went to the city council and we told them that we think another building with another liquor license would be bad for the city and stuff. And they listened and they agreed with us. So they, denied the request, but they [Walgreens] took it up to Phoenix for the, what is it? The alcohol board, or something like that? So, we went up there and, thinking that, because they were giving us all these stories like 'Oh, they never deny. They just want to give them blah blah blah.' But we went up there thinking all these kids from like the Barrio where people say, so it was really rewarding where we stayed there for like seven hours and seeing everybody else's alcohol applications get granted (approved). But we were the one of two that day that were the only one of two that got denied that day. So that was [a] big accomplishment for us.

There was a tremendous feeling of success, especially being aware that it was rare for licenses to be denied. Youth realized that they could make a big difference, and that they were ready to advocate for their city, even by going to the state capital and speaking in front of the state liquor license board. Michal was a part of that mapping project and remembered how it made her feel to become civically engaged in her community:

> When we went to the City Council and went to them about the liquor license, yeah…doing that was a really big thing for us because we were thinking, "Wow, we can really do something our own community." Because back then, we'd think no one wanted to listen to us, they're just kids, ya know? And that made me realize things like, "Wow, this is really helpful, we can really do something."

10.3.1 The Importance of Community Awareness to Create Change

Community awareness of adolescent alcohol use and alcohol availability is key for real change to occur. According to Oscar, community awareness was critical to their success, "*There's a lot more youth involvement because, just everything that's going on now, it's more awareness, like as opposed to five years ago.*" Oscar asserts that increased awareness results in increased involvement. From a CBPR perspective, and one that Oscar agrees with, giving the community an equal voice greatly increases the effectiveness of their efforts.

> …back then if we would have said to the youth 'Oh can you help us out protesting this alcohol request?' We would have gotten like ten and now it was like 50 of us outside of Walgreens protesting and asking them not to do that. So, it's really grown a lot. So, there's more peer pressure in a good way now-a-days. I'm hoping there is, anyway.

The increase in awareness of alcohol norms really has worked well for this community; so much so in fact that the community of South Tucson was able to block a local Walgreens from receiving a liquor license.

10.3.2 Adult-Identified Community Benefits

Adults also identified community benefits from the process of protesting the license. One of the benefits was the ability to go through this process, yet to be able to maintain positive relationships with the businesses. This was achieved because of the campaign message that was agreed up on by all partners, which emphasized the liquor license density, and did not spread negative views of businesses. For example, Michele states, "*As time went on, and even though it was a pretty lengthy process, adults and other key stakeholders, it is a good idea not to have another liquor license, especially with the argument, it did not become so personal, it wasn't just oh those bad kids or those homeless people.*" Michele is commenting here that while the protest of the liquor license took a long time, it was also effective at changing the minds of many adults in the community who were less aware of adolescent alcohol issues. Additionally, with the campaign focusing on "not one more liquor license," the argument was not internal to the youth; it was a message that the community could embrace. Additionally, it did not put any further negative messages into the community about youth drinking or youth who were bad kids; this was very important and conscious to the youth and adults because of the existing negative messages about youth in South Tucson. Josefina, STPC member, also adds "*today there is a positive relationships with Walgreens, (they) are a stakeholder that supports community in South Tucson.*"

One of the benefits identified by adults was that their perspective of the youth in the community changed. It became much more positive in part because youth behaviors challenged their previous low expectations about youth involvement. Michele states, "*What was pleasant too, because it was such a lengthy process, and there were all these things you had to do by a certain time, and make sure you filed with the state and stuff like that and paperwork had to get in, and the teens never wavered in their enthusiasm about going through this, I didn't know how long it would take and if this was going to tail off.*" In effect, Michele was commenting on the ability of the youth to remain focused and to keep the leadership in this long-term strategy. Jaime explained the changes he noticed within the youth:

> For me, work was about the youth...and to watch the youth change and become their own thinkers...and realize their life and how great it is, and show them something new, show them something different, and make them realize how big the world really is and how beautiful it really is and to watch them kind of come into their own.

10.4 Expansion and Institutionalization

It was during this period that the City of South Tucson also made several policy changes in response to the work and the policy advocacy of the youth. Despite their victory over Walgreens, their efforts have since shifted to a new threat that has arisen within the community. Earlier Oscar mentioned K2, a drug that is becoming increasingly popular across the country. Oscar went on to discuss what Y2Y has been doing most recently to try and curtail the use of K2 by youth.

> Cause K2 is kind of a legalized marijuana substance that kids and everybody are smoking now because there's no drug test. You can't really get arrested for it, and it's legal, it's basically like legal marijuana. And it's, synthetic, synthetic something, but it's it does the same effects, if not stronger, and there's been a lot of causes already. I think there are a couple states that banned it already. But we, um, we found out that two smoke shops in South Tucson were selling K2. So we do a presentation, a PowerPoint presentation on all the dangers of K2 and so that's what our next step is. To work on getting a, a ban in the state. Cause we already got a ban in South Tucson.

The result of the work was that the City of South Tucson created several changes to their city code and one new ordinance. In this way, they addressed the concerns of the youth about proximity of alcohol advertising and selling of medical marijuana. Specifically, they created a new section to prohibit the selling of K2 (synthetic marijuana) (see Fig. 10.7, Section 7-34 (e) Restricted Smoking Material) to anyone under 21 years of age. They also responded to the youth-led research and mobilization to create more access to local parks by enforcing a new slum-lord policy that would allow the city to take over abandoned houses where drug-addicted adults would gather. Several of these factors were taken into consideration in the changes to the Neighborhood Preservation City Codes (Fig. 10.7). In the changes to the city code, they also limited alcohol advertising so that it could be not be within 500 feet of youth attractions (see Section 7-34 (c) Outdoor Alcohol Advertising Regulations). All of these new regulations were also associated with enforcement that was assessed as a civic penalty of a fine of $500 per day and a second violation of $1000 per day. They also put into a place a medical marijuana zoning ordinance (Figs. 10.8 and 10.9) that ensured 1000 fee setback from any education or activity facility where children were enrolled; they also had to be over 2000 feet from any other medical marijuana dispensary.

Conclusion

Thus, Michele sums it up "*it was such a big validation to **everybody**, that, again, collectively working together with the youth, with the power in the city of south Tucson, the agency, the university, that collectively we made this body that said if we wanted to we could change it.*" It wasn't just about that one liquor license; it wasn't just about the youth having a success. It was about the community's ability to come together, to work together to create change in this low-income community with so many challenges. Connections between environments, education, and positive youth development are crucial to shifting our focus from simply telling youth to "say no" or only to provide after-school programs, but rather to invest more time and resources into developing community spaces for youth and adult partnerships that are built on research and action in a manner that reflects the key principles of participatory action research. For youth of color, their experiences include structural inequalities and socioeconomic and sociopolitical contexts, which shapes their understanding of health issues and also shapes their recommendations for solutions to health issues with teens (Rubin, 2007; Sherrod, 2007). In the end, it was about one community's ability to recreate their environment into the community that they wanted for themselves and for their families.

SOUTH TUCSON CITY CODE

CHAPTER 7: NEIGHBORHOOD P RESERVATION

Fig. 10.7 Neighborhood preservation city of South Tucson code

SOUTH TUCSON

THE PUEBLO WITHIN A CITY

CITY OF SOUTH TUCSON ORDINANCE NO: 10-03

AN ORDINANCE OF THE CITY OF SOUTH TUCSON, ARIZONA RELATING TO ZONING; APPROVING AMENDMENTS TO CHAPTER 24 ("ZONING") OF THE SOUTH TUCSON CITY CODE, THE ZONING CODE, ADDING DEFINITIONS FOR MEDICAL MARIJUANA DISPENSARIES AND CULTIVATION LOCATIONS UNDER ARTICLE IV ("ZONING DISTRICT REGULATIONS"), DIVISION 13 ("SB-2 BUSINESS DISTRICT") AND DIVISION 17 ("SI-1 LIGHT INDUSTRIAL DISTRICT")

WHEREAS, the City of South Tucson regularly engages in comprehensive land use planning and regulation through the adoption of a general plan, specific plans, and a comprehensive zoning code; and

WHEREAS, the primary purposes of the amendment to Chapter 24, Article IV of the Zoning Code are to preserve and protect the public health, public welfare, and public safety by promoting the location of dispensaries in highly visible zones which leads to more accessible law enforcement, easier access to ill patients, and reduction of the number of patients and caregivers who need to cultivate their own marijuana plants; and

WHEREAS, proposed provisions of Proposition 203 (Arizona Medical Marijuana Act, A.R.S. § 36-2806.01) in the November 2, 2010 election allow cities to enact zoning regulations of medical marijuana dispensaries; and

WHEREAS, the possession, delivery, manufacture, cultivation and sale of marijuana is illegal under both the federal Controlled Substances Act and the Arizona Controlled Substances Act; and

WHEREAS: if adopted, Proposition 203, the Arizona Medical Marijuana Act, may be preempted or limited by the federal Controlled Substances Act or preempted or limited by the Arizona Controlled Substances Act; and

Ord. No. 10-03 Page 1 of 6

Fig. 10.8 City of South Tucson ordinance for medical marijuana zoning to limit proximity to youth attractions

References

Allen, J., Mohatt, G. V., Beehler, S., & Rowe, H. L. (2014). People Awakening: Collaborative research to develop cultural strategies for prevention in community intervention. *American journal of community psychology, 54*(1–2), 100–111.

Berg, M., Coman, E., & Schensul, J. J. (2009). Youth action research for prevention: A multi-level intervention designed to increase efficacy and empowerment among urban youth. *Journal of Community Psychology, 43*(3–4), 345–359.

Burrow-Sanchez, J. J. (2006). Understanding adolescent substance abuse: Prevalence, risk factors, and clinical implications. *Journal of Counseling and Development, 84*, 283–290.

Cahill, C., Rios-Moore, I., & Threatts, T. (2008). Different eyes/open eyes: Community-based participatory action research. In J. Cammarota & M. Fine (Eds.), *Revolutionizing education: Youth participatory action research in motion* (pp. 89–124). New York, NY: Routledge Press.

Cammarota, J., & Fine, M. (2008). *Revolutionizing education: Youth participatory action research in motion*. New York, NY: Routledge Press.

Christens, B. D., & Peterson, N. A. (2012). The role of empowerment in youth development: A study of sociopolitical control as mediator of ecological systems' influence on developmental outcomes. *Journal of Youth and Adolescence, 41*, 623–635.

Dupree, D., Spencer, M. B., & Fegley, S. (2007). Perceived social inequity and responses to conflict among diverse youth of color: The effects of social and physical context on youth behavior and attitudes. In R. K. Silbereisen & R. M. Lerner (Eds.), *Approaches to positive youth development* (pp. 111–133). Los Angeles: Sage Publications.

Flanagan, C. (2003). Developmental roots of political engagement. *Political Science and Politics, 36*(2), 257–261.

Flores Niemann, Y. (2001). Stereotypes about Chicanas and Chicanos implications for counseling. *The Counseling Psychologist, 29*(1), 55–90.

Ginwright, S. (2008). Collective radical imagination: Youth participatory action research and the art of emancipatory knowledge. In J. Cammarota & M. Fine (Eds.), *Revolutionizing education: Youth activism and community change* (pp. 13–22). New York: Routledge.

Ginwright, S., & James, T. (2002). From assets to agents of change: Social justice, organizing, and youth development. *New Directions for Youth Development, 2002*(95), 27–46.

Ginwright, S., & Cammarota, J. (2007). Youth activism in the urban community: Learning critical civic praxis within community organizations. *International Journal of Qualitative Studies in Education, 20*(6), 693–710.

Ginwright, S., Noguera, P., & Cammarota, J. (Eds.). (2006). *Beyond Resistance!: Youth Activism and Community Change: New democratic possibilities for practice and policy for America's youth* (pp. xii–xxii). New York, NY: Routledge Press.

Godfrey, E. B., & Grayman, J. K. (2014). Teaching citizens: The role of open classroom climate in fostering critical consciousness among youth. *Journal of Youth and Adolescence, 43*, 1801–1817.

Males, M. A. (1996). *The scapegoat generation: America's war on adolescents*. Monroe, ME: Common Courage Press.

Martín-Baró, I., Aron, A., & Corne, S. (1994). *Writings for a liberation psychology*. Cambridge, MA: Harvard University Press.

Morgan, W., & Streb, M. (2001). Building citizenship: How student voice in service-learning develops civic values. *Social Science Quarterly, 82*(1), 154–169. doi:10.1111/0038-4941.00014.

Peterson, N. A., Peterson, C. H., Agre, L. A., Christens, B. D., & Morton, C. M. (2011). Measuring youth empowerment: Validation of a sociopolitical control scale for youth in an urban community context. *Journal of Community Psychology, 39*(5), 592–605.

Rodríguez, L. F., & Brown, T. M. (2009). From voice to agency: Guiding principles for participatory action research with youth. *New Directions for Youth Development, 2009*(123), 19–34.

Rubin, B. C. (2007). "There's Still Not Justice": Youth Civic Identity Development Amid Distinct School and Community Contexts. *Teachers College Record, 109*(2), 449–481.

Sanchez-Jankowski, M. (2002). Minority youth and civic engagement: The impact of group relations. *Applied Developmental Science, 6*(4), 237–245.

Sherrod, L. (2007). Civic engagement as an expression of positive youth development. In R. K. Silbereisen & R. M. Lerner (Eds.), *Approaches to positive youth development* (pp. 59–75). Los Angeles: Sage Publications.

Torney-Purta, J., Barber, C. H., & Wilkenfeld, B. (2007). Latino adolescents' civic development in the United States: Research results from the IEA Civic Education Study. *Journal of Youth and Adolescence, 36*(2), 111–125.

Torre, M., & Fine, M. (2006). Researching and resisting: Democratic policy research by and for youth. In S. Ginwright, P. Noguera, & J. Cammarota (Eds.), *Beyond resistance: Youth activism and community change* (pp. 269–285). New York: Routledge.

U.S. Census Burearu. (2010). State and county quick facts. South Tucson, AZ. http://quickfacts.census.gov/qfd/states/04/0468850.html.

Walsh, M., DePaul, J., & Park-Taylor, J. (2009). Prevention as a mechanism for promoting positive development in the context of risk: Principles of best practice. M. Walsh, J. DePaul, J. Park-Taylor, M. E. Kenny (Ed), A. M. Horne (Ed), P. Orpinas (Ed), L. E. Reese (Ed) (2009). Realizing social justice: The challenge of preventive interventions., (pp. 57–78). Washington, DC: American Psychological Association, xviii, 322 pp. http://dx.doi.org/10.1037/11870-003

Watts, R. J., & Flanagan, C. (2007). Pushing the envelope on youth civic engagement: A developmental and liberation psychology perspective. *Journal of Community Psychology, 35*(6), 779–792.

Watts, R. J., & Guessous, O. (2006). Sociopolitical development: The missing link in research and policy on adolescents. In S. Ginwright, P. Noguera, & J. Cammarota (Eds.), *Beyond resistance!: Youth activism and community change: New democratic possibilities for practice and policy for America's youth* (pp. 59–80). New York, NY: Routledge Press.

Yates, M., & Youniss, J. (1996). A developmental perspective on community service in adolescence. *Social Development, 5*(1), 85–111.

Zeldin, S., Christens, B. D., & Powers, J. L. (2013). The psychology and practice of youth-adult partnership: Bridging generations for youth development and community change. *American Journal of Community Psychology, 51*(3–4), 385–397.

Zimmerman, M. A., & Zahniser, J. H. (1991). Refinements of sphere-specific measures of perceived control: Development of a sociopolitical control scale. *Journal of Community Psychology, 19*(2), 189–204.

Chapter 11
Coalition as Conclusion: Building a Functioning Coalition

Andrea Romero, Juvenal Caporale, Elisa Meza, Robby Harris, Josefina Ahumada, Jaime Arrieta, Sofia Blue, Gloria Hamelitz-Lopez, Michele Orduña, Juan "Johnny" Quevedo, Maricruz Romero-Ruiz, and Kimberly Sierra-Cajas

Abstract The purpose of this chapter is to describe the key factors that contributed to the creation, success, and sustainability of the South Tucson Prevention Coalition (STPC) over a period of 8 years. STPC was a diverse coalition whose goal was to prevent underage drinking in one city. Coalition members reflect on their success and describe four factors that contributed to their development. First, they describe how once they understood "We can't do it alone"; their critical consciousness that adolescent alcohol use was influenced by societal context influenced their motivation to work with other agencies. Second, they describe the importance of having a central mission that brings agencies together with a common goal and common passion to help young people. Third, they describe operating guidelines of meetings that contributed to their empowerment. Lastly, they discuss how personalismo, the cultural value of prioritizing positive and trusting relationships, helped them connect with coalition members to sustain their involvement.

Keywords Coalition • Collaboration • Personalismo • Trust • Dialogue

---

A. Romero, Ph.D. (✉)
Family Studies and Human Development, The University of Arizona, 650 North Park Avenue, Tucson, AZ 85719, USA
e-mail: romeroa@u.arizona.edu

J. Caporale, M.A.
Department of Mexican American Studies, The University of Arizona, Tucson, AZ, USA
e-mail: jcaporale@email.arizona.edu

E. Meza, M.S.W.
San Francisco Unified School District, San Francisco, CA, USA
e-mail: mezae520@gmail.com

R. Harris, M.A.
City University of New York, New York, NY, USA
e-mail: robby.d.harris@gmail.com

A.J. Romero (ed.), *Youth-Community Partnerships for Adolescent Alcohol Prevention*, DOI 10.1007/978-3-319-26030-3_11

Community coalitions are now identified by national agencies as a pathway to prevent and reduce adolescent substance use (Rog et al., 2004; SAMHSA, 2015). They are defined as "a group of individuals representing diverse organizations, factions, or constituencies who agree to work together to achieve a common goal." These types of coalitions bring together all people who are committed to improving the lives of the community, which may include any or all people such as insiders and outsiders, professional members, and grassroots leader (SAMHSA, 2015). Longitudinal (2002–2012) analysis of national programs that provided funding for community coalitions demonstrate that 30-day alcohol use by adolescents decreased by 2.8 percentage points among middle school students and 3.8 percentage points among high school students (Drug-Free Communities Support Program, 2012). These results suggest that community coalitions are one effective way to prevent adolescent alcohol use. Community collaboration is one way to leverage existing resources in order to work together to fight one common cause, and coalitions have become increasingly common as a way to address broad social issues. Yet, there is still limited research on how these groups are formed and the most effective processes that lead to functional coalitions (Grekul, 2011). The South Tucson Prevention

J. Ahumada, M.S.W.
School of Social Work, Arizona State University, Mesa, AZ, USA
e-mail: josefina.ahumada@asu.edu

J. Arrieta, M.P.H., C.H.E.S.
Spine Center Navigator, Carondelet Health Network, Tucson, AZ, USA
e-mail: jarrieta1@carondelet.org

S. Blue
Pima County Public Library, Sam Lena Branch, South Tucson, AZ, USA
e-mail: quetzazul@gmail.com

G. Hamelitz-Lopez
John Valenzuela Youth Center, Tucson, AZ, USA
e-mail: gloriahamelitz@hotmail.com

M. Orduña, M.Ed.
House of Neighborly Service, Tucson, AZ, USA
e-mail: miorduna@gmail.com

J.J. Quevedo
Pima Community College, Tucson, AZ, USA
e-mail: Tucsonhigh12@yahoo.com

M. Romero-Ruiz, M.S.
United Way of Tucson and Southern Arizona, Tucson, AZ, USA
e-mail: mrruiz1@gmail.com

K. Sierra-Cajas
Office of Undergraduate Research, The University of Arizona College of Science, Tucson, AZ, USA
e-mail: kjsc@email.arizona.edu

Coalition (STPC) was one of these effective coalitions that worked together over a period of 8 years in a low-income Mexican and Native American community (see Chap. 1 for a community description).

11.1 South Tucson Prevention Coalition Brief Description

STPC members were able to create and maintain a strong coalition that provided vision for advancing community efforts to prevent adolescent alcohol use in the City of South Tucson. Community readiness strategies guided STPC's approach to first raise awareness about community alcohol norms and then move toward collective action to transform the community infrastructure for alcohol availability and alcohol advertising (Oetting, Jumper-Thurman, Plested, & Edwards, 2001; see Chaps. 2 and 11 for details). STPC helped create significant change in the City of South Tucson to prevent adolescent alcohol use. STPC grew their focus from after-school adolescent alcohol prevention to also include community-based events designed to raise awareness of alcohol norms. Through this period of 8 years, the coalition was able to initiate new activities, obtain new funding, grow their membership, analyze new research together, impact alcohol norms, and prevent new liquor licenses. In retrospect, Josefina (Arizona State University Social Work faculty and representative of Southside Presbyterian Church) describes how the coalition was engaged in figuring out how to work together to change the environment in South Tucson, and she states that they accomplished this through two primary strategies: "*(1) youth were supported, . . .adults walked along with them, so that they were growing and developing and getting in touch with their own sense of power, their own sense of being citizens of this community, and they (learned that they) could make changes and they were learning skills about how to lead change (2) the agencies involved were learning about how to work as a collective, in order to, transform agencies that were silo-ed into a working collective. The new grant opportunity challenged them to come up with a campaign that would make a social environmental change in South Tucson.*"

STPC engaged in many activities that have already been identified in other published research as conducive to effective collaborative work. For example, Grekul (2011) identifies the importance of knowledge, community awareness, and support from leaders as essential pillars of community collaboratives. STPC regularly supported additional training opportunities for adult leadership and youth leadership opportunities. These included federal training at CADCA (see Chap. 5 for details), Youth-to-Youth (Y2Y) International Leadership Conference (see Chap. 10 for details), and local cultural competency training. STPC also developed several methods for disseminating data and information to the coalition members, community members, and local government (see Chaps. 8 and 9 for reports). Rog and colleagues (2004) also report that a clear vision and operating guidelines are important to keeping a coalition on track. STPC met once a month to engage in participatory dialogue to review and reflect on progress and also to plan prevention strategies based on joint decision-making. They had a clearly identified mission that guided their discussions and also clear operating procedures for these meetings.

Rog and colleagues (2004) also suggest that diversified funding stabilizes the sustainability of coalitions. STPC had diverse sources of funding over the 8-year period including: two federal grants, faith-based grants, state grants, and community grants. There were different lead agencies for each of these sources of funding (see Chaps. 2 and 8 for more information). However, STPC viewed resources in a very broad manner that did not only focus on external funding but that also included in-kind donations. For example, STPC coalition members made valuable contributions to the coalitions such as offering meeting space, food donations, support and translation services for reports and survey, and rallying many volunteers for events. However, there are still elusive aspects to the process of effectively implementing these principles that we will discuss in the current chapter. Additionally, given the unique demographic context of South Tucson of both Mexican American and Native American groups, we also provide insight through coalition member's comments about how to effectively engage in relationship building through personalismo and trust. The following sections describe the key factors identified by coalition members that contributed to their success. Coalition members give their recommendations for other communities who are considering developing coalitions or who are working to sustain a coalition. We include quotes from key coalition members who participated over several years, including Michele Orduña (STPC coordinator), Josefina Ahumada (Social Worker and representative from Southside Presbyterian Church), Jaime Arrieta (Prevention Specialist), Sofia Blue (Library Associate), Gloria Hamelitz-Lopez (John Valenzuela Youth Center executive director), Kimberly Sierra-Cajas (House of Neighborly Service Executive Director), and Dr. Andrea Romero (university researcher). The chapter is organized around the following topics that were identified by coalition members during a regular STPC monthly meeting (2010).

1. "We can't do it alone": Coalition as Conclusion
   (a) Meaning of membership
   (b) Breaking down silos
2. Common Issue: Mission & Passion
3. Meeting Structure:
   (a) Rotate meetings at each other's agencies
   (b) All participants are equal in meetings
4. Personalismo: Develop personal relationships based on trust over time

11.2 "We Can't Do It Alone": Coalition as Conclusion

The first step towards creating a coalition was to have some level of critical consciousness about adolescent alcohol use as a social issue rooted in community protective and risk factors. Freire (1968) describes critical consciousness as a way to understand the larger context of societal systems and the inherent inequities that impact the issue. He argued that once people reach critical consciousness about an issue, they can gain control over their lives through transforming their society. Critical consciousness is described as the ability to critically analyze one's environment and then act to create social justice-oriented change (Freire, 1968). It is comprised of three factors (1) critical reflection—critical analysis of social environment, (2) sociopolitical efficacy—confidence in ability to create sociopolitical change, and (3) critical action—participation in efforts to change one's environment (Godfrey & Grayman, 2014). Thus, the work of STPC found that the first step toward building coalition was the realization of individuals that the issue at hand was impacted by multiple ecological factors and that in order to solve this issue that one person, one youth, one agency could not do it alone. It was the realization that individuals and agencies needed to work together to solve these issues, because health issues are complex. It was the realization that environmental change is fundamental to individual behavior change, as identified by other researchers (Morales, 2009). In other words, adolescent alcohol use was not just about "saying no" but understanding and changing the community alcohol norms and the community environment in terms of alcohol availability. This is the basis of community transformational resilience, which enhances resilience at a community level by increasing and aligning protective factors while reducing risk factors. Coalition members were dedicated to changing the community to help youth have more opportunities for positive development, but they recognized that they couldn't do it alone. Gloria Hamelitz-Lopez (John Valenzuela Youth Center Executive Director) states: "*We cannot change this entire dynamic of the neighborhood all by yourself. So that was part of the drive (to collaborate). We can really collaborate.*"

Community Readiness Model for Change (Oetting et al., 2001) and Participatory Action Research (McIntyre, 2008) contend that identification of community strengths is essential to effective community-based work. This is similar in the critical consciousness of coalition work. It is fundamental to be able to identify the cooperation of coalition members as a community strength for prevention work. Sofia Blue (librarian): "*I think that the strengths are that all the organizations: the fire department, the city, the police department, the library and a lot of social service agencies seem to be on the same page about it, they seem to be wanting to pitch in, and help out. And I think that's a big strength, and the inter-agency cooperation.*" The way in which Sofia is able to identify several of the core stakeholders and their cooperation as a community strength to prevent adolescent alcohol use is an aspect of the critical consciousness that the issue is affected by multiple factors, and that in order to solve the problem, it will require everyone working together.

Gloria reminds us that in order for the coalition to come together: "*You have to be able to see the big picture.*" One way of staying connected to the big picture of underage drinking was linking to regional and national networks. This was important to the coalition because it reminded coalition members that they were not the only community facing this issue. They also learned new ideas and garnered additional resources from working with larger networks. For example, in one valuable resource for STPC was the partnership with a countywide coalition named the

Community Prevention Coalition (CPC) (funded by a state SPF-SIG and DFC) who supported STPC goals and activities. Michele Orduña (STPC Coordinator) describes how the coalition linked to national efforts to prevent adolescent alcohol use. "*We have tapped into national events as a way to promote local issues, e.g., National Night Out, having larger community events that reached out beyond regular players and finding ways to tap into heritage*." One of the most important benefits of linking to national networks, such as Youth-to-Youth International Leadership Programs, National Night Out, and Drug Free Communities, was that STPC learned that they were actually very successful in their work. It gave them an opportunity for comparison to similar communities who were engaged in the same type of prevention work. The realization that they were doing really well compared to these other groups was something that one person could not tell them. However, witnessing it for themselves transformed their perspective of the coalition and their role in the success.

Kania and Kramer (2011) argue that collective efforts are most successful when individual agendas are abandoned in favor of a collective approach. Jaime, Prevention Specialist, demonstrates how individual ego is placed aside, especially when discussing success of the coalition. Jaime explains the importance of remaining aware of how one's efforts fit into the larger process of change: "*Well, I didn't do it myself. I was just a little small cog in the wheel…and it takes all of those things to make the whole thing function and you just provide whatever you can to make sure that hopefully it works*." His comment is a good reflection of the critical consciousness that the success of STPC should be attributed to the collective, not any one individual or single agency. It is this type of humble response and approach to working with the coalition that ultimately contributed to the success and harmony of large agencies with different agendas being able to work together. Thus, the acceptance of "not being able to do it alone" represents that coalition members agree that it is necessary to have a sense of critical consciousness of underage drinking and being able to see one's role within a larger group process of change.

11.2.1 Coalition Membership

These identified factors clearly speak to the issue of membership, and it is truly the effective participation of members that contributes to overall success. STPC began with a relatively small group of core stakeholders that worked together for 3 years (2002–2005) with moderate success. Yet, after receiving SAMHSA funding for a Drug Free Community (2005), STPC grew from 6 key stakeholders to 20+ individuals who represent multiple community sectors. STPC was a recognized coalition that included many different service agencies, businesses, school, and local government that came together under the umbrella of STPC to focus on promoting a healthy community by preventing or reducing adolescent alcohol use.

Jaime suggests that organizations should "*cast a big net [and] reach out to everybody*." This is a good representation of the STPC approach to membership. They consciously discussed the meaning and limitation of membership. They chose to cast a wide net and to not formalize membership. There was no requirement for members to participate or to formalize their relationship in any way. There were no by-laws or restrictions on voting or participating in discussions or meetings. A brief list of the South Tucson Prevention Coalition members include: South Tucson youth, South Tucson parents, John Valenzuela Youth Center, Southern Arizona AIDS Foundation, Gospel Rescue Mission, Mission View Elementary School, City of South Tucson, Tucson Urban League, Project YES, South Tucson Police, South Tucson Fire, House of Neighborly Services, Youth-to-Youth (Y2Y), Las Cazuelitas, Ochoa Community Magnet Elementary School, Police Explorers, Dr. Andrea Romero, Mexican American Studies, University of Arizona. Youth leaders from the Omeyocan YES and Voz graduates formed the Youth-to-Youth (Y2Y) after-school group and continued to collaborate with South Tucson Prevention Coalition. STPC has also worked closely with the city officials in South Tucson. Kimberly Sierra-Cajas notes that the police involvement in South Tucson is unique compared to similar communities "*Look at what happens when the police do have that connection to the community, when some of them are from the community and when they see the community as being valuable members of society.*" At least twice a year or more, STPC attends a City of South Tucson Council meeting and provides an update of research, accomplishments, and goals. At least one representative from the government regularly attended STPC meetings. The support the local government and Mayor have demonstrated to STPC has been key to our success. Maricruz Romero-Ruiz, STPC Outreach Specialist, describes how the coalition learned to work with the city government, "*The coalition had to be very smart about their approach to working with the city, because they had to constantly get something from the city—they needed to get buy-in. Gloria (JVYC) –kept the back of the coalition—she had dealt with the city government for a number of years—she was very well-informed and had experience in dealing with them. Gloria was amazing, she was a born leader.*" Maricruz identifies how one of the coalition members had a history of working with the city government and how her experiential knowledge helped the coalition have success with the city as well.

However, some coalition members felt that they still fell short in terms of membership, and that there was still more to do, particularly with outreach to more youth and parents. For example, some described how because of neighborhood boundaries and lack of access to transportation among low-income youth they could not always participate. Thus, they felt that some high-risk youth were still not effectively involved or reached by the coalition. In the end, STPC didn't reach many parents, or parents only had intermittent participation with the coalition. Sofia Blue, librarian, agrees "*I think that a lot of what I've seen that we are doing is a lot more geared toward specifically the young people, and I just thought of this now, but maybe we could have more whole families involved in what we do for alcohol abuse prevention we could get more families involved in that … .*" Gloria agreed stating, "*We struggle with getting the adults involved. Big struggle.*" These comments just demonstrate how coalition members were still looking for ways to expand and to further extend their reach into the community.

Grekul (2011) does talk about danger of a collaborative that is too large and unwieldy because it does not offer opportunities for social cohesion and relationship building. They describe how it is common that collaboratives can be "messy" and that progress is often slow or tedious; yet, those who can see the benefit are likely to remain involved (Grekul, 2011). STPC found in their own practice that the core stakeholders regularly attended meetings and actively participated. This approach ensured transparency and openness about coalition activities, and yet, it also ensured that the individuals who participated regularly were those who were most seriously committed to the mission of the coalition. There were other members that only attended meetings once a year, but they always wanted to remain on the email list. Many of these members still participated in annual events, such as National Night Out, but did not always feel that they needed to participate in regular meetings or engage in decision-making. At times even core stakeholders spent more or less time participating in activities; often this was a result of the activities happening in their own agency that at times took precedent. However, the core stakeholders always returned to active participation, and they were always welcomed back into the group.

11.2.2 Breaking Down Silos: Inside and Outside

Even within a core group of stakeholders with critical consciousness, there is a need to break down silos between agencies. Cross-agency work has not been as commonly undertaken; in fact, it is much more likely that similar community-based organizations find that they are competition for funding streams, donors, or participants (Kania & Kramer, 2011). Within STPC, it took time to break down silos between agencies; there were challenges between agencies within the City of South Tucson (see Chap. 5 for details) but also for agencies outside of the City of South Tucson (see Chap. 9 for details). Gloria illustrates how her agency worked to break down barriers within the same community for agencies to work together:

> We had to train our staff and our adults to say no more of the negativity. We want our kids to do these different things and if they go to three different centers that is great. That is great! They should be! And if you want to stay competitive, well then you have to offer the best programs. But you also have to be able to share and promote some of the other activities that kids [from other agencies] are doing… And that becomes scary because of the business aspect. You know, you are required per grant to have eighty kids and stuff like that. So, we kind of knew that there might be an issue there, but it was going to benefit the youth in the end. And what happened was that we did not end up losing kids. They would go and get their tutoring, hang out there, and they would kind of start floating back and forth. Like I said, a lot of that really had to do with the adults. We had to retrain the adults to be more open to that and the kids started following that after a while.

One of the outcomes that is noted here by Gloria is that while there was the concern of loss of participants and loss of funding, the actual result was that her agency did not lose money or youth. In fact, they found that the community benefitted more than they ever expected. They found that youth were able to access more resources, without losing resources or losing connections to agencies where they had first participated. In fact, Kimberly Sierra-Cajas, House of Neighborly Service Executive Director, further describes how this process may have even lead to a more enhanced overall sense of community: "*I definitely think that it was good for the kids to see us working together, the different Safe Havens, because by us kind of eliminating the boundaries that existed between us, that it helped eliminate some of the boundaries for them. So that they could cross agency or have interagency participation in some of our different activities and so maybe encourage it too with the kids and I think this was a big change from what it was like in previous years…So I think that is one big difference is that maybe some communities don't always necessarily encourage their students to participate in other programs. I think that by us all working together we can put on big events like we did and I think made it a lot more like a close knit neighborhood atmosphere even for the parents.*" The internal boundaries between neighborhoods within cities and loyalty to certain agencies can often pose significant barriers to accessing resources, particularly within low-income communities. Thus, this breaking down of silos also became a breaking down of barriers to resources within the community. Kimberly and Gloria note here how the interagency collaboration set an example and role modeled some of this behavior for youth and families who had historically remained within their own neighborhood boundaries. Additionally, they both note that by working together, there were greater community benefits and access to resources.

Kania and Kramer (2011) are correct that encouraging collective impact requires new skills that can help individuals and agencies learn to coordinate resources in order to offer the most comprehensive and cohesive access to community members. They indicate that this process is enhanced when both insiders and outsiders are included in the process. In fact, STPC found that including outsiders was conducive to the development of collaborative work. Kimberly Sierra-Cajas (House of Neighborly Service Executive Director) describes: "*By having STPC there, it helped us to be more collaborative, especially having an outside organization like the University of Arizona involved, and it was helpful. Sometimes in South Tucson you get wrapped up in your own world. It is kind of like having an outside facilitator there. It helped us be more collaborative. So it was just helpful having an outside resource especially. STPC helped take the lead and taking charge of keeping us together.*"

The aspect of neutrality was vital to the continued functioning of the coalition. A fundamental aspect of STPC was that the external funding provided for a coordinator, this person, Michele Orduña, was not connected directly to any previously existing agency. As such, she was a neutral representative whose only agenda was to promote the mission of the coalition. This was important to maintaining the balance within the coalition and to maintaining harmony between the agencies. Michele states: "*I was the glue that kept all the agencies on the same page.*" Additionally, she was skilled at facilitating discussion in order to keep the group on track. The background work that she did to meet with individuals on a one-to-one basis or phone calls helped to keep the core stakeholders on the same page.

Jaime Arrieta (Southern Arizona AIDS Foundation Prevention Specialist) also stressed the importance of the adults who are leading the initiatives getting along and working together toward the larger goals of change. Jaime further explained what this meant for outsiders to the community. He explained that those involved in leading community change have to be genuine and aware of where the larger community is coming from:

> I think everybody in that group just was passionate about making a change and passionate about…coming into this community. Because the first thing you would get (from the community) is: 'But you're not from here. What do you care about this community?' '(he would respond) Well my daughter goes to ballet down the street here and she actually goes to school right next door. Do I live here, no, but this is where I've chosen to raise my child… and it's important to me. There's a big turf thing there. South Tucson is very proud in what they have there . . . it makes it hard sometimes for people to come into a community and want to make some change…you've got to be welcomed. Even though we were all…with the best intentions trying to make things happen…the first bit of resistance was definitely up from the community. …So understanding that community and being patient…and it's been patience and perseverance [from] everybody that sat on the coalition and the youth at the JVYC, and it's like 'we're not going anywhere and this is what we're doing.' And I think once things actually started happening, you know, all of a sudden people started looking.'

Jaime describes very well how he handled questions about his participation and his true intentions. He took the time to explain his background and his relationship to the community. He provides here an excellent example of how to take these types of questions and concerns about the intentions of "outsiders" in stride and how to handle them in a way that can lead to enhanced relationships rather than more resistance. In his comments, he implies that proving his commitment and caring about the community and underage drinking was part of the normal process of coming into a tight-knit community from an outside agency. Particularly for communities that have faced continued injustice and the associated inequities, it is likely that they have reasons to be distrustful of service providers and university researchers; this distrustfulness may manifest in resistance to commitment to involvement in partnership and resistance to supporting health programs that are perceived as originating outside of the local community (Gallardo, 2013). One of the coalition members described how "*Our group comes together well, there are no hidden agendas or camps.*" This comment also recognizes the importance of transparency and clarity of the commitment of all members to the same mission of the coalition. Furthermore, it indicates that the coalition was successful at breaking down silos within the coalition and came together for the common goal of prevention work in South Tucson.

11.2.3 Successful Youth Involvement in Coalitions

Jaime remarked: "*Kids are definitely the most underserved people in the community…and overlooked.*" This unfortunate reality is one that was challenged by the members of the STPC and was slowly being changed in South Tucson. An aspect of breaking down silos that is often overlooked is the inclusion of youth in coalition work; adults most often represent youth programs instead of directly including youth representatives. We argue in this book that youth involvement is critical, particularly when the primary issue is adolescent health. Unfortunately, there are often barriers to youth involvement, such as negative stereotypes or assumptions that youth will lack commitment (Dold & Chapman, 2012). Jaime describes how other adults in the community witnessed STPC success and the outcomes they shared with youth. He indicates that the adults would question "How did you do that? How does that work?" However, it was the adult coalition member's recognition that youth leaders were valued and a community strength that fostered continued involvement. For example, Sofia Blue (librarian) comments "*Youth leaders, they can be invaluable to the rest of the community because they are such a good example of what you can do. (They are) role models because they seem like they are happy, they are having fun, but they are also being productive, and making money, or working on something for their future. I think that just naturally attracts people to them.*" Yet, youth were always involved as part of STPC from the beginning; Michele points out "*We always had youth involved.*"

The youth involvement was a legacy from the work of the Omeyocan YES program youth leaders that advocated for youth representation and youth equality in collaborative decision making (see Chap. 4). Omeyocan YES youth graduates had significant training in participatory dialogue, youth empowerment, prevention knowledge, and leadership skills. The continued role of after-school programing for youth throughout STPC Phase 1 and Phase 2 is important to acknowledge. The continuity of these programs to focus on prevention as well as critical consciousness and leadership were important to sustainability of youth involvement. In fact, it was that youth programming and coalition building were parallel during these periods that contributed significantly to success and sustainability of both activities. Gloria also commented that these programs (Omeyocan YES and Voz) laid the foundation for the coalition success, because it was easier to "build up" from these after-school prevention programs. Juan "Johnny" Quevedo, Y2Y leader, describes the youth role in the coalition, "*The whole purpose of being there, was to get the youth point of view across. They (STPC) didn't have a meeting of just 22 adults and no teenagers. (At the meetings) You were able to discuss what you think and what you feel. It was wonderful to have the coalition expanded outside of just adults. A lot of people who attended those meetings were blown away by what we see and what we know. I appreciate the fact that teens were appreciated and admired. A lot of people could get off track, but it doesn't mean you have to give up on them.*" Juan's comment also indicates that youth who participated felt valued, which further contributed to their desire to be active and equal participants. He also comments that the adult's continued belief and support of all youth was important. The adults tried to continuously send the message that they were not going to give up on the youth in the community.

However, it was the continued interconnection of the programs and other community agencies that created the continued infrastructure for youth leaders to advance their knowledge of prevention. Too often young people graduate from effective after-school prevention programs only to return to communities that lack infrastructure to continue their involvement in prevention activities (Ginwright & Cammarota, 2006) Additionally, youth in low-income and ethnic minority communities face more negative messages and stereotypes or assumptions about their involvement in illegal alcohol and substance use activities. Constantly fighting these criminalized and dehumanizing stereotypes as individuals or in small youth groups can make youth's continued efforts to engage in healthy behaviors even more difficult and frustrating. Some youth may feel that community level change is hopeless without support from adults or that changing their individual behavior is fruitless if people still believe they are using substances. It is these realities of ethnic minority youth that makes the youth involvement and accomplishments of STPC even more powerful.

11.3 Common Issue: Mission and Passion

"We have all come together on behalf of the youth, it is what we have in common, in fact, it is our passion" South Tucson Prevention Coalition Members

The coalition member's collective commitment and agreement on the mission to prevent adolescent underage drinking was central to the success of the STPC. However, initially it was very challenging for the coalition to reach consensus on the specifics of the mission, given there were diverging opinions about whether to focus on alcohol use, substance use, or drunk driving. This decision to narrow the mission was achieved only after one full year of regular monthly meetings and discussion. Kania and Kramer (2011) argue that collective dialogue is necessary to create a common agenda so that all members of the group are on the same page when it comes to the issue that is affecting their community. As a result of this discussion, all participants had an in-depth understanding of the mission and objectives and a clear vision of their role in the collaboration. Additionally, use of a participatory research approach ensured that community members are aware of the program and feel empowered to use the skills they gain through the program. Empowerment can be considered the sense of personal influence over a multitude of forces impacting life situations, such as personal, social, economic, and political (Schulz, Israel, Zimmerman, & Checkoway, 1995). Empowerment of key stakeholders was important from the beginning of the project, development of the mission, and throughout in every activity. A clear vision and achievable objectives allowed STPC to meet their goals as a collective.

Moreover, agreeing on a common agenda helps the collaborative understand the issue and focus their strategies to solve it. Each STPC monthly meeting began with revisiting the mission statement, which served to remind everyone of the common agenda. Moreover, revisiting the mission statement helped to focus the content and direction of their discussions. When the members disagreed about a decision, they went back to this mission statement as a way to refocus. Often the collaborative comes together around one large issue, such as adolescent alcohol prevention that is not likely to be solved in a timely manner. In part because of these natural challenges, Grekul (2011) describes how it is helpful to have immediate and intermediate goals. Thus, immediate tangible goals, such as STPC's town halls or community events, helped the coalition to stay on track and to feel a measure of success. It also helped to have identified intermediate goals, for example, STPC set goals of addressing alcohol norms and alcohol availability, which were measurable in several manners, surveys, observation measures, and policy changes.

And in the end, perhaps the greatest message is the passion of those who participated in this process, for example, Jaime states:

> The biggest thing for me was watching that change and so the work was not always pretty and fun, but that's where I always found myself going back to the youth and the youth were what kept me going and even on the worst day, the youth were always the ones to get me through it.

In retrospect, Josefina Ahumada, Social Worker, Arizona State University representative, Southside Presbyterian Church representative, remarks on the success of working together: "*Community was built, and a group of teens became contagious with a group of adults having a sense of we can make a change.*" Josefina gives credit to the youth for leading the way with their passion and optimism about innovative prevention strategies. Many others agreed as well that youth led the way and helped adults of the community gain new insight and a sense of community and collective efficacy to work together for change. Researchers argue that youth should be seen not only as resources but also as assets for change (Ginwright & James, 2002; Kulbok et al., 2015). However, youth are only involved in approximately 15 % of community-based participatory research published studies (Kulbok et al., 2015), and most youth participatory action research studies primarily focus on youth and adult allies without inclusion of broader community representatives (Ginwright & James, 2002). Through the combined efforts of many individuals, the youth in South Tucson had the opportunity to have a voice and work toward making a change in their community. Despite the passion of members, the enactment of regular coalition activities can be challenging; yet, STPC found that a few key operating principles were highly conducive to building coalition success. They were rotate meeting locations and equal participation for dialogue.

11.3.1 Meeting Structure: Rotate Meeting Location

"We used different locations for our meetings to get to know each other" STPC Coalition member. It was important for individuals to participate in regular meetings and retreats. STPC held all meetings at accessible locations so that all individuals could attend. This level of regular engagement lent to the perception of control and empowerment within the coalition (Schulz et al., 1995). Active engagement is critical to the perception of empowerment at a community level (Schulz et al., 1995). Continued joint decisions to engage in local action were fundamental to benefitting many people across the spectrum of the community. STPC met on a monthly basis in the first year to develop infrastructure organization and develop good meeting and communication habits. These meetings lasted no more than 1 h and 15 min. Ms. Orduña, STPC Coordinator, had significant experience in facilitating large groups of key stakeholders from diverse backgrounds and with different language abilities. She also had relevant training in this area in working with groups, facilitating focus groups and community readiness interviews. She ensured that key

stakeholders were represented at meetings and that all members participated fully in the discussion. She created agendas and kept the meeting on track, while still allowing time and space for open climate dialogue. She made every effort for members to feel respected when they voice diverse opinions. Gloria further commented in regard to challenges to collaborating: "*The adults and egos, take credit for the collaborative event. It makes people not want to join. If other people feel welcome, they are more likely to come back and help out…JVYC…We promote a neutral name and a neutral location, people come around. Kids are easy, adults are difficult.*" This is an important point to consider because in order to keep key stakeholders involved, it was necessary to make all participants feel valued and to feel that the coalition was not being overtaken by a single agency.

11.3.2 All Participants Are Equal: Dialogue and Decision-Making

It was critical to coalition functioning that all coalition members were treated as equals in both dialogue and decision-making of the coalition. For example, Michele states: "*One of the things about the coalition work is that we created this environment where everyone was equal at the table, that was just the way we went about this, that served us well over the long haul—that is how business was conducted" and we didn't have much internal conflict within the coalition.*" An effective approach to participatory dialogue and equal knowledge sharing is the perspective that every participant is an expert in their own manner. The Freirian approach to problem posing was taught in the after-school youth prevention programs and also utilized during coalition meetings, in which issues were brought up as questions for the coalition to critically discuss together through dialogue. Youth participation in the coalition meetings and decision making were excellent opportunities for them to further develop their participatory skills; in other words, the coalition provided a community of practice for their development (Torney-Purta, Barber, & Wilkenfeld, 2007). The coalition worked hard to develop an environment where all the participants were treated in an equal manner with respect for their diverse perspectives. All views were listened and considered in the decision-making. Michele links these operating guidelines to success in decision-making that valued all suggestions equally, including the youth's ideas "*Because of our mentality of how we ran meetings, and how everyone had a voice and everyone had a vote, and it was treated with respect, there was never anyone who said this (Walgreens protest) makes no sense, don't help the teens, they don't know what they are doing, they are not going to continue with it. Everyone said how can we help, what can we do.*"

Jaime states: "*The adults can learn a lot from the youth in the community if they just listen.*" A unique and important aspect of the coalition is that youth were included as equal community members in the coalition. Youth and adults working together can create bidirectional growth, releasing notions of ageism such as "not being old enough" to make informed decisions. It is more crucial than ever to create spaces where adults work alongside youth instead of simply lecturing to them and creating systems of prevention for social issues. Adult partnerships with youth spaces can result in sustainable leadership development, building the capacity of youth to believe in feeling motivated to become the next primary resources for their younger peers. Jaime stressed the importance of dialoguing with youth, colleagues, and the community; he explained that collaboration is crucial for success at every level of the community change process. "*[The youth] have a voice and it can be heard.*" There was still a process of humanization of youth and changes in the perception that youth could be prepared, and capable leaders before community leaders were fully prepared to listen and work equally with youth (see Chaps. 7 and 10).

The regular monthly STPC meetings provided opportunities for an open climate with self-reflection, and collective reflection helped to gain clarity and move the group to the next project or the next action step. The concept of an open climate where all opinions are respected when controversial issues are discussed can help foster the development of critical consciousness among youth or adults (Godfrey & Grayman, 2014). The lack of an open climate can actually have a negative effect when working with ethnic minority youth (Godfrey & Grayman, 2014); given the distrust of ethnic minority communities, the lack of opportunities for discussion or questions may be perceived to be lack of genuine interest. It may also convey lack of transparency which could be translated as hidden agendas. One way in which STPC developed an open climate during the meetings was to focus on dialogue rather than just giving reports without discussion. They learned through a process over several meetings about how to quickly share information and to ask for feedback. The members also became more relaxed and over time came to share their opinions openly. They all learned as a group that this type of dialogue and open climate benefitted the entire group over time.

In STPC meetings, the monthly agenda was created with time for questions and discussion. Although fewer items were discussed, they were discussed more in depth. This required a shift in expectations of the purpose of meetings. Rather than using meeting time to demonstrate accomplishments, meeting time was focused on gaining perspective, reflection, and insight. This was challenging at first, because questions could be perceived to be overly critical and to slow down action-oriented discussions. However, over time the dialogue time became more productive and positive in a manner that was conducive to improving the overall work. Michele opened every meeting reminding everyone that we are all equal in the meeting and that everyone's voice mattered. Setting the tone of discussions and redirecting through the facilitator and the members was important to help keep the coalition on track for open climate and dialogue-based meetings. It was influential that a few older female community professionals often were the pivotal voice to shift the discussion to a positive direction or to rephrase the comments in a productive manner. Their voices were key to ensuring that positive direction of the dialogue. Often they would be the first to voice their comments with first stating something encouraging or supportive. This approach would set the tone for the rest of the members, and also equally distributed the responsibility for facilitation, so that it was not only the project coordinator's influence.

However, good facilitation skills of the project coordinator, Michele Orduña, also helped to keep the coalition on track by setting clear boundaries for what was possible and what was not possible. This was particularly relevant in regard to the use of the available funding. Michele stepped in when dialogue became repetitive; she brought it to a close in a way that summarized the key points, in order to ensure that members knew that their opinions were heard. This was not an easy task, and there were clearly ups and downs over time, and Michele reflects, "*In the five years of the (Drug-Free Community) grant, it was never brought up within the coalition that there was some sort of internal conflict, we didn't always agree with each other, we didn't always want to do the same thing, or the choice the coalition made, but we were always smart enough to agree to disagree, just let it go, no hard feelings.*" Several coalition members indicate the need to see the bigger picture and agree to play a role within a larger coalition that may require giving up ego-driven goals or goals of any individual agency. One of the underlying factors that helped to promote this type of behavior was the personalismo that helped to bond the coalition members together as a cohesive group that was linked through their common mission, passion, and genuine caring for each other and the community.

11.4 Personalismo and Trust over Time

Josefina explains why the coalition worked well together, "*I believe that the team worked well as a result of the trust each person placed in one another. They were respectful of each other and they honored the group's work agreements. 'Personalismo' was a value shared across the group. Personalismo is a cultural value of developing personal relationships and getting to know people, obligation to come back and work together.*" There was a strong sense among the key stakeholders that there was a need for all agencies to be really involved in the community and also to support each other's events. In this way, they worked together on joint projects, but also supported separate activities for each agency, and in the end all participants and the community would benefit from their collective impact. A key point is that *personalismo*, the importance of personal relationships, is an important cultural value in Mexican and Native communities (Marín & Marín, 1991). STPC members understood that many of their efforts and contributions were built around reciprocal relationships that we have built and nurtured over years of commitment. Evidence of the strength of personal relationships in STPC are demonstrated in that the core group of key stakeholders has remained together for over 8 years and that they continued to step up to take more responsibility and leadership. STPC members supported coalition members in the same way that they were asked to support STPC, through support, resources, and active engagement. It was helpful that most of the coalition members were bilingual (English & Spanish) and represented the multicultural nature of South Tucson [Mexico, Native American (Tohono Oodham and Yaqui), and USA]. They also had experience working with Mexican descent and Native American cultures. Maricruz Romero-Ruiz describes her outreach work in the following manner, "*I really enjoyed the work. I really enjoyed working with the agencies—and the library—really quality people—it made my job easy—they were so willing to be a part of the coalition and be part of the community. It helps to identify the people who really care and who are willing to take a leadership role and willing to invest the time. Also, knowing how to approach people and build relationships, it takes time to do those phone calls, and 'charlar (to chat).' It (relationship building) can start off informal, some things happen naturally and that can be stronger. Being able to get involved, find out what they (partners) are doing, what they are all about. The message is that you are interested, that and personal contact to invite them to meetings.*"

Mexican and Native cultural contexts have been found to be more interdependent and to encourage close, positive, and warm personal relationships, through the cultural value of personalismo (Triandis, Marin, Lisansky, & Betancourt, 1984). Personalismo prioritizes personal relationships through personalized communication style that conveys trust, mutual respect, dignity, and self-worth (Altarriba & Santiago-Rivera, 1994; Holloway, Waldrip, & Ickes, 2009; Marín & Marín, 1991; Santiago-Rivera, Arredondo, & Gallardo-Cooper, 2002). This approach reduces power differentials and emphasizes the value of the person as more than the task, which is particularly important when working with populations who often experience prejudice or discrimination where they are treated with less than mutual respect (Gloria & Peregoy, 1996). Within the coalition, personalized communication and interaction ensured equality because it focused on the human rather than the title or job label (Gloria & Peregoy, 1996). Maricruz describes the cultural aspect of her work to build relationships, "*When you have people working in an area where they have a culture that they are familiar with, bicultural/bilingual people, the cultural aspect is second nature. Because you know what this community likes, you follow your instincts. You know that certain things will work. You are doing it naturally because it is part of your culture too. For me, working in the community was very easy because not only am I bilingual, but I am also bicultural. This helped to know how to establish rapport, make them laugh and feel at ease, and that takes time. That is what is hard is relationship building—it is very delicate and cultural norms matte. Being bicultural and being able to identify, you have a sense of how to be flexible to establish rapport.*"

Research has demonstrated that personalismo is linked with enhanced motivation performance and enhanced behavior change in therapy settings for Mexican heritage individuals compared to European American individuals (Sanchez-Burks, Nisbett, & Ybarra, 2000; Savani, Alvarez, Mesquita, & Markus, 2013). Examples of this style of communication to build trust within relationships are to use small talk to develop rapport, self-disclosure of personal background, humor, empathy, and respect (Gallardo, 2013). Failed programs are often attributed to lack of community trust (Alegría, Canino, & Pescosolido, 2009; Thurman et al., 2003), which is one of the reasons that interactions with community that are rooted in trust and mutuality are more likely to lead to sustainable prevention change.

Gloria also comments about using this approach with youth involvement: "*One on one relationship. We push relationship approach.*" She notes the importance of establishing trust and understanding with adolescents in order to tap into true and accurate discussion of use. So, it is not surprising that the youth also internalized this approach to their own motivations and work on prevention. They were strongly linked to other relationships within their community, and this was a powerful motivator for their inspiration to create community change. For example, Michele indicates "*A common thing among the teens when they came up with ideas of things they want to change challenge, they always thought of the kids younger than them, they shouldn't have to see that (alcoholism).*" Josefina also agrees "*Teens were looking out for younger siblings and larger community.*"

Yet, developing respectful relationships takes time; long-term dedication to the issue was a significant benefit to coalition members, especially because at one time or another members may have felt frustrated at the lack of momentum or progress. It was these personal connections and trust that encouraged them to return to the table for coalition meetings. Andrea Romero, university researcher states: "*The process of coalition building can take years in the process. Years of building relationships, one-on-one meetings, and a lot of behind the scene stuff. In other words, coalition building is not an overnight process but one of hard work, dedication, negotiation, and perseverance.*" The long-term perspective was important to the success of STPC; people understood that they were not only participating for a brief period of external funding, but that they were truly committed to the bigger issues within the community. However, the long-term perspective also requires setting smaller milestones and remembering to stop and celebrate when those are achieved. Jaime: "*It's kind of like when you're climbing a big hill, all you really do is look down at the ground. You can't look up because you can't see the top of it but when you look back you look [to see] how far I've come. You forget to turn around and look around…and find something that is working. You've got to remember to every now and then look around and keep an eye out for the change because it might happen and you might not see it.*"

11.5 Conclusion

The goal of this chapter was to present South Tucson Prevention Coalition member's perspectives on the factors that contributed to their success and sustainability. The key factors that identified were first of all the understanding that they could not tackle prevention of underage drinking on their own. The critical consciousness of understanding the societal context of adolescent alcohol use was pivotal to their agreement to participate in a coalition approach and their ability to focus on the big picture, even when unique challenges arose within their agencies. Another central factor for their success was the equal involvement of youth within their coalition; several members identified the passion of the youth as the motivation and inspiration for the adult participation. It was the common commitment to the mission of preventing underage drinking that fueled the coalition member's participation. However, the fundamentals of operating principles of coalition meetings cannot be underestimated, and the members indicated the importance of rotating meetings at each other's agency locations and equality in meetings for dialogue and decision-making. The regular practice of meetings influenced the continued involvement and empowerment of members. Yet, one of the most critical aspects of coalition success in this particular low-income Mexican American and Native American community was that personalismo, valuing of personal relationships, was threaded throughout all interactions between youth, adults, agencies, and community. The genuine value of people in the coalition and support of them as individuals and agencies strengthened the coalition sustainability and healthy functioning to overcome barriers to breaking down silos. The process of creating a new community group can be challenging, yet STPC proves that there are basic techniques that contribute to the successful coalition development and positive results.

References

Drug-Free Communities Support Program. (2012). National Evaluation Report (PDF | 648 KB).

Alegría, M., Canino, G., & Pescosolido, B. (2009). A socio-cultural framework for mental health and substance abuse service disparities. In B. J. Sadock, V. A. Sadock, & P. Ruiz (Eds.), *Comprehensive textbook of psychiatry* (9th ed.). Baltimore, MD: Wolters Kluwer Health Lippincott Williams & Wilkins.

Altarriba, J., & Santiago-Rivera, A. L. (1994). Current perspectives on using linguistic and cultural factors in counseling the Hispanic client. *Professional Psychology: Research and Practice, 25*, 388–397.

Dold, C. J., & Chapman, R. A. (2012). Hearing a voice: Results of a participatory action research study. *Journal of Child and Family Studies, 21*, 512–519.

Freire, P. (1968). *Pedagogy of the oppressed.* New York, NY: Seabury Press.

Gallardo, M. (2013). Context and culture: The initial clinical interview with the Latina/o client. *Journal of Contemporary Psychology, 43*, 43–52.

Ginwright, S., & Cammarota, J. (2006). Introduction. In S. Ginwright, P. Noguera, & J. Cammarota (Eds.), *Beyond resistance!: Youth activism and community change: New democratic possibilities for practice and policy for America's youth* (pp. xii–xxii). New York, NY: Routledge Press.

Ginwright, S., & James, T. (2002). From assets to agents of change: Social justice, organizing, and youth development. *New Directions for Youth Development, 2002*(95), 27–46.

Gloria, A. M., & Peregoy, J. J. (1996). Counseling Latino alcohol and other substance users/abusers: Cultural considerations for counselors. *Journal of Substance Abuse Treatment, 13*(2), 119–126.

Godfrey, E. B., & Grayman, J. K. (2014). Teaching citizens: The role of open classroom climate in fostering critical consciousness among youth. *Journal of Youth and Adolescence, 43*, 1801–1817.

Grekul, J. (2011). Building collective efficacy and sustainability into a community collaborative: Community solution to gang violence. *Journal of Gang Violence, 18*(2), 23–45.

Holloway, R. A., Waldrip, A. M., & Ickes, W. (2009). Evidence that a simpatico self-schema accounts for differences in the self-concepts and social behavior of Latinos versus Whites (and Blacks). *Journal of Personality and Social Psychology, 96*, 1012–1028.

Kania, J., & Kramer, M. (2011). Collective impact. *Stanford Social Innovation Review, Winter*, 36–41.

Kulbok, P. A., Mszaros, P. S., Bond, D. C., Thatcher, E., Park, E., Kimbrell, M., & Smith-Gregory, T. (2015). Youths as partners in a community participatory project for substance use prevention. *Family and Community Health, 38(1),* 3–11.

Marín, G., & Marín, B. V. (1991). *Research with hispanic populations*. Thousand Oaks, CA: Sage Publications.

McIntyre, A. (2008). *Participatory action research*. Thousand Oaks, CA: Sage Publications.

Morales, E. S. (2009). Contextual community prevention theory: Building interventions with community agency collaboration. *American Psychologist, 64*(8), 805–816.

Oetting, E. R., Jumper-Thurman, P., Plested, B., & Edwards, R. W. (2001). Community readiness and health services. *Substance Use and Misuse, 36*(6 &7), 825–843.

Rog, D., Boback, N., Barton-Villagrana, H., Marrone-Bennett, P., Cardwell, J., Hawdon, J. … Reischl, T. (2004). Sustaining collaboratives: cross-site analysis of the National Funding Collaborative on Violence Prevention. *Evaluation and Program Planning, 27*, 249–261.

SAMHSA (2015). *Components of an effective coalition*. http://www.samhsa.gov/capt/tools-learning-resources/components-effective-coalition.

Sanchez-Burks, J., Nisbett, R. E., & Ybarra, O. (2000). Cultural styles, relationship schemas, and prejudice against out-groups. *Journal of Personality and Social Psychology, 79*, 174–189.

Santiago-Rivera, A. L., Arredondo, P., & Gallardo-Cooper, M. (2002). *Counseling Latinos and la familia: A practical guide*. Thousand Oaks, CA: Sage.

Savani, K., Alvarez, A., Mesquita, B., & Markus, H. R. (2013). Feeling close and doing well: The prevalence and motivational effects of interpersonally engaging emotions in Mexican and European American cultural contexts. *International Journal of Psychology, 48*(4), 682–694.

Schulz, A. J., Israel, B. A., Zimmerman, M. A., & Checkoway, B. N. (1995). Empowerment as a multi-level construct: perceived control at the individual, organizational, and community levels. *Health Education Research, 10*(3), 309–327.

Thurman, P. J., Plested, B. A., Edwards, R. W., Foley, R., & Burnside, M. (2003). Community readiness: The journey to community healing. *Journal of Psychoactive Drugs, 35*(1), 27–31.

Torney-Purta, J., Barber, C. H., & Wilkenfeld, B. (2007). Latino adolescents' civic development in the United States: Research results from the IEA Civic Education Study. *Journal of Youth and Adolescence, 36*(2), 111–125.

Triandis, H. C., Marin, G., Lisansky, J., & Betancourt, H. (1984). Simpatia as a cultural script of Hispanics. *Journal of Personality and Social Psychology, 47*, 1363–1375.

Chapter 12
Community Transformational Resilience for Adolescent Alcohol Prevention

Andrea Romero, Elisa Meza, Josefina Ahumada, Michele Orduña, and Juan "Johnny" Quevedo

Abstract The purpose of this chapter is to summarize the work presented in this book about how South Tucson Prevention Coalition created community transformational resilience to prevent adolescent alcohol use. Community transformational resilience is the ability of a collective group to transform their community in a manner that increases protective factors and limits risk factors. Community was created through the building of a coalition based on *personalismo* (value of personal relationships and positive communication) that was comprised of youth, community members, university researchers, and outside agencies. Transformation was built through the process of participatory action research in order to ensure equal participation in dialogue to increase critical consciousness of societal factors for adolescent alcohol use that lead to community-led/youth-led research. Resilience was created because the coalition changed the community environment by increasing community norms of disapproval of adolescent alcohol use and by limiting access to alcohol. Understanding community levels of readiness for change was valuable to creating incremental, yet exponential changes over time to prevent adolescent alcohol use.

A. Romero, Ph.D. (✉)
Family Studies and Human Development, The University of Arizona, 650 N. Park Avenue, Tucson, AZ 85719, USA
e-mail: romeroa@u.arizona.edu

E. Meza, M.S.W.
San Francisco Unified School District, San Francisco, CA, USA
e-mail: mezae520@gmail.com

J. Ahumada, M.S.W.
School of Social Work, Arizona State University, Mesa, AZ, USA
e-mail: josefina.ahumada@asu.edu

M. Orduña, M.Ed.
House of Neighborly Service, Tucson, AZ, USA
e-mail: miorduna@gmail.com

J.J. Quevedo
Pima Community College, Tucson, AZ, USA
e-mail: Tucsonhigh12@yahoo.com

A.J. Romero (ed.), *Youth-Community Partnerships for Adolescent Alcohol Prevention*, DOI 10.1007/978-3-319-26030-3_12

Keywords Community transformational resilience • Resilience • Prevention • Underage Drinking

Underage drinking continues to be a health concern among adolescents; in 2013 approximately 35 % of United States high school age youth drank alcohol in the past 30 days (Centers for Disease Control and Prevention, 2013). Although it is commonly acknowledged that adolescence is a period of experimentation (Burrow-Sanchez, 2006), it is illegal for youth under the age of 21 years old to drink alcohol, and there are many other risk factors associated with adolescent alcohol use, including problems with brain development, increase risk for physical and sexual assault, serious alcohol-related injuries, and even death (alcohol associated car accidents, homicides, suicide, alcohol poisoning, or injuries) (National Institute on Alcohol and Alcohol Abuse, 2015). The extant research on adolescent alcohol use has identified that risk factors (increase likelihood of use) and protective factors (decrease likelihood of use) occur at both the individual level and context level (Burrow-Sanchez, 2006). Context level factors include policies that deal with alcohol/substance use, availability of substances, and community norms (Burrow-Sanchez, 2006). It is acknowledged that the interaction between the individual and the community can promote or inhibit healthy behaviors (Bronfenbrenner, 1986); however, there is still much work to be done to understand community-level factors for adolescent health. Ethnic minority youth living in poverty impacted neighborhoods experience environments with the fewest amount of resources and the greatest amount of neighborhood hazards linked with higher rates of alcohol and substance use (Kirmayer, Gone, & Moses, 2014). However, we chose to not view youth as victims of their communities; rather, we took a resilience perspective to our prevention strategies that considered not only individual level resilience of youth but also collective aspects of community-level resilience (Sousa, Haj-Yahia, Feldman, & Lee, 2013).

The South Tucson Prevention Coalition (STPC) was a coalition that served the City of South Tucson. *The mission of the Coalition was to prevent substance use among adolescents (age 9–15 years) in the City of South Tucson. The long-term goals were (1) to expand and strengthen collaboration among Coalition members to support prevention and reduction of youth alcohol use; (2) to prevent or delay adolescent first use of alcohol through perception of risk and harm from drugs and disapproval of drug use by peers family and; (3) promote data driven prevention services for alcohol use among youth.* The Coalition's plan to reduce underage drinking included conducting an in-depth assessment of the community, including: (1) age of onset for alcohol and illicit drug use, (2) past 30-day use frequency, (3) perception of risk or harm, and (4) perception of disapproval of use by peers and adults. STPC members worked closely with the evaluator to create, organize, and implement the needs assessment and on-going evaluation. The coalition participated in coalition building activities, which promoted a community-level readiness for change. STPC coalition members were strongly engaged in efforts to prevent or delay youth substance use as a method of achieving community empowerment and promoting the health of adults and families in the long term for the South Tucson community. One of the goals of is to provide a place-specific focus that allows for practical translation of prevention practice. Thus, local practitioners can improve their own practices and policies (Grekul, 2011). Community collaboratives are one way to leverage existing resources in order to work together to fight one common cause, and they have become increasingly common as a way to address broad social issues. Yet, there is still limited research on how these groups are formed and the most effective processes that lead to functional collaboratives (Grekul, 2011). We feel that the descriptions in this book provide new insight into how to create and sustain functioning coalitions. To begin with (1) inclusion of youth as equals in prevention strategy development, (2) personalismo or relationship-based approach, (3) importance of specificity and clarity in mission, and (4) linking strategy to readiness level of community.

In this chapter, we summarize the previous chapters that describe coalition building, youth and community collaborations, youth and community-led research, community-level strategies to raise awareness and to change alcohol norms, and prevention of new liquor licenses. In overview, we discuss the major themes and lessons learned that contributed to the development of community transformational resilience by the South Tucson Prevention Coalition (STPC). We describe community transformational resilience more in depth and summarize how the major themes of the book contribute to this concept. This chapter will be organized around these themes of (1) Developing Community, (2) Transformational Capacity, and (3) Resilience. First, we will describe the nuances and key elements that contributed to the successful development of community through a personalismo-based approach to coalition building with youth, community leaders, university researchers, and outside agencies. Second, we will describe how the process of participatory action research led to the development of critical consciousness and a unified approach to collective action for community transformation. Third, we will discuss the key components of how community transformational resilience can help promote positive youth development and inhibit alcohol use through increasing resources, alignment of resources, building on community cultural assets, and proactively addressing governmental decisions on community infrastructure.

12.1 Community Transformational Resilience

Resilience theory is one way to understand how individuals living with adversity are able to overcome challenges (Luthar, Cicchetti, & Becker, 2000). Early definitions of resilience focused only on internal individual level characteristics (Luthar et al., 2000). However, many researchers have contested original views of resilience that focus primarily on individual-level factors because they overlook the important shaping context of political and structural systems and unequal infrastructures associated with poverty (Pearson, Pearce, & Kingham, 2013; Ungar et al., 2007). More recent definitions of resilience based on qualitative and quantitative research with international samples of adolescents indicate that resilience is an interaction between the individual and their environment (Ungar & Liebenberg, 2011).

Longstanding historical inequities rooted in generational poverty and historical discrimination against ethnic minority groups, including Native American and Mexican Americans, require substantial changes in the current structural factors (Kirmayer et al., 2014). The disruption of those longstanding structures may be the pathway to healing community health behaviors in a way that is sustainable in the social environment. For example, a study of neighborhood resilience in New Zealand focused on explaining the contradictory finding of low mortality in areas of high social deprivation, and they found that resilience was associated with densely populated areas which had less access to unhealthy living, specifically with less access to alcohol (Pearson et al., 2013). When youth are supported by community members and their environment to choose positive health behaviors, they are more likely to stay on positive development trajectories.

In this book, we take that definition even a little further to focus on **Community Transformational Resilience**, *which we define here as a community's ability to overcome adversity through changing their community infrastructure in ways that can promote positive youth development by increasing the number of resources and access to resources while also limiting accessibility to risky behaviors*. To a certain degree, this concept is built upon the concepts of transformational resistance that describe how Latino student use critical consciousness to push back against oppressive institutional systems (Solorzano & Bernal, 2001; Yosso, 2005). However, with community transformational resilience, we argue that collectives can come together to create changes in those systems in order to develop resilience that will impact many individuals within their community and if sustained will affect more than one generation of youth. This dynamic exchange between adolescents and their environment for healthy behaviors is much more likely to be sustainable (Kirmayer et al., 2014).

Community transformational resilience is one way to increase protective factors by aligning ecological contexts to provide more options for healthy development for young people (Kirmayer et al., 2014). Based on the research presented in this book, we identify the following process that led to this type of resilience (1) building community based on personalismo, (2) critical consciousness of existing oppressions and inequities based on participatory action research, and (3) commitment to collective action to create change in the ecological context for the purpose of social justice. We argue that STPC demonstrated how this process lead to the capacity to change the norms within the community in relevant and meaningful ways. In order to create changes in community infrastructure, communities need to mobilize and work together because it needs multiple sectors of the community in order to create large-scale changes. We also define community transformational resilience outcomes as community wide changes that (1) add new protective factors, (2) remove risk factors, (3) align existing resources, and (4) create new relationships among community member and agencies. For example, STPC added new protective factors such as after-school prevention programs, youth-led after-school programs, grants, coalition building, community events, research, and new avenues for advocacy. These positive and protective factors also seemed to lead to changes in the way that the community saw themselves and especially the way that they viewed youth within their community.

12.2 Asset Focused and Solution Oriented

The concept of community transformational resilience is also distinguished from previous work on collective resilience that examines emergency situations. In the current conceptualization, we are focused on communities who are dealing with chronic stressors associated with generations of poverty embedded communities. Thus, these communities are dealing with the accumulation of historical trauma and structural inequities that are often not quite the same as emergency situations; however, in some ways it may be even more challenging with these communities to build up hope and capacity after generations of witnessing lack of support. Josefina describes this as, "*Sometimes when people look at the City of South Tucson, what they see is Latino, the majority of residents live below the federal poverty level, and they see what people don't have, unemployed, underemployed, homeless folks who walk through the city. They see all these negative things, poor ethnic brown community, and yet out of that are all these wonderful jewels, these assets.*" Josefina's comment reflects what several other coalition members, especially youth, have identified in previous chapters, the negative stereotypes and assumptions about a low-income ethnic minority community. However, so many of the coalition members used this as a motivator to represent a positive view of their community, and it reinforced their desire to build on the strengths and assets that they viewed from within their community.

While many researchers have implicated the sociopolitical context as an important factor for health, particularly among low income minority populations, there are still few projects that aim to transform this context (Sousa et al., 2013). This begs the question of understanding how to create resilience within communities through transformation, not only how to identify those that are resilient already (Chaskin, 2008). From this approach, the default victimization and deficit models of minority communities are not assumed; rather they are seen as sources of potential agency and assets for change. Yet, the community readiness model reminds us that change often is slow and incremental, and that we cannot assume that all community members will be ready to accept change or to even accept that there is a problem. Thus, community transformational resilience is focused not only on building community relationships, but in actually changing the ecological structure of communities in a manner that it creates new sources of protective factors rooted in community cultural strengths and in ways that limit the self-identified risk factors specific to the unique community environment.

One of the things that is unique about this concept is that the community itself is seen as a source of resilience, no matter what the current resources and challenges are that exist. Community members are seen as active agents of change to be involved in the recovery and transformation of their own community. This perspective is not only based on preexisting relationships and resources, but instead indicates that new sources of coordination and cooperation can be developed that can transform the community structure. There was a change in the work of STPC such that youth were once seen as "the problem" and now were viewed as not only assets, but "the solution." For example, Josefina Ahumada (STPC Coalition member) states: "*84 % or more are Latino, the assets of the community are the teens, and adults, and being proud of your culture, family and wanting to be protective of your family, and not having your little brothers/sisters to be exposed to drinking*." The youth momentum inspired the adults to also see the opportunity for change within their own community; this was a key source of critical consciousness that humanized the community, while acknowledging the existing inequities such that individuals felt hopeful about creating change.

12.3 Community

In this book, we discuss a very specific place-based approach over several years to address adolescent alcohol prevention. Place-based approaches have been indicated as important and targeted ways to integrate community involvement (Florin & Wandersman, 1990). Community involvement has been found to be particularly important to effective prevention strategies with low income and ethnic minority communities; however, truly in-depth community involvement continues to prove to be challenging (Grekul, 2011). By focusing on a regional location, it is possible to build on the unique strengths and assets of that community. Moreover, place-based approaches can be effective if they build on community assets, such as preexisting regional identities and local commitment to resources. Clearly recognized communities with distinguishable boundaries allow prevention strategies to consider multiple levels of ecodevelopmental contexts in their environmental prevention strategies. In this way, researchers and prevention specialists can consider the nuanced complexities of communities, which is more likely to lead to the development of sustainable prevention infrastructure. However, even with place-based strategies, it cannot be assumed that an interconnected and unified community already exists. In most cases, there is still a need to build community and, in fact, can be even more challenging because of historical divisions or conflicts within the community.

There are many ways to define community; in the current study we defined community boundaries based on our place-based approach to work with the City of South Tucson (Fielding & Anderson, 2008). An aspect of the decision for the place-based strategy was also the strong sense of connection that many community members feel to this small city. Michele Orduña, STPC Coordinator, "*The people who live in the city of south Tucson, have a strong sense of place, of community, they are proud of it, there is a strong cultural tie to there, here is a sense of belonging if you come from South Tucson, it has still that village mentality, these are my people.*" However, actually developing a community of practice to lead the alcohol prevention efforts was a significant amount of work that was done through the creation of the coalition, STPC. Despite the clear city boundaries, there was not a preexisting "community" who was linked through a common mission to address adolescent alcohol prevention. One of the lessons learned by STPC was that by defining community broadly, as those people who were invested and cared about the youth of their community, they were more likely to create changes within their community. This meant that STPC included not only community insiders but also outsiders, such as outside prevention agencies and also university researchers. Solidarity among individuals can promote positive adjustment, particularly in response to chronic and accumulated stressors, such as the lack of resources within poverty impacted environments (Ebersöhn, 2014). Ethnic enclaves may increase intragroup marginalization, but may also contribute to positive views of one's ethnic group because of more immediate role models and support for a positive ethnic identity, more access to traditions and heritage language—may enhance the appreciation for one's culture and associated norms, values, behaviors, traditions, and language.

12.4 Personalismo

The development of a cohesive group of individuals and agencies required a significant amount of breaking down silos and learning to work together as equal participants with a common mission of preventing underage drinking. The community coalition was built on the basis of a *personalismo*-relationship-based philosophy. *Personalismo* is a cultural value that prioritizes personal relationships through a personalized communication style that conveys and develops mutual trust, dignity, and self-worth (Altarriba & Santiago-Rivera, 1994; Holloway, Waldrip & Ickes, 2009; Marin & Marin, 1991; Santiago-Rivera et al., 2002). The *personalismo* approach is even more valued and appreciated by communities of color who have experienced historical trauma and current discrimination. This approach values the individuals more than tasks, and it helped to maintain the orientation of the coalition on the mission of helping youth, so that personal egos and agency agendas were put aside at times for the good of the youth in the community. The mutual trust developed among coalition members was evidenced through their support of each other's programs and events. In this way, they were able to align and connect community resources and enhance community access to existing resources in a manner that had not previously been achieved.

Personalismo is based on positive and supportive relationships among community members and community agencies. Walsh (2002) also refers to relational resilience that is rooted in aspects of positive and harmonious relationships that lend themselves to collaborative problem solving. A resilience promoting aspect of the development of community relationships is that individuals are likely to develop a heightened concern for others within their own community, particularly an enhanced concern for adolescents (Drury, Cocking, & Reicher, 2009). Thus, this collective sense of mutuality and trust may be more likely to lead to collective efficacy or the confidence that a group can work together to improve their community (Sousa et al., 2013).

Collective efficacy is defined as perceived collective capacity to take action on shared community issues of social, economic, or political relevance (Collins, Watling Neal, & Neal, 2014). Collins and colleagues (2014) find that more civic engagement is linked with more collective efficacy and more bonding social capital.

This shared belief in community capacity has been identified as a key factor that links to action. Thus, they argue that the neighborhood is a key setting for enhancing collective efficacy through relationship building. These concepts of collective efficacy are more about the perception that one's community may do something, but is not necessarily about organizing and working together to change the existing system. Collective efficacy is one possible outcome of coalition work; it is the belief that a community can come together through mutual trust in order to intervene for the common good (Sampson, Raudenbush & Earls, 1997). Collective efficacy is the belief that a community can work together and is prepared to engage in shared efforts in order to intervene for overall community improvement (Sampson, 2001). The belief that a group can make an impact is at the heart of the concept of collective efficacy, the belief that a community can work together for change, and a belief in the agency of a community is one of the first steps towards taking collective action (Watts & Guessous, 2006).

12.5 Transformation

Critical consciousness is specific to understanding that health occurs within an ecological context and can be linked to action-oriented collective problem solving, which can help to transform the community infrastructure. Freirian approaches to raise consciousness can humanize individuals and their affiliated group that has been negatively stereotyped and dehumanized; moreover it can help increase understanding of how structural inequalities contribute to the current health problems faced by their community (Hernández, 2002). Community can be instrumental to promote healing in minority communities by reconstructing positive relationships based on personalismo (Hernández, 2002). However, relationships that lead to unity and social support are not sufficient for community transformational resilience; it also requires action to create change in the shared ecology; otherwise the community will continue to be constantly under attack from oppressive structures. For example, youth may have social support, but will continue to encounter risk factors, such as permissive community norms for alcohol use and alcohol availability. Juan "Johnny" Quevedo, Y2Y leader, describe it best as, "*When we came together, we did things, we did amazing things. It helps to be sure where you are from and what is around you, whether it is good or bad, if it is good and then go out there and talk about it, if it is bad, go out there and do some action, take care of your own place, take care of who you are. Never, never stay quiet.*" Critical consciousness is important to increase the understanding that individual health behaviors are influenced by factors in the ecological context that impact everyone within that community. Moreover, there is a need to raise awareness that adolescent health behaviors matter to everyone in the community, not only because of the potential consequences that may occur with risky health behaviors but also because positive youth development can help youth transition to become healthy and successful adults who can help improve the communities that they come from.

However, as Juan states, in the end it is really the praxis, the move to action; the move to transform the inequities is what is essential to any prevention work.

12.6 Resilience Community Outcomes

While teens and community members both recognized adolescent drinking as a problem for the health, well-being, and future success of their community, they also repeatedly stated "*We can't do it alone.*" They knew that the scope of this issue was extended far beyond youth and far beyond individuals. Moreover, and more importantly, they recognized that in order to solve this problem, that any one group could not successfully do it alone—it was going to require many sectors of the community to work together in order to create significant community change for the youth today and the youth that would follow them. A resilience-based approach is strengths based and highlights the importance of building skills and capacity to be critically conscious of the systemic nature of adversity and the skills to be able to change these systems and the knowledge of means through which to create change in systems. This is much more than just adapting to adversity of negotiating hardship, but working to reduce the risks in the ecological context. Community resilience includes the presence of hope as well as unity among community members, and that is what we clearly saw evidenced in the work of South Tucson Prevention Coalition (Hernández, 2002).

Olsson, Bond, Burns, Vella-Broderick, and Sawyer (2003) define resilience as a dynamic process that involves interaction between the individual and their environment where in both there are risk and protective aspects. It also represents overcoming adversity, which can result in an outcome of resilience, resilience as a developmental process to adapt and resilience as a multifactorial concept (layers). Resilience is not about being invincible to stress, but rather the ability to develop in healthy ways even while under great hardship. It also includes the outcomes wherein overcoming adversity creates new skills and strengths or enhances existing strengths and skills. Resilient outcomes are usually the ability to remain functional and focus on mental health, performance, and social competence. This focus on multiple outcomes has muddied the waters in regard to the conceptualization of resilience. In terms of mental health, a resilient person may show high levels of distress, but still be highly functioning—this is where it is messy to use emotional distress as a marker of resilience. In thinking of resilience as a process, the positive resilience promoting factors include individual, family, and community aspects. Most of the work done to create resilience in social environments has focused on the school environment and the aspects of supportive peers and teacher/adult mentors. However, there is some evidence that supportive communities (outside of school) also serve to promote resilience. Zolkoski and Bullock (2012) describe individual level sources of resilience as well as family and community. To demonstrate resilience, one must first face adversity, but resilience is not a unidimensional construct; it is composed of positive outcomes that result across multiple aspects of life over time and is routed in several skills and protective factors.

Resilience is not a static notion that simply exists, but one with dynamic interactions. New collaborations with individuals will lead to new levels of development within the environment, and importantly within the lives of all partners (Walsh, DePaul, & Park-Taylor, 2009). Fielding and Anderson (2008) describe three ways to create collective aspects of resilience, risk reduction or prevention, asset enhancement, or facilitation of protective mechanisms in ecodevelopmental contexts of family, school, and community. Chaskin (2008) also suggests that community resilience can be found through regrouping efforts to reorganize existing resources, redevelopment to promote change, or resistance to change the nature of the health issue. Thus, he suggests to invest in human capital as well as organizational infrastructure to promote any or all of these forms of community resilience. Ebersöhn (2014) calls for a collectivist and transactional–ecological view of resilience that focuses on relationships as positive resources that can further enable resilience through accessing existing resources.

Sometimes, the changes in resilience are harder to identify and even harder to begin to measure and track. Michele describes some of the changes in the youth that she saw over time: Michele Orduña, STPC Coordinator: "*I have kept in distant touch with some of them, and I can really see that they continue to hold some of those things true within themselves; it is really hard to change, even in your environment even if you want to; they are not held up to a standard that they are idols, but we all know those of us that worked with those teens—that we have experienced something together, and we have this knowledge that you have done this—and that is a lasting thing, that that those teens have—they have this knowledge that this is a lasting thing, some have gone on to graduate from high school—and that is challenge in this community—and the majority of them have jobs—which is a major thing—a few have gone on to college—I think we had something to do with that. I think these teens hold their heads high, I would like to think we had something to do with that, we are not the only fact, but we had something to do with that, and I like to see them every once in a while.*" In fact, it may be exactly this sense of empowerment and self-worth that was sustained among the young people and the community members as well.

12.7 Lessons Learned about Youth Involvement

There were many lessons learned during the years of work of the South Tucson Prevention Coalition. However, here we will focus on a few key lessons that were particularly pivotal to move the community towards change or the lessons that seemed to transcend more than one phase or more than one activity.

Given the appropriate tools and support, youth can provide inspiring assets to their community, no matter what toxic factors exist in their environment. By embracing youth in the efforts for team building and collaboration, communities can enhance youth positive development and their growth as leaders (Larson, 2007). By connecting youth with adults in their communities, youth can develop a greater capacity to navigate shifts in society in order to avoid risky behaviors and to transition into successful adult leaders. However, this requires dedication of resources to building youth resiliency, empowerment, and voice. Rather than perceiving youth as victims of the existing economic and political forces surrounding their development, they are perceived as able to improve their own community through leveraging the access and capacity that they already have at hand within their families, schools, peers, community centers, and city. As such, youth are not seen as the problem, but rather as active, involved community members instead of passive recipients of society (Noguera & Cannella, 2006).

However, youth-led work should not be romanticized; most individuals who work with youth would agree that there is need for adult participation (Noguera & Cannella, 2006). There are few models for adults who may not already be consciousness about youth's ability to be agentic in positive change. In the South Tucson Prevention Coalition, youth worked with youth and adult allies in small settings to develop critical consciousness and to engage in YPAR activities; however, one of the things that made STPC unique was that youth were then integrated within an adult coalition. This was not an easy task because not all adults in the coalition were allies or critically conscious about youth development. Certainly, the youth development programs rooted in Freirian models were fundamental to develop critical consciousness and foster leadership among youth before and during their participation with adults. Yet, it was the adults who were often surprised by the level of participation by the youth and their honesty in discussions about youth alcohol and substance use. At first adults expected youth to carry out the adult decisions, or they expected that they would not participate in discussion or decision making. At first some of these meetings were challenging for all participants, youth, and adults. However, the adults that continued to participate began to change their perspectives and their expectations of youth. They found that the youth voice added value to the conversation and to the planning of activities. They found that youth often had innovative takes on ideas for strategies and solutions that had not been previously considered by adult leaders. Although the primary goal of the coalition was to focus on preventing underage drinking, a consequence of our YPAR approach was that they gained critical consciousness about the humanity and equality of youth in their own community.

Change does not happen all at once; the community readiness model for change was helpful to understand the steps that lead to larger community changes. For example, the importance of community awareness of adolescent alcohol use as a problem was essential not only to coalition member involvement but also to creating a broader community-level readiness to be ready to support prevention programs as well as limiting alcohol availability. Also, the understanding that change happens in incremental steps was important for the coalition members to be patient and to not give up their prevention efforts with their community. By creating change in the existing infrastructure, community members may actually further increase their sense of efficacy and hopefulness for future projects. For example, Josefina Ahumada, Social Worker and STPC member, describes how "*When it comes to communicating with the larger community, or getting the larger community to respect us, sometimes there has been some pessimism about that, and I think that the teens had a way of breaking through that, and saying hey, we can go to Phoenix, we can speak to these power brokers and make a change.*" This is an insightful and important comment about the transformative nature of including youth who have fresh perspectives. Youth may be more optimistic than some adults who have worked in low income communities for a long time, because adults who have seen failed programs may become pessimistic. Thus, youth involvement can help maintain a positive outlook of the future and invigorate community-based initiatives with a youthful hopefulness.

12.8 Conclusion

Transforming community-level resilience is a seismic change that requires a community to reconsider how they view themselves, their community, and their ability to change their community into what they want it to be (Cahill, 2008). In the chapters, there are several comments about how the adults and youth had moments when they gained a critical awareness of youth alcohol use and also moments when they became conscious that working together as a community could be transformative. In fact, this book demonstrated how one community nurtured their interconnectedness, their humanity, and in the process developed critical consciousness that enabled their ability to change their community to become healthier for youth and adults by implementing community transformational alcohol prevention strategies. The results of South Tucson Prevention Coalition encourage communities to fight poverty structural factors that negatively contribute to the development of their young people. STPC demonstrates that youth and adults can effectively work together to obtain funding, collect data, dialogue, and develop collective decisions to engage in collective action to change ecological risk factors within their communities. The end result of STPC was community transformational resilience that was created as a result of systemic changes to promote adolescent health in a sustainable manner. This was done in such a way to maintain and develop youth participation in the existing local political system rather than in defiance; while it was a form of disruption of the previous status quo, it was done in partnership with community leaders and adult allies.

References

Altarriba, J., & Santiago-Rivera, A. L. (1994). Current perspectives on using linguistic and cultural factors in counseling the Hispanic client. Professional Psychology: *Research and Practice, 25*(4), 388.

Bronfenbrenner, U. (1986). Ecology of the family as a context for human development: Research perspectives. *Developmental psychology, 22*(6), 723.

Burrow-Sanchez, J. J. (2006). Understanding adolescent substance abuse: Prevalence, risk factors, and clinical implications. *Journal of Counseling and Development, 84*, 283–290.

Cahill, M. (2008). Community collaboratives addressing youth gangs: Interim findings from the Gang Reduction Program.

Centers for Disease Control and Prevention. (2013) Youth Risk Behavior Survey. Available at: www.cdc.gov/yrbs. Accessed on (7-27-15).

Chaskin, R. J. (2008). Resilience, community, and resilient communities: Conditioning contexts and collective action. *Child Care in Practice, 14*(1), 65–74.

Collins, C. R., Watling Neal, J., & Neal, Z. P. (2014). Transforming individual civic engagement into community collective efficacy: The role of bonding social capital. *American Journal of Community Psychology, 54*, 328–336.

Drury, J., Cocking, C., & Reicher, S. (2009). The nature of collective resilience: Survivor reactions to the 2005 London bombings. *International Journal of Mass Emergencies and Disasters, 27*(1), 66–95.

Ebersöhn, L. (2014). Adding 'flock' to 'fight and flight': A honeycomb of resilience where supply of relationships meets demand for support. *Journal of Psychology in Africa, 22*(1), 29–42.

Fielding, A., & Anderson, J. (2008). *Working with refugee communities to build collective resilience*. Perth: Association for Services to Torture and Trauma Survivors.

Florin, P., & Wandersman, A. (1990). An introduction to citizen participation, voluntary organizations and community development: insights for empowerment through research. *American Journal of Community Psychology, 18*(1), 41–52.

Grekul, J. (2011). Building collective efficacy and sustainability into a community collaborative: Community Solution to Gang Violence. *Journal of Gang Violence, 18*(2), 23–45.

Hernández, P. (2002). Resilience in families and communities: Latin American contributions from the psychology of liberation. *The Family Journal, 10*(3), 334–343. doi:10.1177/106680702010003011.

Holloway, R. A., Waldrip, A. M., & Ickes, W. (2009). Evidence that a simpático self-schema accounts for differences in the self-concepts and social behavior of Latinos versus Whites (and Blacks). *Journal of personality and social psychology, 96*(5), 1012.

Kirmayer, L. J., Gone, J. P., & Moses, J. (2014). Rethinking historical trauma. *Transcultural Psychiatry, 51*(3), 299–319. doi:10.1177/1363461514536358.

Larson, R. W. (2007). From 'I' to 'We': Development of the capacity for teamwork in youth programs. In R. K. Silbereisen & R. M. Lerner (Eds.), *Approaches to positive youth development* (pp. 59–75). Los Angeles: Sage Publications.

Luthar, S. S., Cicchetti, D., & Becker, B. (2000). The construct of resilience: A critical evaluation and guidelines for future work. *Child development, 71*(3), 543–562.

Marín, G., & Marín, B. V. (1991). *Research with hispanic populations*. Thousand Oaks, CA: Sage Publications.

National Institute on Alcohol and Alcohol Abuse. (2015). Underage Drinking. http://pubs.niaaa.nih.gov/publications/UnderageDrinking/Underage_Fact.pdf

Noguera, P., & Cannella, C. M. (2006). Youth agency, resistance, and civic activism: The public commitment to social justice. Beyond Resistance! Youth Activism and Community Change: New Democratic Possibilities for Practice and Policy for America's Youth, 333–347.

Olsson, C. A., Bond, L., Burns, J. M., Vella-Broderick, D. A., & Sawyer, S. (2003). Adolescent resilience: A concept analysis. *Journal of Adolescence, 26*, 1–11.

Pearson, A. L., Pearce, J., & Kingham, S. (2013). Deprived yet healthy: Neighbourhood-level resilience in New Zealand. *Social Science & Medicine, 91*, 238–245.

Sampson, R. J., Raudenbush, S. W., & Earls, F. (1997). Neighborhoods and violent crime: A multilevel study of collective efficacy. *Science, 277*(5328), 918–924.

Sampson, R. J. (2001). How do communities undergird or undermine human development? Relevant contexts and social mechanisms. Does it take a village? Community effects on children, adolescents, and families, 3–30.

Santiago-Rivera, A. L., Arredondo, P., & Gallardo-Cooper, M. (2002). *Counseling Latinos and la familia: A practical guide*. Thousand Oaks, CA: Sage.

Solorzano, D. G., & Bernal, D. D. (2001). Examining transformational resistance through a critical race and LatCrit theory framework: Chicana and Chicano students in an urban context. *Urban Education, 36*(3), 308–342. doi:10.1177/0042085901363002.

Sousa, C. A., Haj-Yahia, M. M., Feldman, G., & Lee, J. (2013). Individual and collective dimensions of resilience within political violence. *Trauma, Violence and Abuse, 14*(3), 235–254. doi:10.1177/1524838013493520.

Ungar, M., Brown, M., Liebenberg, L., Othman, R., Kwong, W. M., Armstrong, M., et al. (2007). Unique pathways to resilience across cultures. *Adolescence, 42*(166), 287–310.

Ungar, M., & Liebenberg, L. (2011). Assessing resilience across cultures using mixed methods: Construction of the child and youth resilience measure. *Journal of Mixed Methods Research, 5*(2), 126–149.

Walsh, F. (2002). A family resilience framework: Innovative practice applications. *Family relations, 51*(2), 130–137.

Watts, R. J., & Guessous, O. (2006). Sociopolitical development: The missing link in research and policy on adolescents. *Beyond resistance*, 59–80.

Walsh, M., DePaul, J., & Park-Taylor, J. (2009). Prevention as a mechanism for promoting positive development in the context of risk: Principles of best practice. In M. Walsh, J. DePaul, J. K. Park-Taylor, E. Maureen, A. M. Horne, P. Orpinas, Reese, L. E. (Eds.), *Realizing social justice: The challenge of preventive interventions* (pp. 57–78). Washington, DC: American Psychological Association, xviii, 322pp. http://dx.doi.org/10.1037/11870-003

Yosso, T. J. (2005). Whose culture has capital? A critical race theory discussion of community cultural wealth. *Race ethnicity and education, 8*(1), 69–91.

Zolkoski, S. M., & Bullock, L. M. (2012). Resilience in children and youth: A review. *Child and Youth Services Review, 34*, 2295–2303.

Index

A.J. Romero (ed.), *Youth-Community Partnerships for Adolescent Alcohol Prevention*, DOI 10.1007/978-3-319-26030-3